The Fluid Nature of Being

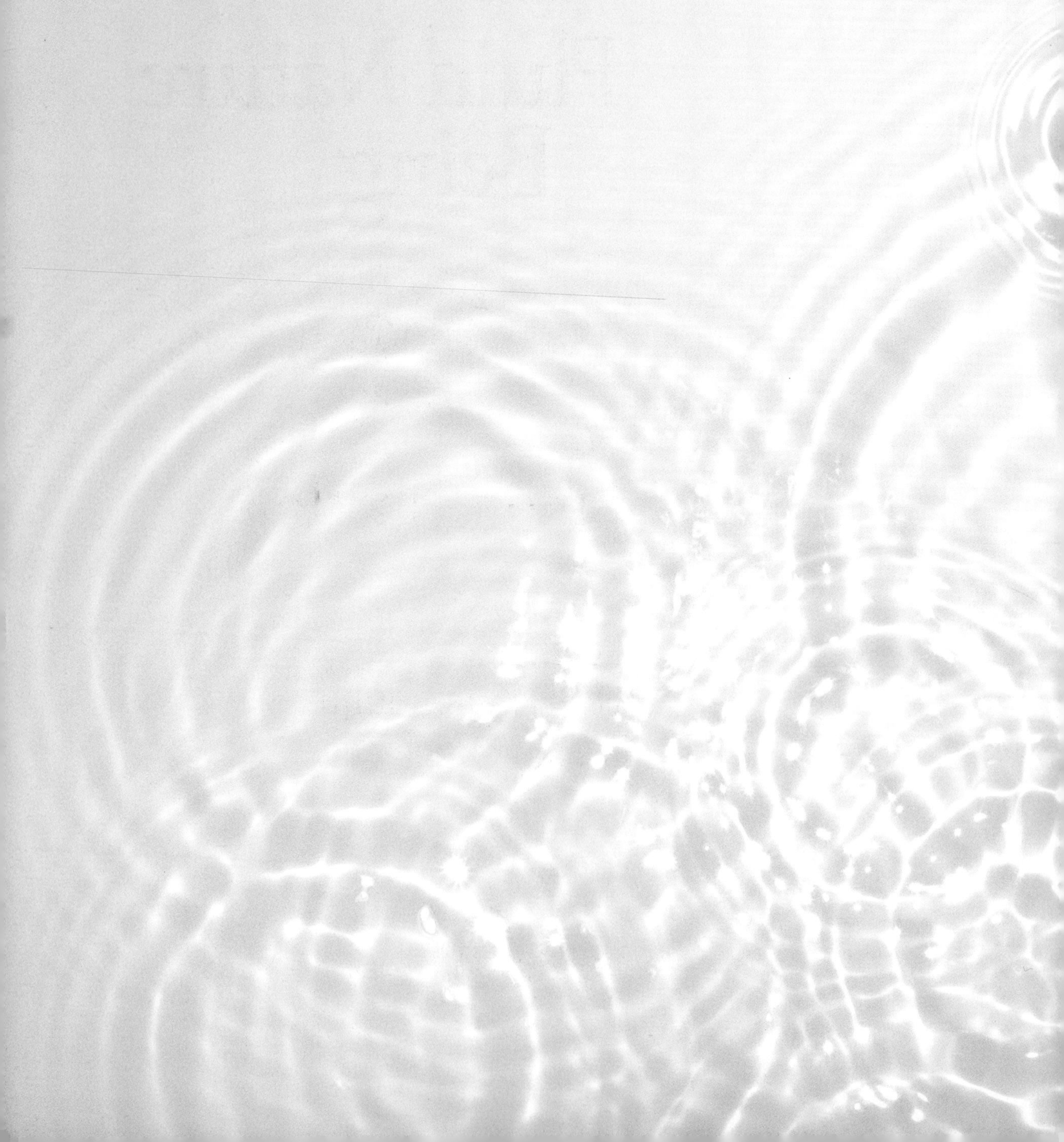

The Fluid Nature of Being

Embodied practices for healing and wholeness

Editor
Linda Hartley

Forewords
Don Hanlon Johnson
Martha Eddy

HANDSPRING
PUBLISHING

First published in Great Britain in 2022 by Handspring Publishing, an imprint of Jessica Kingsley Publishers
An imprint of Hodder & Stoughton Ltd
An Hachette UK Company

1

Notice
Neither the Publisher nor the Authors assume any responsibility for any loss or injury and/or damage to persons or property arising out of or relating to any use of the material contained in this book. It is the responsibility of the treating practitioner, relying on independent expertise and knowledge of the patient, to determine the best treatment and method of application for the patient.

All reasonable efforts have been made to obtain copyright clearance for illustrations in the book for which the authors or publishers do not own the rights. If you believe that one of your illustrations has been used without such clearance, please contact the publishers and we will ensure that appropriate credit is given in the next reprint.

This book is a guide for personal exploration and is in no way meant to substitute for any type of medical advice – allopathic, Western, Eastern, Indian. It can complement a healing protocol. Ultimately all movement ideas are to be visited with gentleness allowing your body responses and related sensations to guide you.

A CIP catalogue record for this title is available from the British Library and the Library of Congress

ISBN 978 1 91342 6 491
eISBN 978 1 91342 6 507

Printed and bound in Great Britain by Bell & Bain Limited

Jessica Kingsley Publishers' policy is to use papers that are natural, renewable and recyclable products and made from wood grown in sustainable forests. The logging and manufacturing processes are expected to conform to the environmental regulations of the country of origin.

Handspring Publishing
Carmelite House
50 Victoria Embankment
London EC4Y 0DZ
www.handspringpublishing.com

Commissioning Editor Sarena Wolfaard
Project Manager Morven Dean
Copy Editor Wendy Lee
Designer Bruce Hogarth
Indexer Aptara, India
Typesetter Amnet, India

The
Publisher's
policy is to use
paper manufactured
from sustainable forests

Contents

Dedication

Dedicated to our dear friend and colleague Ania Witkowska, who left too soon.

About the Editor

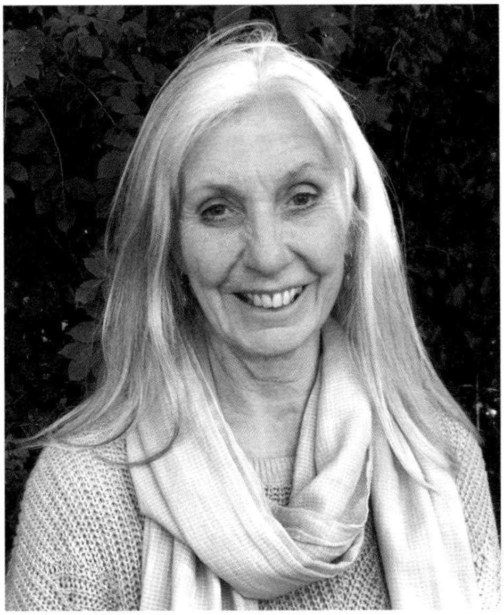

Linda Hartley, MA, RSMT, BMCA reg, Dip Psych CTP, has studied, practiced, and taught in the fields of somatic movement and dance, somatic and transpersonal psychotherapy, and Authentic Movement for almost five decades. In 1990 she founded what became the Institute for Integrative Bodywork & Movement Therapy, and has been developing and running a 3-year Diploma Program in Germany, the UK, Lithuania, and Russia since that time. Based on the practice and principles of Body-Mind Centering®, and integrating in-depth studies in Authentic Movement and Somatic Psychology, IBMT is an International Somatic Movement Education and Therapy Association (ISMETA) Approved Training Program.

Linda's studies in the somatic dance approach of Release Work (Mary O'Donnell Fulkerson), T'ai Chi Ch'uan, and Buddhist meditation, and the Process Oriented Psychology of Arnold Mindell have also informed the development of a holistic approach to learning, growth, and healing. She practiced for 30 years as a somatic movement therapist and somatic and transpersonal psychotherapist, and has taught for numerous organizations across the UK and Europe.

Currently, Linda focuses her time on her writing and teaching the Discipline of Authentic Movement in North Norfolk, UK, where she now lives.

She is the author of several books, including *Wisdom of the Body Moving* (1995), *Servants of the Sacred Dream* (2001), *Somatic Psychology: Body, Mind and Meaning* (2004), and *Contemporary Body Psychotherapy: The Chiron Approach* (Editor, 2009). Information about these and some of her articles and chapter contributions can be found at https://www.lindahartley.co.uk/index.html.

Foreword

I am honored to lend my hand to the welcoming of new life, the birth of this book. Being a midwife to "game-change" is awe-inspiring. Tonight, under the full moon, human life spawns concern in me as I read about femicide in Mexico. Yet, the somatic field and this book give rise to solutions, the good news being that somatic movement is touching psyche and body amongst the women there who are scared by day-to-day occurrences and possible death. Somatic movement is powerful: it relieves body and soul in its educative process, perhaps not always preventing violence but ameliorating its effects. This is a book about pathways to change, specifically the routes of Integrative Bodywork and Movement Therapy (IBMT).

Through myriad paths this book provides a "tending toward" what is still somewhat unknown. It offers gateways to new routes, like neural circuits being set down and, through practice, becoming habituated. It communicates new possibilities for artists, educators, and therapists. New circuits are laid out through thought patterns – sensory experiences – and movement responses. Experiencing the knowledge held within these pages helps myelinate new cultural options. The expanding choices validate the exploratory. At our Moving On Center, we talk about engaging the improvisational mind. This mind thinks outside of the box only because of necessity – one must be quite creative to survive when living on the margins. It would be interesting to know if that is why these pathways have yet to become "the norm." Sadly, I believe it is because people who are able to live in relative comfort prefer not to rustle the status quo, which – more often than not – is unaware of the interconnectedness of all beings. To widen choice, reset neural networks, and stabilize one's options, we need to focus on the improvisational aspect of attuning with the moment, deeply awakening to self and our dependency on our beloved surroundings. With reading and doing, feeling and sensing, we can make these options more normal.

Linda Hartley has been birthing newness for decades, midwifing embodied shifts in consciousness through her books and educational systems. She has a long history of supporting the emergence of what was once a new field: Somatic Movement Education and Therapy (SME&T). She is of a new generation and an older one too. This book represents the solidifying of the new, its maturation, sitting within a new genre that comes with the passing of time. IBMT is a grandchild of various influencers – Body-Mind Centering®, Authentic Movement, Somatic Psychology – a third generation of Somatic Movement practices if one begins when the field began to be called somatic. If you take a more expansive decolonial perspective, it has grown over thousands of years, and is returning to its roots.

In recognizing generations, one can look back and forward at the same time. In *The Fluid Nature of Being* the newness, which is rooted in the past, different ways of being in the world – with movement, touch, embodiment, the wholeness of psyche and body – are integrated. There is an invitation to dive in, to investigate.

I've known Linda since 1980, and it gives me great honor to salute the majesty and depth of this book. We first met as colleagues, training together in Body-Mind Centering®, and I continued to admire her when we lived on different continents. I was touched and supported by her published words. She wrote a book about somatic movement long before it was fashionable, about the work we studied together, our shared body of knowledge – BMC. Those of us teaching BMC could use her *Wisdom of the Body Moving* as a textbook because of its logic and sequential unfolding. When Linda moved into making connections with the somatic psychology field, she opened yet another door. Her educational program, like many SME&T systems, includes touch and movement and her work was among the earliest movement systems to convey the importance of not just the body, but movement, in psychotherapeutic work. In my book *Mindful Movement*, Linda is placed in the third generation. We sit together as part of what I dubbed "the amalgam generation," bringing together different influences.

Foreword *continued*

In Linda's case, the amalgam is somatic movement (BMC), somatic movement with overlaps to Dance/Movement Therapy (Authentic Movement) and psychotherapy (Somatic Psychology). This blending of approaches resonates throughout the pages of this book, crafted with tender care. And the creative investigation of soma is repeated, this time through the next generation, with her group of scholars of IBMT, the body – the mind – the spirit accessed and integrated.

It begins with the body – not just the human body but that of our mother, the body called the Earth – and how we as humans can relate to it. Food comes into the body and is sourced from our mother. The umbilicus of our biological parent provides sustenance that begins our journey in life. The book spirals out from here to infant development, children with disabilities, and special ways of learning and being, perhaps even the indigo child. It moves into the relational for adults as well, rooted in early childhood attachment patterns and allowing the expression of dance as performance or personal artistry to speak. The experience of being and the exchange of being seen and allowing for responsivity are both valued. Further exploration includes the psychodynamic work of transference and counter-transference, viewed from the experience of the witness, the caring and compassionate holder of suffering and pain.

There is no one better than Linda and the people she has touched to share this range of somatic work. Her maturity and depth of "wisdom of the body moving" have spiraled out into the world. Now we have a resource for these times. The roles of the artist as healer, healer as educator, educator as artist come alive through IBMT and *The Fluid Nature of Being*. These interconnections are delightful and can be experienced in sequence or like a dip in the ocean on a day when you most need fluid support. These words provide a chance for each of us, as readers, to deepen in our own aliveness.

Martha Eddy CMA, DEP, CTBMD, MFLCI, RSMT, EdD

Founder and Director of BodyMind Dancing & Dynamic Embodiment SMT

Director of Programming and Research

www.MovingforLife.org

DrMarthaEddy.com

March 2022

Foreword

Conversation: Towards a Science of Subjectivity

In the isolations and fragmentations during this COVID-19-ridden epoch, where is it possible to engage with others in the kinds of meaningful dialogues that work towards resolving some of the serious issues that face us, such as global warming, nuclear proliferation, social justice, dealing with health issues, and many others? A century-old text, *The Mass Psychology of Fascism* by Wilhelm Reich,[1] has gained new relevance in the face of these upheavals. In this idiosyncratic document of one who suffered through various forms of fascism and unbridled authoritarianism until he died in a US penitentiary for transporting health devices across state borders, Reich raises the question of whether or not there exist any models of a successful egalitarian society that might serve as guides to creating more. He argues that one place to examine are those communities organized to alleviate the extremes of human suffering: emergency medical workers; people caring for the elderly, disabled, and the dying; therapists; health researchers; and firemen. His reasoning is that the intensity of the suffering in these cases is so compelling and immediate that it trumps more ethereal qualities of ideological beliefs and personal obsessions. This collection is an example of what he was proposing: a large community of highly skilled professionals, focused on various demands for healing, engaging in communal reflection about how to move forward in creating a more humane world.

Integrative Bodywork & Movement Therapy is the concept that gathers these writers, weaving together two longstanding communities of healing practice created by visionary elders: Body-Mind Centering® by Bonnie Bainbridge Cohen, and the version of Authentic Movement developed by Janet Adler. This weaving is a generative example of how a group of diverse people, mature, skilled in their particular works, devoted to healing the wounds that lurk everywhere, can form a collaborative document that enables their works to become more widely accessible by taking on the difficult task of articulating what they are actually doing and achieving.

This particular community of writers also fills a gap in much of the social science literature, which is the absence of art. Poetry, painting, literature, music, drama, and dance reveal dimensions of bodily life that are not touched by the biological sciences. These authors each represent a seamless blending of artistic form, radical inquiry, and disciplined practice.

For that reason, this publication represents, along with a handful of other similar collections, early stages in the construction of a desperately needed science of subjectivity, a methodical articulation of the strategies and underlying principles required to refine the realm of immediate direct experience, taken in its own right, not as something to be objectified, or reduced to the operational categories of the biological sciences. On the threshold of the waves of horror set afoot in the 1930s, Edmund Husserl, the founder of Phenomenology, argued that unless we can advance such a science, yielding a more effective understanding of subjective pathologies like violence, hatred, and denial, we are doomed.[2] At this moment, nearly a century later, thanks to the science of objectivity, we are about to be able to view the origins of the Universe through the James Webb telescope, while at the same time we cannot begin to handle the increasing violence between peoples, the destruction of the environment that enlivens us, and a host of other subject pathologies.

1 Wilhelm Reich, *The Mass Psychology of Fascism*, trans. Vincent R. Carafagno (New York: Farrar, Straus & Giroux, 1980).

2 Edmund Husserl, *The Crisis of European Science and Transcendental Phenomenology*, trans. D. Carr (Evanston, IL: Northwestern Univ Press, 1970).

Foreword *continued*

Developing a reliable science of the subject presents two very difficult challenges that account for its feeble progress:

- How to handle self-deception and bias. In objective sciences, the purging of these confounders is handled by measurement and mathematical formulation, the very reason for their amazing successes in the ancient searches for truth. A science of the subject requires methods for emerging from a self-enclosed reporting of purely personal experiences in diaries and memoirs. In this work at hand, the very act of putting words to the page where unknown others will read them is a fundamental act of moving into a more reliable realm of clarity about the truths of one's own work.
- How to gather experiential patterns that are intelligible instead of collections of individual events. Here you have such with Body-Mind Centering and Authentic Movement, which enjoy a robust literature defining the patterns being learned within those schools that, when practiced over time, generate experiences of a specific kind (e.g. breathing, sensing, or posture), and carefully articulated documents of many individuals sharing these experiences. In addition to the accumulation of such basic data of patterned direct experiences, there are mediating layers of dreams and imaginative imagery.

For those reasons, this document, as well as a number of similar documents, are something like field notes towards a science of subjectivity, like Darwin's notes on the various species he observed on his generative voyage to the Galapagos on the H.M.S. Beagle or his children playing in their home. In an emergent notion of intellectual work, the gathering of this and other such documents elicits by its very nature more abstract and general notions based on these accounts. Reliability of claims grows out of that foundation instead of dangling out in ethereal dissociation.

I would add to Reich's examples of egalitarian communities successfully joining to work together, those groups who join in longstanding research projects, tracking a particular inquiry through many refinements of data gathering and interpretation. A stunning example in the present is the James Webb telescope, which at this moment is heading a million miles out to its eventual resting place. It is the latest stage in at least a 5000-year-old search into the nature of the cosmos originating in the ancient observatories at sites like Stonehenge, transmitted through the inventions of Tycho Brahe, Galileo, down to the Hubble. The Webb is the work of thousands of highly skilled technicians and designers working over 20 years to insure the success of a complex enormous object that will not permit any repairs because it will be so far out of human reach.

This volume represents a more modest instance of this old human impulse to make sense of how to navigate this vast mystery in which we live.

Don Hanlon Johnson PhD

Professor, Somatics

California Institute of Integral Studies

California, USA

January 2022

About the Contributors

Mari Winkelman MA (Dance and Somatic Wellbeing), Dip Psychosynthesis Counselling, Dip IBMT, AHPP reg Psychotherapeutic Counsellor, RSMT (ISMETA)
IBMT therapist and educator in private practice; ongoing commitment to social and environmental justice movements, as a person and as a professional

Rachel Lambert MA, Dip IBMT
Foraging guide and award-winning author on nature, wild food and cooking. Founder of www.wildwalks-southwest.co.uk

Mari Joyce BA (Hons) (Art), Cert IBMT, RCST, Dip MTI
Somatic therapist in private practice marijoycebodywork.co.uk; Songwriter/musician marijoyce.com

Raima Drąsutytė MA (Arts and Sculpture), Cert IBMT
Visual and performance artist; IBMT practitioner in private practice; former IBMT Programme Co-ordinator, Lithuania

Beverley Nolan Dip IBMT, E-RYT500, RSME/T (ISMETA)
Founding Director of Barefoot Body Training (Yoga & Somatics); IBMT Practitioner; former IBMT Faculty member; Yoga United Education Guest Tutor (Experiential Anatomy and Therapeutic Presence)

Anna Titova Dip IBMT, RSME (ISMETA), BMGT
Somatic BODY practitioner; Director of Somatic BODY program, Moscow; Lecturer, Institute of Osteopathy, Moscow
www.annatitova.com
www.somaticbody.ru

Frauke Burchards Dip IBMT, RSMT (ISMETA)
Physiotherapist; Dance Artist; IBMT Faculty member

Anna Feoktistova Dip IBMT, RSME/T (ISMETA)
Somatic therapist and somatic movement educator; Assistant organizer, IBMT Moscow
www.somaticana.ru

Penny Collinson MA by Research, Dip IBMT, FHEA
1998-2021 Senior lecturer at UCLan, Preston, UK; Steering group member and Research Development Panel member of the Knowing Body Network; External Examiner Institute for Integrative Bodywork & Movement Therapy

Heike Kuhlmann MA (Choreography/Performance Studies), Dip IBMT, RSDME (ISMETA), Body-Mind Centering® SME, Dip Physical Education & Biology
Faculty member: Somatische Akademie, Berlin - Somatic Basic training; EMERGE, somatics in dance; CARE, somatically grounded early childhood education
www.heikekuhlmann.net

Paul Beaumont BA Hons (Social Policy & Administration), Dip Counselling, Dip IBMT, RSMT (ISMETA) Dip Creative Approaches to Supervision
Somatic Movement Therapist and Supervisor; IBMT Faculty member; Director of IBMT Training Programme, UK
www.paulbeaumont.net

Daria Shamina MA (Social Psychology), Dip IBMT
Psychotherapist; Psychologist at the studio of practical psychology 'Empathy'; Assistant organizer, IBMT Moscow

Anna Khasina Dip MSU Clinical Psychology, Cert IBMT, ISP, MGI (standard EAGT), APS Bodynamic
Therapist, supervisor, trainer in Body Gestalt; Member of professional Gestalt community; Family therapist; Specialist in dance-movement therapy

Maren Hillert Dip IBMT, RSMT (ISMETA), Registered Heilpraktikerin (Berlin), Dip Ing (Landscape Planning), Cert Aguahara Practitioner (Bodywork and Dance in water)
Creative Dance Pedagogue; Somatic Movement Therapist; former IBMT Faculty member www.maren-hillert.de

About the Contributors *continued*

Jane Okondo MA (Dance and Somatic Wellbeing), Dip IBMT, RSME/T (ISMETA), RCST, SEP
Somatic Movement Therapist and Somatic Experiencing Practitioner; Discipline of Authentic Movement and Continuum Teacher; IBMT Faculty member; Director of IBMT Training Programme, UK

Barbara Teresa Erber MSc (Dance Movement Psychotherapy) RDMP, Dip IBMT
Movement psychotherapist; PhD candidate, University of Edinburgh
www.barbara-erber.com

Leticia Santafé MA (Acting, Theatre and Performance), Dip IBMT, Body-Mind Centering® IDME, RSME (ISMETA)
Somatic Voice/Body Movement Educator; Founder and Director of Formacion SOMart: Voice and Somatic Movement Education for the Arts in Spain; Fulbright Award in the Performing Arts, New York; Linklater Designated Voice Teacher, New York.
www.formacionsomart.com
www.centrovozenmovimiento.com

Maria Grudskaya Dip IBMT, RSMT/E (ISMETA)
Dance Artist and Educator; IBMT practitioner; IBMT Faculty member; Director of IBMT Training Programme, Moscow

Gaelin Little MA (Creative Practice: Dance Professional Pathway), Dip IBMT, RSMT and SMDE (ISMETA)
Artistic Co-director of dance quartet Eleven Farrer House www.elevenfarrerhouse.com and Compass Dance www.compass.dance

Aistė Kriukelytė MA, Dip IBMT, member Lithuanian Dance Movement Therapy Association
Dance Artist and Educator; IBMT practitioner; Guest Lecturer, Lithuanian Academy of Music and Theatre
www.judetigera.lt

Agnietė Laurinaitytė MA (Psychology), BA (Music), Cert IBMT
Author, poet, singer; Leader of retreats and Satsangs; IBMT Practitioner in private practice; Director of IBMT Training Programme, Lithuania

Preface

The Fluid Nature of Being is a collection of writings by practitioners of Integrative Bodywork and Movement Therapy (IBMT), an approach to somatic movement education and therapy. The cultivation of consciously embodied movement is at the heart of somatic movement practice. Through embodiment practices, *soma* – the subjectively experienced sense of embodied self – becomes a vital, living reality and a foundation through which a healthy relationship to others, to nature, and to life as a whole can be nourished.

The Fluid Nature of Being describes the practice, thinking, research, and creative work of 21 IBMT practitioners. Each has also trained in other disciplines and their writing weaves together their broader learning, passion, and professional practice within the IBMT approach to somatic work. In this volume we offer a collection of expressions with a rich diversity of themes and styles, bringing these voices from a new generation of somatic movement practitioners, writers, and leaders to a wider audience.

An experiential training is always an **initiation**, where often deep and profound embodied learning and change take place. To honor the impact their personal encounters with IBMT have had on them, some of the writers refer back to experiences as trainees, writing in a moving and convincing way *from*, rather than *about*, their experience of somatic practice. Some offer explorations for the reader to try, or client case material that gives a sense of their inner process as a practitioner. In this way, I hope the reader will receive a deep and embodied sense of IBMT somatic practice, one which touches them in a sensory and feeling way, as well as intellectually.

The book covers topics such as IBMT in therapy, education, early years learning, dance, and theater; the integration of this approach to somatics with psychotherapy, psychoanalytic thinking, and somatic trauma therapy; and the connection between individual healing and the healing of the Earth and nature during this time of planetary crisis.

My own training in the fields of somatic dance, somatic movement education and therapy, and Authentic Movement has been primarily with Mary O'Donnell Fulkerson, Bonnie Bainbridge Cohen, and Janet Adler, along with many others. Their inspiring teaching, together with training and practice in transpersonal and body-oriented psychotherapy, has led me to develop an integrative approach to health and wellbeing rooted in the belief that we each hold within us the seeds for our own growth and healing. I have been developing and teaching professional training programs in IBMT since 1990. Programs have been offered in the UK, Germany, Lithuania, and Russia, and this collection reflects the international scope of our practice, with contributors from several countries.

There are many aspects of IBMT practice described in this book that are shared with somatic practices in general, though there are also aspects which are specific to this approach. The IBMT Program uniquely integrates in-depth studies in Somatic Psychology and the Discipline of Authentic Movement into a foundation of Body-Mind Centering® training. At the core of the practice is the quest to deepen connection with self, and from there, connection with others and the world around us. While there are many interventions available to the practitioner, practice is client-led and sensitive to the needs and circumstances of the moment-to-moment arising of process, within the client and through the relationship between client and practitioner. Therapeutic and educational process is a co-creation, a shared journey of discovery rather than an expert-led treatment, so that the student or client is empowered to access their own inner authority, agency, and wisdom.

Body-Mind Centering offers innumerable principles, practices, and somatic skills which can serve as keys to unlocking a person's potential for healing and integration. Students and clients learn to attend to a wide range of subtle nuances of expression that the bodymind reveals, from cellular motility to an immense variety of qualities of movement that specific body tissues, organs, and systems express. The study of embryology, the development of infant movement patterns, and the embodied learning of the anatomical body systems through focused awareness, touch, mindful movement, voice, and creative expression, form the basis of this core aspect of the work. Through these processes we seek to increase integration, support, flow, and ease within a student's or client's bodymind, seeing body and mind as an intrinsically connected and constantly interacting whole.

Accessing the somatic key which will unlock this particular person's potential for healing in this specific moment requires attentive listening and witnessing on the part of the teacher or therapist. The ability to witness in an open, receptive, non-judgmental, and compassionate way is learned through study and practice in the Discipline of Authentic Movement; developing the capacity to witness with clarity and compassion enables practitioners to deepen their capacity to be with all that their students and clients may bring.

The development of embodied presence, and its application in embodied relating, are core to the practice of IBMT. We address blocks to this process through the study of our own psychological patterning: through an approach that is rooted in somatic practice we explore psychological models to better understand our own resistances, limitations, qualities, strengths, and growing edges as practitioners, as well as those of our clients. Somatic Psychology offers maps and pathways to guide us through this process of discovery and integration. It offers understanding and interventions that can help to orient and hold a client's process when challenging emotions and psychological patterns are evoked through somatic practice.

The book is intended for practitioners and students of somatics and related fields of practice, including body-based psychotherapies, bodywork, dance movement therapy, and eco-psychotherapy; yoga, dance, and the creative arts; and therapists, educators, and parents interested in somatic approaches to early years learning. It is hoped that there will be much to interest the lay reader and student too. Our wish is that these writings might inform, inspire, encourage, and make you curious to explore further.

Although the majority of the contributors to the book are women, IBMT and somatics in general are practiced by all genders. In these chapters, unless a specific gender is indicated, the authors' intention is to include all, and we hope every reader will feel this, whether the designation *he, she*, or *they* is used.

Whether you choose to follow the narrative of the book set out here, or dip into the sections that invite you most strongly, perhaps you will find places to pause, breathe, experiment, and taste some of the expressions of somatic practice offered here. May this have benefit for you, and for those with whom you work and engage.

Linda Hartley

Norfolk, UK

January 2022

Acknowledgments

We thank all those who have come to learn and practice with us over the years. To my own students and clients, from whom I have learned so much, and the students and clients of each contributor to this book – thank you for trusting us and courageously diving into this wondrous adventure of embodied learning. Through each of you the work continues to grow and unfold.

I am, as always, deeply grateful to all my teachers and colleagues, who have given so much inspiration and support over many years. Very special thanks to Bonnie Bainbridge Cohen, whose extraordinary pioneering work is at the root of the practice of IBMT, which we write about here, and to Janet Adler, whose dedication to the exploration of conscious embodiment continues to inspire and open hearts.

Heartfelt thanks to friends and family who stayed close while this book was coming into being, during the long journey through a pandemic and at a time when what we human beings need and love most – direct embodied connection with one another – was severely curtailed. In particular I am grateful to Brue Richardson, Liz McCormick, Gillian Mortimer, Pauline Sayhi, Hannah Birley, Caroline Randell and Cherry Cooke.

Thank you to Sarena Wolfaard and the team at Handspring Publishing for bringing this book into the world. It has been a pleasure to work with them.

And finally, my personal gratitude goes to each contributor to this book for their creativity and the hard work of translating their skill, insight, and love of somatic practice into language. When brought together, each unique voice helps create something that is rich and whole.

Integrative Bodywork & Movement Therapy professional training programs:

http://www.ibmt.co.uk www.ibmt.co.uk – Devon, England

http://www.ibmtrussia.ru www.ibmtrussia.ru – Moscow, Russia

http://www.ibmt.lt www.ibmt.lt – Vilnius, Lithuania

Introduction Linda Hartley

During the period that this book was coming into being, the world was plunged into crises on many levels. A pandemic caused our human community to be largely shut down, and we were impelled to turn inwards while also looking out, wide and long, at the conditions we have collectively created in our world and the kind of future we want to see. Threats and injustices in the ecological, climate, social, racial, and political spheres finally began to be acknowledged more fully and publicly; moving beyond the concerns of minority groups and campaigns, they could no longer be ignored.

Living at a threshold moment in time brings added urgency to what we do. I believe, as some of the contributors to this book describe, that somatics has an important part to play in the re-envisioning and regeneration of the world that so many of us want to see. We are part of a much wider movement of regeneration and add our voice as one small but integral contribution to the collective turning towards respectful, sustainable, and compassionate ways of relating – to our own inner self, to each other, and to our home, the Earth. When we touch into our own authentic embodied self, with care, respect, curiosity, and compassion for our suffering and limitations, we cannot help but become more attuned to and concerned about the natural world we inhabit.

Somatic work cannot be only for personal betterment or it might risk becoming something of a narcissistic affair. Its true potential is to open us to ever-widening circles of connection and relatedness. The book begins by introducing this wider context. In the first part, **Body, Earth, Nature, and Connection**, four contributors explore this theme. Mari Winkelman writes about the ways in which environmental, social, and political injustices have resulted from human beings' separation from our "organismic intelligence." She argues passionately for somatic practice as a resource to help rebalance our relationship, as human beings, to Gaia – the potential for reconnection to our nature as embodied beings who participate in planetary healing and wellbeing. This vision is further developed through Rachel Lambert's description of intimate encounters with the natural world. She describes how, via somatic practices of opening through skin and senses and her observations of nature as a wild food forager, she finds personal healing through a deepening connection to the nature within herself and, simultaneously, in the world around her. In Chapter 3, Mari Joyce describes the practice and Discipline of Authentic Movement as a way to connect more deeply to self, to the collective body of humanity, and to the wider non-human and natural world of which we are part. Personal notes from studio practice open out into reflections on the place of this discipline in relation to Buddhist practice, ecological movements, and personal and planetary healing at a time of crisis. The first part of the book ends with a visual account of a performance project co-created by Raima Drąsutytė, where a group of women respond to the exploitation that results from commercial drilling and excavating activities. The performance is both a peaceful protest and a practice through which the women reaffirm their connection to the earth.

Movement, in all its many forms, is life; there is no life without movement, however subtle this might be. Where there is movement, there life is growing. Parts 2 and 3 of the book explore the theme of **Moving into Life** from several different perspectives. In the first of these parts, themes circle around the somatic exploration of embryology, beginning with Beverley Nolan's fascinating refolding of development back to its origins in the moment of conception, to the vibratory nature of beginnings. Here, she finds resonance, an intersection, between yogic philosophy, science, and somatic exploration of the developmental journey.

Introduction *continued*

Anna Titova then unfolds the journey forwards, describing how the fascial network and the Navel Radiation pattern provide the substance and means by which movement originates and the embryo develops. She weaves together modern scientific and philosophical ideas with ancient cultural practices that view the umbilical cord and placenta as a source of wisdom and home to the soul. The exploration of embryology concludes with Frauke Burchards' description, in words and photographs, of the creation of a dance performance inspired by the embryological journey. Her visual and literary images map the miraculous folding and unfolding that is the movement of emergence into human form.

The second part of **Moving into Life** begins by looking at the birth process from the mother's perspective. First, Anna Feoktistova describes somatic practices that have informed and supported her during the stages of being pregnant, giving birth, and recovery after birth. Her personal discoveries have led to offering this work to other mothers-to-be and new mothers; most of the somatic practices she shares are highly relevant to those who are not pregnant too. Penny Collinson continues the theme of birth from the mother's perspective as she revisits her experience of birthing her second child. From a somatic exploration that revealed unexpected responses to the trauma of the actual birth, then a creative process of dedicated studio practice to uncover the memories still held in her own body, she reflects on the nature of healing through somatic practice and embodied imagination, and how her own journey of discovery and healing might support that of her daughter too. Following on from birth, Heike Kuhlmann guides us through the process of infant movement development and offers insight into how these early experiences develop the child's brain and their sense of self. She demonstrates theory with descriptions of her movement practice with children, and Contact Improvisation classes for caregivers and children together, which support the repatterning of relationship as well as movement in both. Paul Beaumont continues the theme of working with children and young people as he describes his work with those who have been adopted. He offers examples of sessions that demonstrate his integrative approach, using somatic and developmental movement, play, witnessing skills from Authentic Movement, and the Integrative Bodywork and Movement Therapy (IBMT) approach to somatic psychology to unfold his process of supporting these young people to grow and heal.

In the following two parts of the book, six practitioners describe various **Therapeutic Applications**. They weave into their work theory and practice from other disciplines that they are also trained in, creating a rich tapestry of therapeutic approaches with core IBMT principles and practices at their heart. Daria Shamina opens with a discussion of the nature of the Circle: as the container of life at the cellular and embryonic level, this fundamental form is found in many cultures as a symbol that holds healing processes. Her practice integrates Authentic Movement, the "Mandala" method, somatic work with the body systems, and a psychodynamic understanding of the infant–parent and client–therapist relationship. In Chapter 13, Anna Khasina further develops some themes touched on, as she explores somatic counter-transference and resonance within psychodynamically informed somatic therapy. She elucidates theory with several examples from her practice, describing her internal process of cultivating awareness of the counter-transference through witnessing her own sensations, feelings, images, and movement impulses. The focus of Maren Hillert's work is on balancing the autonomic nervous system, which, as she describes, becomes easily imbalanced in our fast-paced, industrialized culture where people are drawn away from their own natural rhythms of rest and activity. She describes the ways in which she supports students and clients to access the healing quality of the parasympathetic state as a basis for listening to their own needs and restoring balance. This work of "resourcing" lays the ground for the next part of the book, where three different approaches to working with an autonomic nervous system that has been overwhelmed by the reactivation of trauma are described.

Jane Okondo begins the second part of **Therapeutic Applications** by describing the use of somatic bodywork and movement in healing from trauma. In her practice she integrates Peter Levine's Somatic Experiencing with IBMT bodywork and movement practices; her description includes theory and examples of client sessions, giving the reader a clear and subtly nuanced sense of the healing potential of this way of working. Integrating IBMT and Dance Movement Psychotherapy, Barbara Erber focuses on Authentic Movement as a powerful way to address post-traumatic stress in clinical practice. She describes theory which relates chronic pain with unresolved trauma, interweaving examples from her own personal healing journey as well as from her clinical practice, where she specializes in addressing chronic pain through Authentic Movement. Theatre director, performer, and teacher Leticia Santafé then offers a creative perspective on the emergence and resolution of trauma: she describes her personal experience of confronting trauma within the context of theatrical performance, and the work that this has led her to develop as she integrates IBMT with Linklater voicework and the training of actors, whose profession necessitates entering the often-traumatized worlds of the characters they inhabit.

As with many somatic movement practices, IBMT's creative, open, and process-oriented approach to embodiment attracts many dancers and artists. The final part of the book explores the interface between **Somatic Movement and Dance Research**, including a discussion of the similarities and differences between therapeutic, artistic, and spiritual practice within dance. Maria Grudskaya introduces this enquiry as she navigates a path between somatic exploration in educational and therapeutic contexts, and somatic dance as "Poetic Movement." Like other contributors to this collection, she names the importance of the inner witness, exploring the place of the witness in the process of dance making and performance, and enquiring into how the inner witness might function differently in the contexts of therapeutic and artistic work. Gaelin Little continues the research into "the porous membrane between therapeutic, educational, artistic, and spiritual contexts" as she describes the resonant space, a transitional place, like the membrane of the cell, where form emerges from emptiness and all is still possible. She brings the practice of the loving witness to the process of dance making, enabling the depth and authenticity of somatic practice to be present within the artistic process. In the final chapter, Aistė Kriukelytė also explores the interface between art and therapy through a research project in which she, with a colleague, offers a dance to one person, a gift for that individual alone. Recipients' responses and her own experiences reveal issues of vulnerability, safety, and connection, and questions about these themes in relation to early attachment and developmental trauma are touched on. The research project also opened up a timely question for the fields of dance and somatics alike: this time of the pandemic has gathered many practitioners to reformulate teaching, therapeutic practice, and performance for online forums. The question she introduces is one

Introduction *continued*

that, having been initiated in this time of necessity, I imagine will be explored long into the future: what is lost, and what might also be gained, within the field of embodied practice when it is occurring online instead of face to face, body next to body, in the movement studio or practice room?

A new step in the development of embodied practice has emerged, where our relationship with and through technology becomes another vital ingredient to consider. And we, as practitioners of embodied awareness, also know the irrefutable value of being in the physical presence of another, of experiencing connection through our living, breathing cells and tissues, communicating and responding in a myriad of non-verbal ways that allow us to come to know ourselves, the other, and our world with the immediacy and intimacy of direct experience.

Following Aistė Kriukelytė's gift of a dance, the book concludes with a gift to the reader of three poems from IBMT practitioners and singer–songwriters Mari Joyce and Agnietė Laurinaitytė.

Each contributor to this book has developed their responses to IBMT practice in their own unique ways. The work is not about teaching set protocols for practice, but rather about learning principles and processes that support the creation of a space in which each person can become more truly and authentically themself. When the core of self is touched, creativity can flourish and individual pathways of expression are revealed. In response, their offerings have taken many different forms and directions, reflecting the open and inclusive nature of this work. The interplay of form with formlessness, key skills and knowledge with open enquiry into the "fluid, impermanent nature of being human" (Collinson, in this collection) in an ever-changing world, is the challenge we engage with when we enter embodied relationship with our students, clients, or audience, inviting curiosity, exploration, and courage to go beyond the known and familiar, where we might discover something that feels truly authentic and sustaining, and of real value to ourselves and others.

Part 1

Body, Earth, Nature, and Connection

Gaia Body

Mari Winkelman

1

The invitation to contribute to this book has come at a time when I have been longing to write something about the profound impact of embodied practice in my life: to express how restorative the notion of relational, organismic intelligence can feel, at times of socio-political imbalance and human cultural trauma. Integrative Bodywork and Movement Therapy (IBMT), as a training and a practice, has fundamentally changed the way I perceive and orientate my life through my body systems and senses. Through my struggles with sensitivity to pain in my own body and in the world, I have developed empowering relationships to cycles of life and death in natural living systems. Linda Hartley's book, *Somatic Psychology: Body, Mind and Meaning* (2004), opened my heart and mind to the deep importance of becoming embodied in order to understand life within me and around me, and I visit some of the ground she covered in this book almost two decades ago because it is still so very relevant and guides my inner compass.

The story in this chapter is about how I have awoken to my embodied sensitivity at midlife in the last decade. I came to life anew again, falling in love with intensity and sensitivity in new ways, recognizing deeper values to guide me in life, and I had to meet the struggles to let go of old habits, hurts, and defenses within myself. I then began to learn about the ever more vivid backdrop of our global malaise and I could not avoid feeling terrified about it. There have been some intense moments of reckoning with the impact of dominant colonial forces of humanity on our living planet in this time of capitalist collapse, climate change, human oppression, and ecological degradation from human activity. There are great numbers of refugees created by political abuses and mismanagement of resources. Media manipulation confuses our orientation to our own higher values and democratic power. More and more revelations emerge of systematic oppression of people who do not conform to arbitrarily chosen yet socially enforced physical or sexual norms, or whose religion or political values threaten a dominant status quo. A pandemic chronic health crisis of obesity and pain exists in countries who have wealth to resource and heal but do not, and most recently a pandemic virus has spread easily within our "global village." Within this frightening time, there is also a powerful, compassionately heartful, intentionally embodied uprising by many thousands of ordinary people wanting to heal the wounds, and this calls me deeply to connect in all ways possible.

My Journey

I am a wounded healer who has spent the first quarter-century of life as a confused mind, rejecting my body while trying to make my way in a magnificent yet desperately wounded world. I am a middle-aged white, childless, queer woman, who has always felt challenged by my body image because I felt as if I did not naturally represent the ideals of a patriarchal, white, capitalist, colonial conditioning and did not know where I belonged. I was feeling sodden, depressed, despairing of humanity and my own failures to progress in the world. I felt I had not succeeded in becoming a psychotherapist, failed at a significant relationship, and was trying to find my way to the truth of my vocation and reason for living. I had been through a few rebirths already: a recovery from bulimia, training as a psychotherapeutic counsellor, a change in sexual identity, to name a few. I arrived into the IBMT training group in 2009 with my body despairing, lost in a geographical transition, seeking home and guidance, and desperate for an inward journey that would help me find myself anew.

When I completed the IBMT diploma and qualified in 2016, I emerged into the world with renewed willingness to pursue my vocation as a therapist and with a refined ability to perceive the world from my body. The IBMT womb gestated me as I was arriving more and more in my body and my vocation, as well as in my adult understanding of my belonging and impact on the world. I had done so much healing work on myself and wanted desperately to offer healing in the world in so many ways. And yet I felt so raw and did not know if or how I could make it further into the world. This chapter visits some of the key themes in this journey and a legacy with which I still live.

Outer and Inner Worlds

Before I began my training with IBMT, I saw the world "out there" and appreciated nature in many ways, as I enjoyed passing through environments and landscapes. I had not understood my body as a living organism beyond my thoughts and ideas.

The term "Gaia" was coined in relation to our physical planet Earth in 1972 by James Lovelock. Gaia refers to Earth as a living planet with interrelated life support systems, much like those that occur in our bodies (Lovelock 2000). Hartley illustrates the interconnection between our bodies and our worlds:

> *within the membranous boundary of our skin, we find a microcosm of the universe, and also of the social and political systems existing within our world ... Each cell, each organ, and each tissue layer is different but equally important and necessary to the wellbeing of the whole.*
>
> Hartley (2004: 166)

I have learned, by becoming more in touch with my embodied systemic knowledge, that my Earthly home, Gaia, is just like my body home: organismic, alert and responsive to me and my impact upon "her." I feel how I care within me about what is happening around me; and my practice is a homecoming to living within my body on this Earth. I am a microcosm of Gaia, just as my cells are a microcosm of me. There is a searing feeling of intimate connection in a vast ecosystem between my cells and the universe, sharing an experience of life.

"In coming into our body we become connected to our greater home, the Earth; we become a part of the earth and she a part of us" (Hartley 1995: xxi). This is the world of my longing, by living this practice and sharing it with others. Indeed, in my movement groups I feel a profound sense of community of bodyminds awakening and sharing intimately our embodied experiences in ways that do not happen "out there" in the everyday world, yet I hope it will eventually become more commonplace.

Cultural Paradox – Threshold

Gaia is an organism; our bodies are organisms. Given the context of human confusion and wounding within all dimensions of Gaia, in which my experience unfolds, there are paradoxes inherent in the living of the embodied paradigm. I am born of this wounded world, but it is hard to belong without regular immersions in the natural environment, which, as a species, we are killing off. Without this organismic backdrop, how do I make sense of my own organism? In reality, I have descended from a lineage of European body oppression, shame, and subordination to the power of the intellect and a land-owning elite human subgroup, and have been seduced by the dominant cultural norms of numbing my sensitivity to survive in environments and relationships which honor neither my organismic body nor Gaia.

Practicing embodiment makes me sensitive to feeling my own, and the collective, wounds of separation from our "greater home, the Earth." How can I and we tolerate feeling these wounds and avoid diversions into the desensitized culture? How can I develop resources to restore health to myself and to my world? A decade on, I live with a strong dilemma around holding focus on pioneering an embodied culture and resisting the disconfirming messages of my cultural conditioning. I wrote about this dilemma as I entered the IBMT training environment for the first time:

> **I walk into the training room and see most people sitting or lying on the floor, some in touch or contact with each other. It feels familiar, relaxed, yet I feel dissonance and confusion, as I am meeting another culture to the one I have been living in, and to which my mind and body, unconsciously, have an attachment. My sense is of immersion in a slower state. I feel this in my movement and notice that, while initially I am powerfully drawn into this scene, a minute later, I feel I don't belong here ... I feel disorientated and not sure where to put myself.**

This experience continues to accompany me as I transition in and out of body-sensitive group retreats and trainings. I have come to recognize the confusion that comes from the fact that I am primarily in my external senses and habituated thoughts in a space where the intention is to be more in touch with the responsiveness to internal senses. From our organs, our perceptions of reality are different. I realize that this cultural undoing and reforming of my embodied perception is fundamental for my living relationally with wounding, and for being with change in myself and in the world, but it is deeply unfamiliar and therefore exciting and scary at the same time! During my training years, it was rare for me as a white person to find this embodied culture amongst my white cultured family, workspaces, and community. I used to long for it each time I returned home.

A Practice

If you would like, I will give you an experience of relating from your inner world to your outer world, which will influence how you feel as you choose to continue afterwards to read, or not. You can take this in part by part, and take time to gather a feeling and sense of your inner experience and allow thoughts, images, and beliefs that come from here into your consciousness.

In an embodied culture, we relate in this way to our inner and outer environments with interoception – sensitivity to inner movements of our organs; proprioception – the movement senses in our joints and vestibular system; and exteroception – the senses of sight, hearing, smell, taste, and touch.

> **Check you are comfortable and uninterrupted.**
>
> **First, I point you to the proprioceptive sense for a moment. Focus on the feeling of your ribs and diaphragm as you breathe a few breaths. Can you feel your posture, your relationship to the ground, and whether you are in balance? Close your eyes and bring your attention inside, while noticing the feeling of this movement as proprioception.**
>
> **Now let us go to the interoceptive senses of digestion or awareness of other organs in your body. What do you feel in your belly? Try moving your hand into and out of contact with your belly to see if you sense the impact from inside. Again, close your eyes and perhaps place a hand over your belly to focus your attention.**

Chapter 1

And next, using your exteroceptors, look and listen around you, smelling the air to bring yourself out into the exterior space. What do you think, feel, and believe?

How do the inner worlds connect or relate with each other?

The exercise may have left you feeling out of touch with reading and more in touch with feeling what has been going on for you in your body, and perhaps at times attracted by your everyday thoughts. How is it to find yourself there? You can practice going in, coming out, and bringing with you aspects of each world into the other and see what happens.

White colonial dominant culture values cognition, science, and patriarchal authority which is imposed in generalizations by experts, over the individual's "irrational" and "intuitive" embodied perspectives. My own experience is that I do not recognize myself in these generalizations or they reflect only one part of my experience. I enjoyed reading that there is an alternative model which validates engaging our body senses in receiving and transmitting information and co-creating meaning through lived experience between bodies:

Enactivism … is a theory wherein human mental/emotional/physical experience can now be understood as dependent upon our conscious and unconscious bodily experience. The term "participatory sense-making" means that as human beings, we make sense of the world and of our relationships inter-acting in it, with our body.

(Galbusera and Fuchs n.d.)

To participate in my body's experiences of thriving and of imbalance, I need to feel the sensory signals which indicate inner fullness and upwelling of joy, but also to feel pain and discomfort. When I am in joy, I do well when I allow this joy to carry me towards fulfillment of the ideas and relationships. And when I am in pain, I need to adjust my activity and environment to facilitate my body's healing process. When I encounter my own pain instead of numbing it, I grow resilient and can also take in more of the pain I witness in our world. IBMT offers an ongoing enquiry from the most basic practice I offered you above, and from the deepening into my own body I befriend the pleasure and the pain and integrate this basic awareness into my everyday life.

Recent neuroscience shows how the ventral vagus nerve modulates our physiology and our emotions in our bodies via the "social engagement system." That is to say, our experience of connection to ourselves and each other happens through qualities of eye contact, vocal tone, facial expression, gestures and behavior, as well as via words spoken in relationship (Porges 2011). More is written about the vagus nerve in later chapters, but I want to name it here because it governs our sense of safety and threat. It seems that even when there is pain and hardship, co-regulatory relationships can make the hardships surmountable and joy can be experienced in moments along the way. I wonder what experiences of co-regulation come to your mind when you read this. Many intuitive models of health and therapy, including IBMT, put the principles of co-regulatory relationship between practitioner and patient/client at the heart of the healing work, which enables the therapist to help her client to navigate the pain and retrieve the joy.

Existing Culture, Emergent Culture, Paradox

Having experienced my living anatomical body, I feel the allopathic approach is like seeing only the tip of the iceberg. How would it be if we could accurately locate and describe our internal processes from the sensations we felt, if we could recognize how our digestive and immune systems were interrelated, and how these affected our mood? How would we feel if we could self-assess foods, activities, and environments that would support our interrelated systems to rebalance naturally?

The interconnection between our Gaia bodies and our Gaia world was essential for somatic practice, pioneered by white-bodied dancers, healers, and therapists. Somatic therapies developed by white Westerners evolved largely from travels, studies, and engagement with indigenous community practices of healing, relating, and tending life on all levels in embodied ritual and collective relational experiences. These were observations of human movement by people who were not medically trained, but who had been taught to work with creativity and health in the human being and were interested and curious about how body and mind were connected.

The lineages of teachers preceding Hartley reminded her of ancient truths from the holistic health traditions of Asian countries and cultures: interrelated systems of body and nature, cultures of community, and respect for all life. Western medical science developed observational understanding of human anatomy and functions, and this enabled Westerners to interpret the detailed "fabric" of the body. Combined with Eastern intuitive practices and languages, as more white Western people found health from somatic practices, these lineages have evolved vocabulary and somatic languages for expressing and teaching embodiment. Two of Hartley's primary teachers, Bonnie Bainbridge Cohen (1993) and Janet Adler (2002), have provided the foundational practices and language for IBMT, her unique integrative, relational, somatic practice.

As a therapist, dancer, and educator, Hartley models her integrative practice in a way of teaching that I call "transmission." She brings forth the fullness of sensitivity in a body in her physical presence, her tone of voice, and her method of experiential education. She speaks at a slower pace and brings movement and gesture to her words, inviting sensitivity in her students and clients. In the presence of Hartley, I can actually feel the impact of her sensitivity in my own body when I relax and my curiosity opens to my anatomical senses and how they influence my movement.

Experiencing myself as embodied changes my own feeling of presence, and my perception of myself and my environment changes. Tactile and interoceptive senses offer counter-balances to visual and auditory senses. My values change from being outcome-driven to caring more about how I feel into processes, and this shift changes how I understand my personal impact and contributions to humanity and the natural world. I internally feel my interconnection in the world more fully as I move between environments and relationships, so I recognize that, in the relational exchange between me and the world, what I do or do not do, and the qualities of my presence, matter much more.

IBMT and a New Paradigm for Gaia

IBMT is a somatic therapy which asks us to let go of our habitual identity and give ourselves more wholly to open enquiry into the world of sensation and movement within our body. We witness curiously the moment-by-moment sensory-motor processes of our bodies without judgment, and in returning again and again over time to these natural, emergent senses and movements we find familiarity *and* novelty within our embodied experience. We reflect on the discoveries and draw, write, speak our new experiences together, making meaning that includes our bodies' subjectivity. Thus, IBMT integrates rational and intuitive frameworks for us

Chapter 1

to make meaning of our experience, while honoring the mysterious unknown and emergent aspects of our experience that motivate our enquiry about life in a body.

I transition between the worlds ... back in my dance between my conditioning – which is busy with thoughts and activity, and dependent on a capitalist economic structure – and the new emergent culture of embodied community that I am inhabiting and co-creating. As I become a facilitator of this practice for others, I encounter my own internalized dismissal of this paradigm: "*it's not a priority for most people, it's self-indulgent and subjective and can only really be received by those who've already opened their minds in this way.*" At the same time, *my* bodymind *needs* this – I *have* to offer it! I can be guided by my desires, longings, and fears to release, relief, pleasure, and timeless space to witness my natural rhythms, but it is a very intimate experience and can be difficult to put in words or share with others. Even though I am pulled back into my conditioned habits in my everyday life, over time I remember how it feels to be liberated into my embodied senses, and this remembering keeps me returning to nature and including attention within my body in my everyday life. Hartley and the IBMT practitioner community hold the cultural space for me to keep returning to my body, to keep inventing or evolving language to describe my experience and to help me to meet, allow, and reclaim my bodily orientations.

I discuss below some of the most important parts of the IBMT culture and language which have influenced my perspectives on our world so much.

Wisdom in Our Cells

Our world needs a deeper democracy that only organisms can know. With environmental imbalance now at catastrophic levels, with pandemics on the increase and national health crises building, it is clear that, having only partial "awakeness" to our situation, we need to wake up more of our senses and become more responsive. This depth requires us to slow our processes down enough to allow us to witness and support our bodies to inform our orientations to life.

Our cells are organisms, impacted by our outer as well as our inner environments, so the state of our cellular mind is profoundly affected by the dominant culture in which we live. On the most basic level, our cells orient us to gravity, they breathe us, they metabolize the food we ingest, and they adapt over time to regulate our bodies in our specific environments. The cellular membrane negotiates with the world outside the cell – as does our skin – to maintain homeostatic balance between the outside world and the conditions in our bodies.

Each cell in our body has living intelligence. It is capable of knowing itself, initiating action, and communicating with all other cells. The individual cell and the community of cells (tissue, organ, body) exist as separate entities and as one whole at the same moment. Cellular embodiment is a state in which all cells have equal opportunity for expression, receptivity, and cooperation.

(Bainbridge Cohen 2017)

I remember loving being in cellular processes within the IBMT training where I could feel these states of at-easement and activation unfolding in my body, mostly simultaneously in different areas. Mainly, I loved being invited and appreciated for allowing myself to engage the bodily adjustments in movement and in my attention which these impulses were requesting, and the deep unwinding of my knots of expectation and habit that are my social conditioning. This was the **Being** and allowing of my cellular body process for which modern life does not make space. I realized that I need this connection to cellular consciousness to notice my conditioning and return to a simple relationship with my body: a time that was spontaneous and unsocialized, yet deeply safe and choiceful. This reweaving allowed me insights as I cared more about pacing that respects my tissues, rather than my mental aspirations and strivings to get things done, to achieve the perfect body, or to be seen performing "beautiful" movements.

The unassuming and deeply curious mind of the cells felt joyful and permissive of physical separateness or connection between bodies with an overall sense of interconnection and belonging. This is influenced by what I feel is my membrane intelligence, seeking out connection and resource, and avoiding too much challenge. In the practice of embodying our cells we are invited to stay at the edge with curiosity, attending to sensation, while staying aware deep within to inform our membrane's actions and receive the responses.

Exploring the cellular mind shows us experientially that we are uniquely complete as organisms. We tend to gravitate towards our needs and away from threats when we have freedom to do so. This is what informs our embodied intelligence and is integral to our sense of self, belonging in an environmental and communal context. As the quote above illustrates, from our cellular authenticity we claim an authority that is ours. An inherent paradox is that we need respect for our individuality but we also need connection to each other; we share resources with others and need to take care of the collective community so that we can also thrive. Our bodies demonstrate this paradox well: when in health, our cells are being themselves and are innately in service of the whole body. When stress and illness come along, the interdependent systems of cells do not function well and our whole body system can be overwhelmed.

Because the membrane is so essential to cellular orientation, we become very interested in touch relationship and interconnection that informs the nervous system. In time, it will be revealed how the physical distancing enforced during the Covid-19 pandemic will influence our cellular mind and our nervous system, and how we may adapt to find ways of touching our own bodies with intentions of care and nourishment to feed support to our own cells and nervous system.

From Microcosm to Macrocosm

We all develop from a single cell into complexity with trillions of cells, each empowered with more specialist but cooperative life-support purposes and resources. The same simple principles of cooperation and homeostasis translate into more complex interrelated systems. Our brains are not designed for us to be aware of the whole of them all of the time, but we can increase our awareness in order to support our bodies' internal systems of regulation.

White supremacist, capitalist culture encourages us to stray even further from awareness of these processes in our bodies, instead keeping us mentally busy with complex social and economic systems that we have to navigate. Culturally, our sensitive skin, the membrane we might be organismically informed by, is deemed more important as a visual presentation of our worth to others than as a channel of intelligence for our bodily wellbeing. In cultures dominated by white supremacist norms and values, "white" skin is valued over darker skins, while within "white," there are several tones that are definitely not white but exist in a hierarchy where privilege and priority are assumed in so many ways within social and political contexts. This is a profoundly harmful legacy of, and challenge to, our colonial past that renders our bodies as commodities, rather than living systems. We adapt to the restrictions of commodification by desensitizing our skin, buying products, and managing our sensitivity rather than revealing it. However, this cannot be sustained, and just as the skin "breaks out" when we have a build-up of toxins, or emotions, people rise up to break out of the oppressive system when limits feel too much to bear by those affected. Black Lives Matter (2013) and Extinction Rebellion (2018) are two major uprisings that emerged globally in 2019–20 and are set to stay until balance can be restored, or further enforcement of the cultural order ensues to the detriment of our human sentient wisdom.

We urgently need structures and a culture that facilitates our inner sensory reference and connection. Martha Eddy reviews a variety of aspects of "bodymind": thinking, cellular intelligence, and nervous system patterning and repatterning through experiences of movement: "The 'alive body' is capable of healing and self-regulation because the soma perceives itself and makes decisions" (2016: 16). The patterns in our nervous systems come from our socialized behaviors and beliefs, which require us to sacrifice some of our unique original ways of being in order to conform. IBMT invites and permits us to return to our unique original form – the cell – and to imagine and move into the open-mind orienting behavior to respond to here-and-now conditions, rather than the predictive reactions based on our patterns.

Finding Freedom in Movement

As we come into the world, we are allowed a certain amount of freedom just to "be ourselves," as long as our needs are met well enough by our carers/parents and our environments. Increasingly, in a more crowded and ideologically polarized world, less freedom is allowed for each of us, and it is only the ones who can be independent of culture or systems who can explore this freedom. Being ourselves involves authentic and self-regulating movement in our bodies, which comes from connection to our needs, desires, and ideas. Freedom to move is essential for our health and wellbeing. Interestingly, often on vacation or in retreat, we are drawn to nature and draw closer to our animal nature, closer to the ground. I remember vividly my grief in remembering my animal ancestry and my embodied biography, coming to terms with how my biography impacted on my animal nature, suppressing my wild nature. My liberation was through devoted practice in the Infant Movement Development module (Hartley 2010), and repeating the developmental vertebrate, reptilian, and mammalian movement sequences until they felt more natural to me.

Dr Daniel Stern (Stern 1985) researched and wrote about the development of the human nervous system and sense of self, and situated the formative interrelationship of movement and mind centrally in this process of development. Since we know about neuroplasticity as an inherent capacity in our nervous system, we know that revisiting these stages can identify and rework our stuck or harmful patterns of sensing and moving, and we can take part in reforming our own mind as we live on. As Hartley has written:

> *Where movement is both free and integrated, there life will be felt to flow freely and strongly. This freedom and integration is a gift of our journey; as we explore in detail this complex and wondrous body, our life-force and thus our essential wisdom become more available to us.*
>
> (Hartley 1995: xix)

In the experiential anatomy of the Body Systems module (Hartley 2014–16), I found my pacing and connection to my experience in my digestive system. I could validate my rhythm and cycle of hunger and satiety but then my struggle was to find my way to belong with others, as the group was held to a rhythm of mealtimes, into which I did not fit. I encountered my belief that we cannot coexist when our needs are different and explored my feelings about being different, eating at different times within the daily routine. I was welcomed in this difference and I could shift my sense of authority and belonging into balance.

Meeting Myself in the World of My Longing

During my IBMT training I discovered a way into the world of my longing which has been a parallel process with my reawakening into relationship with the natural and human world. This is the living process of relationship that I feel passionate about making more visible and felt in microcosmic and macrocosmic dimensions.

Above, I reflected on aspects of IBMT, which have taught me about the organismic living mind in my body. Through the practice of Authentic Movement as taught by Hartley, herself a student of Adler (2002), with eyes closed I have learned how it changes me to let my body senses move me, and to bear witness to myself in my somatic movement. Then, with eyes open, I have learned to include my inner experience, as I am, in witnessing other movers. I have learned about embodied relationship through being in the mysterious emergent process of tracking sensory experience, discovering cultural meaning, and awareness of the impact of my witnessing and being witnessed in the world.

How could this practice help inform and create the world of my longing? I recently was able to glimpse a facet that let me see and feel how this could happen. I had a very powerful experience of the impact of ritual witnessing on a public environment in this way in 2019 as I donned the Red Rebel (2019) robes and make-up and processed through London and Bristol, bearing witness to the scenes being played out by Extinction Rebellion activists, the general public, and the state law enforcement.

As Red Rebels, we directed our focus to feeling embodied in our movement, being responsive with gestures in ritual form to what we saw and putting ourselves outside of the social conditioning of the

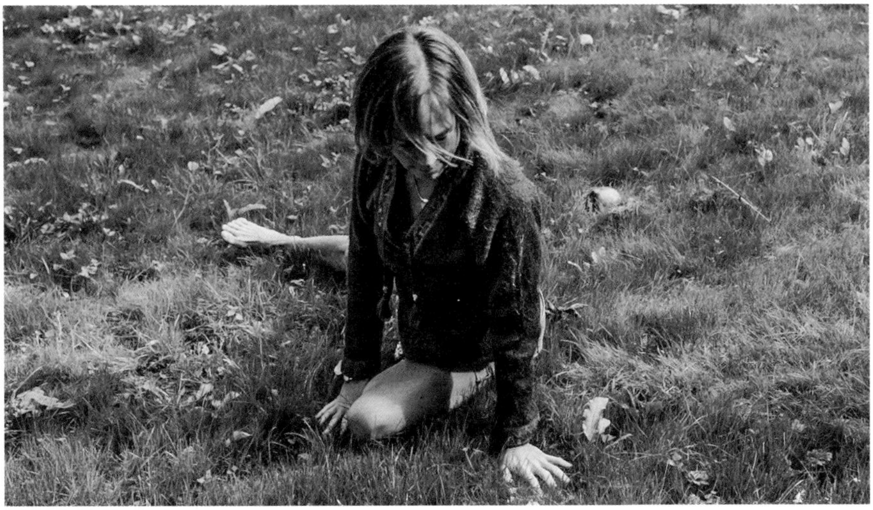

Mover: Mari Winkelman. Photographer: Nikoletta Monyok, 2020

bodies around us. We were visibly moving against a mass movement of public and traffic, outside of the socialized and traffic rules, yet also held within the codes of the Extinction Rebellion (2019) uprising, magnetizing attention and sentiment by modeling our own feelings and movement as free, semi-choreographed, and contextually responsive.

I was experiencing the way in which my embodiment practice, often so introspective and self-sensing, was informing my participation in action that was connecting my bodymind to the bodyminds of the other Red Rebels, as we gave our embodied attention to the external environment with great care. We were enacting and facilitating a collective response to the crisis unfolding in our natural world, which has been a direct result of human carelessness and excessive plundering of resources. This is where enactivism meets activism! We moved as a shoal of fish would move, or a flock of birds. The capacity to move others and be moved as a group is reliant on an expansion of awareness in the heart and belly organs, which extends beyond the skin. The impact we had on people was powerful, and different depending on which "side" of the dominant culture they were on: most did not really *know* how to respond to us. However, they could not avoid a response, and it was instinctual and often deeply moving emotionally.

In my therapeutic work, I enter another facet of the world of my longing: a world where relational attunement through our bodies is normal, essential to communication, and truth is allowed to emerge as it often does, not perfectly practiced but clumsily, slowly, confusingly, and then clearly through the connection to our body intelligence. As I attune to my own breath and inner sensations, I am noting how my clients and movement participants are attuning to theirs – or not – and supporting them to notice more, become more conscious of their body senses.

As humans, we are designed to attune our nervous systems to each other via the vagus nerve. We often do this unconsciously, attuning or misattuning to each other, but without vocabulary or confidence to articulate our body experiences. Our bodies are suppressed, then, and we continue to submit to the words and concepts being fed to us by our cultural media: perfect visual forms, conformity to social codes, or the pressures of our financial needs and relationships. This suppression has increasingly pervaded our culture and been absorbed by our individual bodies, causing confusion or mental and physical illness in more and more of our national urban populations.

For urban populations, somatic therapy and somatic movement practice can offer windows through which to facilitate individual and mutual enquiry into the experiences of our bodies. From there, we can participate in co-regulation and ability to "see" and feel ourselves and each other more clearly. In seeing and feeling ourselves from our bodies, we gain knowledge about deeper individual and communal truths about our interconnections, interrelationships with nature's creatures and ecosystems, and mysteries of healing when we are more embedded in our natural habitats, which have been overlooked, denied, and kept out of the dominant urban commercial culture. I long for somatic therapy to be more commonly offered alongside medical interventions, to open more of us to these truths and empower more of us to participate in our own health, and care for each other and our environments.

As I continue to value my organismic body, including my somatic experience in negotiating life choices, I am sometimes defined by my bones, sometimes by my skin, sometimes by my energy field. I feel that I belong on an Earth that is Gaia and am part of the great living community of beings. I would love for more people to experience this sense of their bodies and interrelationships with the living world.

I find myself "zooming in" and "zooming out" with my attention, from microcosm to macrocosm, noticing dominant patterns, and seeing/feeling beyond them towards that which my somatic mind wants to guide me. At one point it is towards an inspiring new initiative to provide organic vegetables to a community; at another moment I divert towards a terror of war that I cannot ignore; and at yet another it is towards a tiny beetle on the bark of a tree which is magnificently living its tiny life – tiny only in my humanly conditioned eyes, but magnificent in my Gaia mind. I do this zooming in and out to see the world in parallel processes – where I am drawn by what I feel within.

The human world I live in is full of healing and wounds, full of paradoxes, seemingly created and experienced by humans who have left their bodies behind to forget and bury personal and ancestral traumas, and to follow the intoxications of their aspirations and hedonism. I have experienced this personally as an intoxicated human and as a sentient being who feels the wounding this creates. The rest of the living world has to feel the impact of unconsciously wounded behavior. As I encounter my inner struggles with an embodied life, I recognize the struggle we are all waging to let go of our addictions to numbing ourselves so that we can cope in this oppressive and over-stimulating, homogenizing colonizer culture.

"Theories and interpretations are not much help in the terrifying depths of the psyche. A psychotherapist's own experience of being wounded is what helps her face the suffering client in simple relatedness" (Larisey 2012: 13). The facets mentioned above are ways of moving through the struggle of the modern world into ways of being in healing. Body, emotion, truth, and seeing clearly are the rewards I have gained from my own struggles. As babies, most of us struggle through the birth canal, though many are interfered with in this process – cesarean and forceps delivery – and these efforts strengthen our muscles, bones, and determination to find a way out. My struggles have indeed strengthened or diverted me in necessary ways for me to find and express my truth in the world.

The dominant culture and systems of living have become so hurtful for many, so that life can be easier for a few. How do we stay resourced and willing to live through this time? How do our bodies respond and how do we embrace this reality together, when there seems to be so much fear, anger, and conflict between people?

I cannot offer answers or resolutions for those questions, but I can offer what I love about the cultural space held by IBMT and would wish to sow more into the world of my longing: the return to our organismic intelligence which knows interconnected thriving. There may be leaders, but nobody is the expert because enquiry is a method of learning which facilitates a deepening of democracy, and thus we can return again and again to the question and notice how we respond to it in different times.

The new paradigm I dream of is building resilience and valuing sensitivity at the edges, just as in a cellular organism. Sensitivity matters, and witnessing our world sensitively can help us through our cerebral conundrums and biased polarizations that lead to oppression of the many by the few. These values support a curious connection in difference and collaborative meaning-making that is adaptive to changing contexts. It is the *moments* of meaning-*making* that are important, rather than holding on rigidly to the meanings themselves. My sense is that this relational sensitivity is what Gaia wants for all of us. The potency of small things matters as much as the larger events in our world ecosystem. In this version of our world, the health of our organismic bodies matters and they are our truly smart homes. When more of us learn to empower our sensitive smartness and act in collaborative connection toward our collective sharing and thriving, those in the capitalist power hubs may feel able to let go of their dominant separation from the rest of us and rejoin Gaia.

With love and thanks to Linda and all my peers and buddies for rebirthing me and accompanying me on this journey into a new world.

Glossary

Bodymind: a facet of mind that includes interoception, proprioception, and exteroception. Using the term "bodymind" enables us to share our experience outside of "consensual reality" by bridging into purely subjective sensory experiences in "bodymind reality." By naming this essential realm of experience, we can open minds to diversity of experience, validate subjectivity, and facilitate understanding about how we qualify and quantify our experiences of life so differently while inhabiting the same planet.

Body systems: the name given to distinct, yet interrelated and interdependent fluid and tissue processes of the body: for example, the skeletomuscular system, the lymphatic system. There are many subsystems within each "body system," as categorized by Body-Mind Centering®. This is for the purpose of the experiential study of our complex bodies, enabling us to focus on a system within the whole for detail and qualities of experience.

Embodied: taken to mean attentive and responsive to experience within my own body, and thereby inhabiting my body. To embody a "body system" or "body part" is to bring my attentiveness and responsiveness to that system or body part, to inhabit that system or part.

Exteroception: orientates our perception to our eyes, ears, nose, tongue, and touch receptors in our skin.

Interoception: orientates our perception towards sensations in our organs and awareness of our inner fluid movements, indicating experience being communicated from our nervous system.

Organismic: an adjective imbuing a process or experience with the immediacy of an organism's sensitive receptivity and responsiveness.

Proprioception: orientates our perception towards sensations in our skeletomuscular joints and tendons, and the sense of balance from the vestibular canals in our inner ears. These sensors indicate which parts of our bodies are in movement, and quantifies these movements and our body's relationship to the vertical and horizontal planes. When our eyes are closed, our proprioception guides us in our movement.

Social engagement system: an anatomical system identified by Stephen Porges and others, whereby the vagus nerve, which regulates our state of activity and rest, metabolism, and recuperation, connects with our auditory and visual nerves and facilitates relational interactions to navigate consensus and bonding with other humans and mammals. The social engagement system is found in social animals but the human and primate social engagement systems are more advanced, with nuanced tones and visual cues in eyes, mouth, and body gestures.

Video link

Cellular Self Human Organism –
A Short Film, 2020
Film Maker: Nikoletta Monyok; Sound Artist: Russell Evan

Becoming Nature

Rachel Lambert

2

I am nature. As a human being I am a natural organism within the pulsing, living organism of the earth. How much do I know and experience this in my bones, though, or is it just an interesting concept? In this chapter I explore questions of what it means to be a fully-fledged human being, and the role of presence, acceptance, and change. I also ask how somatics can support natural processes and how nature can support the practice of somatics.

Soma means the experience of the body from within, and the practice of somatics is the process of sensing into, or the felt-sense of, the body or bodymind.

My writing is informed by my time in nature, experiential somatics including Authentic Movement, foraging, observing animals, and my continuing evolution as a human being. The text is interspersed with my own nature writing and excerpts from my movement journal.

The Separation of Human and Nature

Earthling, earthly being, natura,
natal, native, birth, humus, ground,
of the earth, humble.

These are some of the origins of the word "human" – born of the earth. Speak to any indigenous (meaning living naturally or having always lived in a place) person or tribe and their connection to nature is innate, unquestioned, and an integral part of their existence. For many of us living now, however, this connection does not come naturally. Instead, nature can feel alien and just an idea.

We have transitioned as a society from forager to farmer, from soil to concrete, from manual to mechanized, from heart to head. Our relationship to ourselves and our surroundings has changed considerably; one such change is an increased sense of disconnection from nature. When I think about being human, I look to my relationship with nature as a guide. Here I share some of my explorations, questions, and observations.

A Nature Being

I am lying on the undulating ground of the Cornish moors; an easterly breeze is whipping around me, yet my attention is mostly on the pleasure of nature's mattress, soft grasses growing over clumps of uneven earth; my body empathizes, then colludes. My head, freed from its normal responsibilities, lies heavily on my makeshift mattress and becomes pure matter once again.

It is often time outside that gives me the space and support to settle into myself. Out in the environment of animals, birds, sky, earth, vegetation, and minerals, my body remembers how to be a sensing animal again. In this way, nature is my teacher; just as somatics has given me the tools to arrive in my body, the natural environment reflects back my own nature through its elemental essence.

My body feels cold with that whipping easterly, yet still I feel my skin soften and open as it receives the support of the ground, and the ground, faithfully, meets my body. I am reminded of Annie Brook's book, *From Conception to Crawling* (2001), and her experience of **comfort** as the precursor to human conception: comfort as laying the foundation for a soul to come in, for arrival. On that soft ground I allowed myself to find comfort.

Arrival has not always been easy for me. In truth, my history tells that I am better at running away! I remember Linda Hartley's invitation to me to "find my nature within," to find a way to be with myself rather than running away to the nature outside of myself. I now feel the two can support each other – the nature within and outside of me.

Embodying the porous, sensing surface of my skin, allowing my body fluids to be both suspended and supported by the earth below me, to feel into the vibrant weightiness of my blood – rich, dark, and full. Connecting to the location of my bones and how they relate to gravity and, in turn, with my bones more present, how my muscles can relax a little more. Enjoying my brain as an organ, a sack of matter and not just a thinking vehicle that could potentially take me into or out of myself. These are my somatic tools for assisting my physical, mental, and emotional arrival into the here-and-now.

Sensing as Nature Intended

I watch my dog sigh as he finishes a long, satisfying stretch in the sun. I observe the poised bud of a daffodil flowerhead, knowing that, any hour soon, it will gracefully pop open and bloom. I sit up against the bark of a solid yet flexible tree, its age and wisdom talking to me in ways that words cannot. I know its roots, entangled with a network of mycelium below me, will be communicating with other trees about threats and fine-tuning their immune responses, naturally – sensing, not through a brain, as such, but through a broader intelligence. The inspiration of animals, plants, and trees with their abilities to thrive, adapt, communicate, and respond to life, moment by moment.

In her book, *Molecules of Emotion* (1999), Candace Pert outlines her scientific research identifying neuropeptides throughout the body, not just in the brain. Her findings provide the first hard evidence of the bodymind: an intelligent network that extends throughout the body and is not limited to the brain. Intelligence versus intellect: I see this aptitude echoed through the natural world, compared to the human animal, in whom the higher brain has been elevated, or perhaps disproportionally developed.

In my practice of Authentic Movement, I have learned how to trust the wisdom of my body-mind again. The practice has taught me to listen sensitively to my body, dropping below my mind, thoughts, judgments, or "shoulds." Sitting, I wait for an impetus to move, listening and allowing my body to respond to its own knowing without the overbearing authority of my thinking mind. I am often surprised at the results. Compassionately, I witness myself, or am witnessed by another. I learn about my timings, my longings, my ability to attend to what is needed in the moment, to find resolution or discover another door that needs opening.

I am kneeling. My head is lifting upwards in a continual figure of eight, I am enjoying the rhythm and pattern. My nose is drawing down towards the ground and touching the sheepskin rug in front of me. My chin is edging forwards and my mouth finds my hand. Comfort. I am sucking the side of my hand and feel true comfort.

(Excerpt from my Authentic Movement practice journal)

Bonnie Bainbridge Cohen, the founder of Body-Mind Centering®, argues that movement "is the first perception to develop and therefore the most important for survival" (2008: 114-15). She is referring to the fact that the first cranial nerves to myelinate in an embryo are the vestibular nerves, which regulate movement. Her work acknowledges the profound significance of movement for experiencing oneself and the world: a value that can be lost when the rational, analytical brain is considered more worthy of being listened to. My experience of my body through movement, touch, and sensing is that it/I can intelligently perceive constant

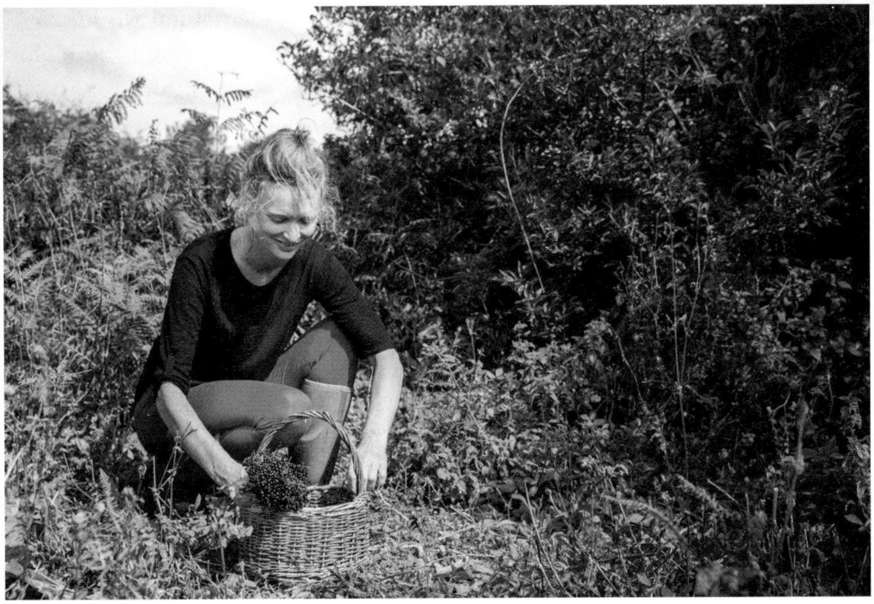

Forager/mover: Rachel Lambert. Photographer: Elliott White

reflections of self and other. I am reminded of a line from a Leonard Cohen song (1984), expressing a numbness of feeling and so trying to touch instead. Touch and movement offer a way to access feelings, sensations, and insights that awaken the natural intelligence in us all.

I step over the stone stile into the field, my head full of important things. I barely hear the grass. I feel the wind but do not let her in, despite her embracing caresses. I see the plants – sorrel, nettles, and plantains – but only as distant friends with whom I long to reconnect. I continue moving, one foot in front of the other, waiting for the important things to dissolve as my senses awaken. I walk until my mind finds humility and takes its place as a devotee of my sensing, joyful body – until I soften into being.

What Part of Nature Am I?

My human body is made up of trillions of cells, all individually functioning yet also communicating as one. The outer layer of my human form is the skin: a semi-permeable membrane, with me on the inside and the world on the outside. Yet there is a constant exchange of atoms, cells, bacteria, fluids, minerals, and vitamins between my body and the environment. As I drop my attention into the substance of my body and connect to the natural organism that I am, I allow myself to connect to myself as this semi-permeable being.

The largest element my body mass contains is water, produced from the plant life and marine algae that I love to eat and watch move in the ocean or on the earth around me. In turn, the trees, seaweeds, and phytoplankton absorb carbon dioxide from the deoxygenated air that I breathe out. In and out, exchanging, giving, and receiving, naturally. What is on the outside comes in, and what is on the inside goes out, literally, on every breath. I breathe in and absorb the element of oxygen from nature, and breathe out the element of carbon dioxide back into nature.

Chapter 2

In these reflective moments, I find no words to describe these wonders of life. Instead, I find a kind of peace, a sensation of fizziness inside me, an excitement and ecstasy that there is something bigger than me, that I am an integral part of the natural ecosystem. At various points in my somatic and nature-based career I have tried developing exercises to facilitate a deep knowing of this connection, knitting together exercises that straddle concepts with practical experiences. I have tried to be clever, disclose my knowledge and understanding, and facilitate something wonderful in people. Yet I also know that this cannot really be taught, only experienced. It is only really known from deep within our bones, or perhaps deep within our lungs, oxygenated cells, or alveoli, where those oxygen and carbon dioxide gases are exchanged.

This also alludes to the question how much of me is really "human" or what a human body is really made up of. It is thought that only around half of our bodies consists of human cells; the rest exists as microbes – bacteria, viruses, and fungi. Our relationship with these non-human microbes within us helps create and greatly influences our humanness, as do the microbes and life around us. Becoming human is perhaps more about receiving and giving rather than trying to contain or separate ourselves.

I am reminded of many moments in my Authentic Movement practice where I have witnessed or participated in a synchronicity between people which seems to speak of an invisible intelligence connecting us:

> **I am a witness. I am sitting in a circle and observing three movers in the space. One is sitting, knees up, touching her toes delicately. The second is standing with her weight on her right leg and the third is also standing, turned away from the other two with her head dropped downwards and her hands held together in front of her chest. Spontaneously and without awareness of each other, the three movers each lift their left arm towards the ceiling. I feel amazed and sense myself gasp. I imagine an invisible force connecting these movers to each other and the space. I am smiling.**

(Excerpt from my Authentic Movement practice journal)

Cows, Skin, and the Environment

A few years ago, I was preparing my teaching material on the skin – the boundary between "I" and the environment. I decided to take myself, with my notes and thoughts, to the field behind my house and allow my skin and the environment to be my inspiration.

It was such a joy to walk across the field, dropping into my body and allowing my attention to go to my skin and my surroundings. I went to my favorite spot on the far side of the field, where a rounded rock protrudes out of the earth, just big enough to drape myself over. It looked so inviting and I nuzzled down. The stone and the earth felt so comfortable and welcoming. Had I not noticed that before or was it that my attention was now on my skin – a place of receptivity, of meeting my environment and allowing it to meet me?

I was so enjoying feeling, sensing, touching, and writing about the skin that it took me some time to notice that my environment was changing. A large herd of cows, with their young, were munching their way across the land. The calves started to buck and run across the field; it felt as special as witnessing a herd of wild deer. I drank the scene in with my eyes and stayed present with my skin as a receptive membrane, sensing and welcoming my environment. Slowly, a few of the calves ventured forward alone, with their elders not far behind, allowing the meeting with something close to grace, I thought. I heard their breath, sensed their presence and intrigue, a large snout edging its way towards mine. Somewhere between intrigue and being ready to bolt, the exchange lasted a few moments.

The skin is a semi-permeable membrane and, on my rock, I was somatically exploring what it felt like to be porous: to let the love and the heavenly, magical world in while simultaneously having a clear boundary to keep out unwanted elements. Then the cows came. Those big, hefty bodies who protect their young as a herd – I had previously admired their guarding watch as their calves rested or frolicked. I had passed them many times in the last couple of weeks, yet this was the first time they were coming to me. From the perception of my skin, I put my trust in my senses and stayed present.

Through the sensing organ of my skin, I met the cows. I felt received by them and I hope they felt welcomed by me. Through my somatic awareness, it felt easier to connect to these four-legged friends, as if body sensation and feeling were more in tune with their language, enabling me to become a better human animal, perhaps, and a more harmonious part of nature.

The Natural Evolution of Change

From the moment of human conception, a mighty journey begins: cells multiply, specialize, and organize themselves into the imprint of a small human being. From birth to 2 years old the learning is intense and constant, with an innate, evolutionary impetus to develop – nothing to force, just allow.

To be present is not to do nothing; it is to allow the natural process of change and growth to unfold. Buddhism and meditation practice have been teaching this for thousands of years. Using body awareness and taking time to notice feelings and sensations can be useful tools for change. Christina Feldman is an experienced meditation teacher and co-founder of Gaia House Retreat Centre in Devon, UK, a center offering silent meditation retreats in the Buddhist tradition, which welcomes people of every age, ethnicity, cultural heritage, religious background, socio-economic group, sexual orientation, and gender identity (https://gaiahouse.co.uk). She believes that being attentive to the present is, in its very essence, a process of assisting change with great care and kindness:

Through attention we learn the skill of being whole-heartedly present with great sensitivity. Every moment of dissolving habit with clear attentiveness is a moment of fostering sensitivity and a clear connection with the present moment.

(Feldman 1998: 118)

Feldman clearly links being present and attentive to dissolving habit – not just blindly going on as we normally do. Similarly, Peter Levine, in his book *Waking the Tiger: Healing Trauma* (1997), discusses the value of somatically connecting to one's present experience to transform trauma into healing. Levine identifies the stress response (to traumatic events) of freezing as a place that people often get stuck, where the natural movement towards healing is frozen and change is on hold. By focusing on body sensation and how the body unconsciously wants to move, Levine explains how we can assist it in its natural leaning towards health. Here, change towards health is, again, not directed, but rather a process of allowing the automatic body responses to unfold.

Unfortunately, the human brain can obscure this natural process. A common belief is that judgment and guilt can be motivators for change – "I feel so bad I have to change." However, I also feel that judgment can greatly inhibit change.

Chapter 2

In the Chinese art of T'ai Chi there is a saying: "the chi (energy) goes where the mind flows" (Liang 1977: 70). I find this saying really helpful and it reminds me to watch my thoughts and come back into my body, rather than becoming too lost in my head.

I am running along the seafront, smelling the sea and hearing the gentle waves rolling in; it feels good to be outdoors and to experience my heart rate increase and my breathing find a steady, deeper rhythm. I do not run far and I am overtaken by several "serious" runners. Occasionally, I judge myself for this, repeating phrases in my head such as "I should try harder, I should run harder, run further, I should take this more seriously." I have a sinking feeling in my heart and belly – a heaviness in my legs, even – and my motivation to run again is tainted with dread.

On other days I accept my limitations and run free, acknowledging when my body is tired and turning towards home. I enjoy the fact that I can find a pace that suits me and that others are faster, fitter, or just different from me. I return home elated, feeling kind towards myself and motivated to get on with my day. For me, when I judge myself, my ability to change or even continue feels stifled. By comparison, when I accept myself, change feels easier and natural, and my enthusiasm for it bubbles up in me.

I watch a crow pick at the remains of a sticky-furred rabbit at the side of the road. I see a weighted wave crash down on an unbalanced surfer. I witness the river swell and overflow, claiming muddy banks and tree roots within an expanding watery domain. Nature does not judge; it just is. Perhaps becoming nature means to bypass judgment for acceptance, with no force, no belittling or scoring.

Change, according to Bainbridge Cohen, is a fine balance of moving through feeling, sensing, and action that enables the flow of change to exist: not holding, not staying still, not perpetually acting/doing but flowing through these stages in a real, embodied way. Through somatics, body awareness, and the teachings of nature, the body's organic movement and wisdom could be its highest self: nature.

Awakening to the Collective Body: Authentic Movement as a Path to Wholeness

3

Mari Joyce

A thunderclap under the clear blue sky
All beings on earth open their eyes;
Everything under heaven bows together;
Mount Sumeru leaps up and dances.

Wu-men, H., *The Gateless Gate*

Now it can dawn on us: we are our world knowing itself.

Joanna Macy, *World as Lover, World as Self*

In this chapter I explore how the practice of Authentic Movement can support us in navigating uncertainty and meeting emergent processes as they arise, opening us out to new pathways for healing, integration, and wholeness, at the level of the individual and collective. Authentic Movement is an embodiment practice in which we track our experiences of sensing, feeling, and moving through the body, allowing for a gradual process of integration of unconscious material at the level of the individual. Through cultivating the art of clear seeing and relational presence, we learn to take in another as she is, free of the obscurations of our judgment and projection. As a therapeutic and spiritual practice, Authentic Movement supports the cultivation of awareness and compassion, with which we may open to widening circles of connectedness, to include not only self and other, but also the collective body.

Throughout this chapter I share examples of personal practice relating to different aspects touched on in this writing, and include images taken from a video I created with dancers Gaelin Little and Cat Westwood (see the link at the end of the chapter). I hope that these may offer a different felt way of accessing the material explored here.

I begin by exploring "The Journey of Descent," that process of dropping down to meet the undercurrents of what is arising, at the level of individual and collective process work. I next turn towards the themes of healing and embodiment as I relate to them in my own practice as a somatic therapist. I then come to the practice of Authentic Movement, to describe its form and some different aspects of the practice. I look at Authentic Movement as an embodied relational practice, in which the deepening of our own embodied connection can open us out to ever-widening circles of relationship, which include self, other, and the world.

The practice supports us to widen our sense of self, potentially to include the collective body and more-than-human realm (Abram 1996), opening us to an experience of what the deep ecologist Arne Næss has described as "the ecological self" (Næss 1985). At a time when it becomes clearer than ever that our actions necessitate the consideration of our wider community, may these practices support us in our ability to relate to our bodies and the Earth with greater reverence, care, and compassion. May we feel our place in the wider dance of creation and connection, to participate in the co-creation of "the more beautiful world our hearts know is possible" (Eisenstein 2013).

The Journey of Descent

Spiraling rivulets dance before my eyes. Whirling eddies that shift and meander through the river bed. My heart follows these journeys, soaring and drifting with the continual letting go of water. I feel my body as the container of the earthen

Chapter 3

banks, and the flow of experience like this water, continually arising and passing away. The words of the eight-century Tibetan Buddhist teacher Padmasambhava come to mind, which resonate for me, now more than ever, as we move through the darkness of challenging times: "I do not know. I do not have. I do not understand." I feel the water as a blessing, calling me to presence and inviting connection.

During the year in which I write, we are living through unprecedented times. We are moving through a pandemic in which millions are currently in lockdown around the world, many experiencing acute fear, loneliness, and loss, or facing illness and death alone, or working in hospitals, pushed to their limit and carrying the grief of collective suffering. We have also witnessed the ongoing violence of institutional and systemic racism, as we mourned the lives of George Floyd, Breonna Taylor, and the many other victims of murder and police brutality. And we continue to live with the ever-present threat of ecological collapse, as we enter what scientists speak of as the sixth mass extinction. As I write these words and connect with these painful realities, I notice the need to orient to embodied resources to be able to stay present. I allow a slowing and settling, to feel my body and the depth of feeling moving through. I orient to my outbreath and sensations of release and letting go, which open me to the support of the earth below.

We are witnessing the unfolding of a collective process of surrender, as we meet these deeper realities of uncertainty and impermanence, so evident at this time. The normality of everyday life has fallen away, no longer holding the illusion of solidity. There is, all at once, a challenge and a gift in meeting these realities, for in the midst of great unrest lies the hidden opportunity to begin the work of healing. My perspective of healing work is that which facilitates a return to wholeness and connectedness, rather than an approach of "fixing" or "making better."

The journey of healing often begins with "the dark night of the soul," in which we encounter our suffering and shadow aspects in what can be described as a journey of descent. This very human process can be seen at once as an initiation and an invitation, a call to awakening (Hartley 2001;

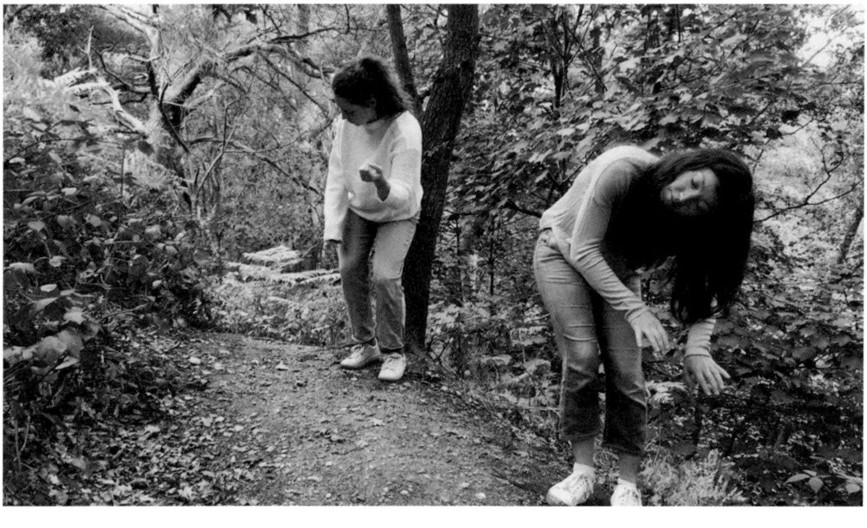

Dancers: Gaelin Little and Cat Westwood. Photographer: Mari Joyce

Moore 2005). To hear that call, we may be required to listen quietly and deeply, against the din of the busy world and a culture hooked on numbing and tuning out. At other times, this call may come crashing into our lives, unmistakable and impossible to ignore, perhaps in the form of great crisis, death, a breakup or breakdown. Thomas Moore perfectly describes these specific processes:

During the dark night there is no choice but to surrender control, give in to unknowing, and stop and listen to whatever signals of wisdom might come along. It's a time of enforced retreat and perhaps unwilling withdrawal. The dark night is more than a learning experience; it's a profound initiation into a realm that nothing in the culture, so preoccupied with external concerns and material success, prepares you for.

(Moore 2005: 8)

We might speak of this journey as "the path of the wounded healer," or as the quest of soul retrieval. However we choose to frame it, this is a journey of making whole. Martin Shaw points to it in the myth of the "wild twin": a lost part of ourselves that holds all we have relegated to shadow and cast out. We endlessly seek it, and it in turn is always trying to speak to us, whether in the language of myth and dream, in the cry of a dark night, or in the call of the world around us:

In the labour of becoming a human, you have to earnestly search this character out … If there was something you were here to do in these few, brief years, you can be sure that the wild twin is holding the key.

(Shaw 2020: 10)

Coming Home to the Body

In my practice as a somatic therapist my aim is simply to accompany people on their journeys of meeting their embodied experience. The root of the word therapy goes back to the Greek *therapeia*, which means to care for or tend to another soul. This work of soul tending requires us to meet ourselves as we are with awareness and compassion, and often involves a process of dropping down into our embodied experience, to traverse our oceanic depths of feeling and sensation. The archetypal image of the labyrinth speaks to me of this process, in which we move through the darkness of unknown landscapes, open to whatever we may encounter, including those aspects kept in shadow (represented as the minotaur within Greek mythology). When we travel with the thread of awareness, a return journey is made possible. We witness this in the fine red thread gifted to Theseus by Ariadne as he traversed unknown paths in the darkness of the Cretan labyrinth. We can see the thread as the art of witnessing, which allows us to shine the light of awareness in the depths of our inner experience, for the sake of integration, wholeness, and homecoming.

Throughout this chapter I will be using the term "embodiment," by which I mean our lived experience through and from the body, rather than *about* the body. The online Merriam Webster dictionary defines embodiment as "the act of embodying," as well as "the state of being embodied," which tells us that it is a participatory process, an enquiry into bodily experiences that is concerned with how we live and inhabit the world, through our senses. Marion Woodman describes bodywork as "soulwork" and says that we must be in contact with our inner world if we wish to live a rich life.

Soulwork demands that we come back into relationship with those parts that we have lost contact with. At the heart of the divided self and our dualistic culture lies our split from the body. We can see the body as the site of the unconscious itself, holding all that we relegate from our sense of self.

Chapter 3

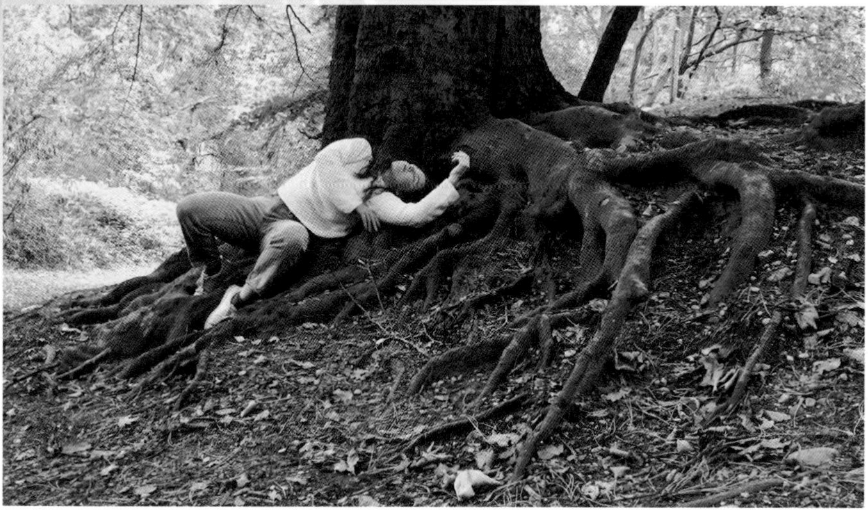

Dancer: Gaelin Little. Photographer: Mari Joyce

John P. Conger explores this in *Jung and Reich: The Body as Shadow*, stating that "without the body, the wisdom of the larger self cannot be known" (2005: 183). The Cartesian culture in which we live has long divided body from mind, and matter from spirit, elevating scientific knowledge over embodied understanding. These emphases can leave us in danger of being bereft from the wilds of our lived experience, and the subtle undercurrents which can speak to us through both the personal and the collective body. Reconnecting to ourselves in this way is a process of remembering, gathering up the lost and forgotten parts. Attending to our experience with awareness and compassion, we find pathways of connection that can bring us back into relationship with ourselves as individuals and as part of a wider whole.

As a somatic therapist, I work with the body as the ground of process work, listening to the subtle signals of gesture, rhythm, and impulse through the body. Beneath symptoms, illness and disease lie conversations that are trying to happen through the body. When we attend to our embodied experience in this way we can witness a deeper wisdom from the body, which has its own knowing about what needs to unfold. To work in this way requires that we slow down, to come into present-time awareness and be able to orient to the dynamic flow of sensation and feeling moving through us from one moment to the next. We can do this in simple ways throughout the day, by orienting to sensations that speak of the support of ground or the shifting rhythms of our breath. Can we allow time to settle? Like a shy bird, we may need to wait with some patience and curiosity, as our felt experience makes itself known to us. Can we simply meet whatever is present here, orienting to sensations and feelings within the body with a gentle curiosity? My work is deeply underpinned by the practice of Authentic Movement, which I will now describe.

Authentic Movement

Authentic Movement is a contemplative movement practice originated by Mary Starks Whitehouse and further developed in the Discipline of Authentic Movement by Janet Adler. The ground form of this work is the dyad structure of mover and witness. The practice takes place in the ritual context of a moving and witnessing circle, in which the mover steps into the circle with eyes closed, free to follow arising impulses, while the space is held by the witnesses for an agreed amount of time. The other aspect of the practice takes place within the speaking and listening circle, in which the mover takes time to speak about her experience after returning from the moving circle.

The mover is encouraged to ground her experiences within the context of her sensations, feelings, and gestures while moving, rather than stories *about* her experience. Mover and witness wish to stay as close to the mover's embodied experience as possible, and so speak in the present tense to support this. The witness offers the possibility of sharing her own experience while witnessing, which is grounded in her own felt sense of observing the mover. In being witnessed, the mover begins to cultivate her own inner witness, as she meets the depths of her own inner process with growing awareness and compassion. Adler writes:

The intrapersonal work concerns the forming of the inner witness. The presence of the outer witness can become a compassionate model for the aspect of the mover that is becoming conscious of her own experience.

(Adler 2002: 6)

Early on in practice, the mover may find that gestures and movements are predominantly unconscious and she may remember very little of her experience. The witness supports a filling out in the mover's awareness and recollection. Receiving witnessing can feel like being offered precious gifts, as aspects of the movers' experience are reflected back to them through verbal sharing, all in a deeply accepting and compassionate field of relationship. The witness holds a safe space through clarity of presence and embodiment, allowing depth of material to be processed and integrated.

The heart of the practice is about the longing, as well as the fear, to see ourselves clearly. We repeatedly discover that such an experience of clarity is deeply and inextricably related to the gift of being seen clearly by another and, just as importantly, related to the gift of seeing another clearly.

(Adler 1999a: 194)

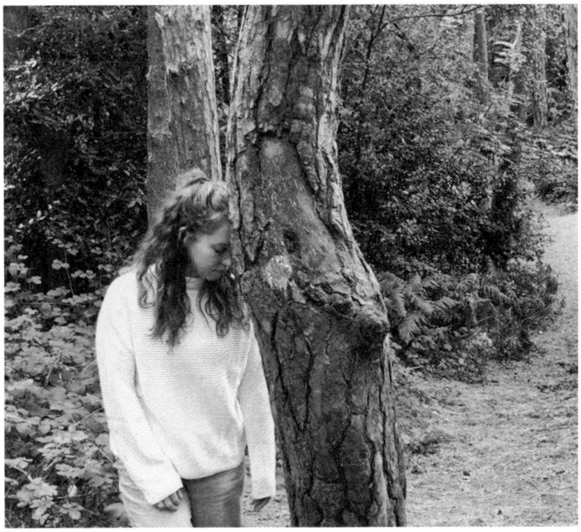

Dancer: Gaelin Little. Photographer: Mari Joyce

Within the practice of Authentic Movement, we may experience a deep longing to be seen and received by a compassionate witness, echoing our needs for a "good enough" holding field in our early development. I first came to the practice of Authentic Movement full of curiosity and a longing for connection with myself and others. Closing my eyes, moving into the container of the circle, I discover that my early experiences were often around the theme of longing for connection, to myself, other, and the wider ground and space.

My experience in the practice, and my learnings from the Integrative Bodywork and Movement Therapy (IBMT) diploma, have given me an

Chapter 3

appreciation of Authentic Movement as a practice grounded in our capacity for embodied relational presence, the whole practice rooted in the process of awakening witness consciousness through the body. As we work, we connect to a growing sense of embodied resources – experiences in which we feel safe and supported, and have a sense of pleasure through the body, and in relationship to other bodies and the ground.

The aliveness of beings and bodies. We meet and bend and ricochet and settle, turning over and over countless times, finding each other like billowing leaves or laundry or delicate ornate clockwork, finding a thousand places of rest. I cannot see our arrangement, but feel the touching of hands, and feet and heads turning over each other. The places I anchor into ground. The soft and gentle knowledge of safety and trust.

An element within the practice which continues to intrigue me is its ability to hold mysterious moments of connection and synchronicity. I have experienced this many times, as a mover and as a witness. Each time feels like an affirmation of the mystery and the clarity of how our experiences are unfolding within the container of a unified relational field. Two movers align themselves precisely, moving together with mirroring gestures, creating something that becomes more than each alone. These moments of synchronous atunement are often hard to give words to, but arise in the moment with a quality of mysterious unfolding. They speak of an inherent connectedness, and seem to arise when we allow a letting go of volition and surrender to not knowing.

The Art of Not Knowing

Within the practice of Authentic Movement we drop into a particular state of being in which we wait and allow ourselves to be moved by an impulse. This aspect lies at the heart of the practice and is a key to opening to the possibility of "being moved." Mary Starks Whitehouse describes this in the following passage:

[T]he open waiting, which is also a kind of listening to the body, an emptiness in which something can happen. You wait until you feel a change – the body sinks or begins to tip, the head slowly lowers or rolls to one side. As you feel it begin, you follow where it leads, like following a pathway that opens up before you as you step.

(Starks Whitehouse 1999: 53)

These words offer a vibrant example of the way in which we can potentially navigate the unknown in Authentic Movement, through a process of listening and tending to our arising experience. We shift our state of consciousness to one of receptivity, to meet emergent processes as they unfold. As we work with the practice over longer periods of time, we may deepen our ability to surrender to not knowing, relinquishing the grasping of the rational mind for solid ground, certainty, and control. We open instead to a wider and more expansive state of consciousness, akin to states found in meditation practice in which we witness the arising and passing away of experience. In engaging this way, we are cultivating the art of not knowing, aligning ourselves with a deeper reality of how things really are, which is inherently uncertain.

This aspect of practice speaks to me of Buddhist teachings on impermanence, which point to the reality that all things change. One aspect of this is loss, but another is renewal and rebirth, and the recognition that change, growth, and awakening are possible. The teaching of emptiness means specifically that all things are empty of a fixed self

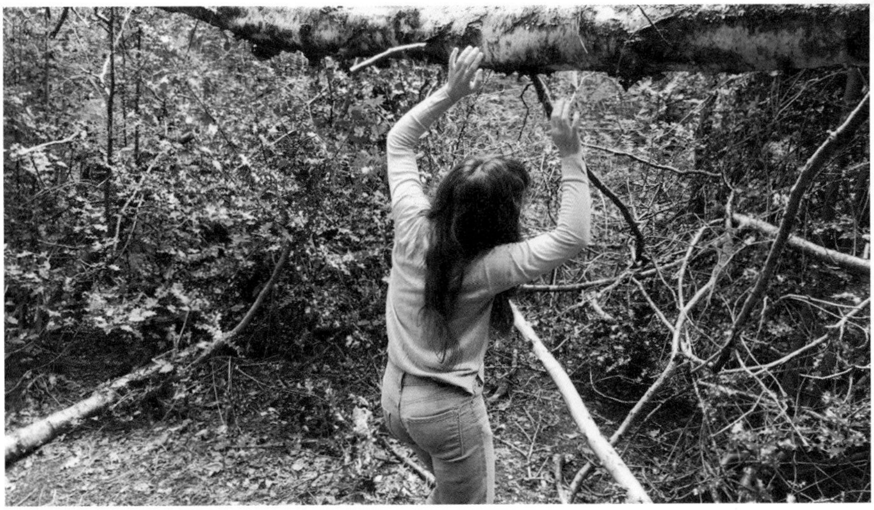

Dancer: Cat Westwood. Photographer: Mari Joyce

– nothing exists in isolation but rather is part of a broader web of interconnection or interbeing. To open to our experience with a genuine spirit of surrender and acceptance involves meeting these realities.

I enter the circle backwards. I need to find a way to experience anew, to meet the familiar with whole-body openness and listening. I invite myself to let go of knowing, and in this moment experience an opening out through my heart and chest. I feel my body like a gateway, open to receive. I feel my bones, bare and open to the sky. Heart and mind empty, waiting. Full of longing for the light to enter me, to touch those parts hidden in shadow.

The practice of Authentic Movement allows us to grow a compassionate enough inner witness to hold the experiences of life, as we meet them. In this sense, the work truly becomes a discipline, a commitment to keep shining the light of awareness and warmth of compassion on all that arises in our experience. Living in this time of collective crisis, it seems that we are so often swinging between overwhelm and compassion fatigue, and patterns of numbing and closing off. But we do not get to simply shut off from our pain without also closing off to our joy and aliveness. Authentic Movement supports us to cultivate resources for somatic knowing, embodied relational presence, and compassion, to meet what arises. Cultivating these inner tools feels more needed than ever at this time, as we continue to move through the unknown.

The Longing for Wholeness

Gradually, the work opens out to include a connection not only in relation to self and other, but also to the collective as a wider whole. Taking our place in the collective, we open to an experience of self and other as both separate and profoundly interconnected. Through Authentic Movement practice, we can discover new potential for wholeness as we move out beyond experiencing an isolated sense of self. At the relational level, witnessing another as she is, without additional layers of judgment or preconception, we may experience a moment of grace, also seeing ourselves with greater clarity.

Chapter 3

"Seeing another as she is – Loving her – enables me to see myself as I am" (Adler 1999b: 154).

Each of us holds the very human need to feel part of something bigger than ourselves. Janet Adler speaks of her own longing for embodied knowing, not just conceptual understanding, of "the web of interconnectedness": "It is not enough when the development of the self excludes an integrated relationship to the whole" (Adler 1999a: 191). Maldoma Somé from the Dagara tribe writes beautifully of this, describing his own experiences of being part of the collective of his tribe: "I understood that what makes a village a village is the underlying presence of the unfathomable joy in being connected to everyone and everything" (Somé 1994: 301).

The wholeness of the collective echoes wholeness at both micro- and macrocosmic levels. We can see the earth in the body, the body in the earth, and how the collective spans from cellular to planetary bodies. We can also include the very elements that make up our planet – the earth and air and water which we share – which also make up our physical bodies. Circles within circles of life, arising and passing away in rhythms of renewal and regeneration. Holding a transpersonal perspective, we can place human consciousness within the wider field of collective consciousness. In this light, we can hold a curiosity about our ability to listen and recognize how the earth body is speaking to us. I am curious about the notion of the Earth's own intentions for healing. If we are that part of the Earth made conscious, what responsibility lies with us, as caretakers of "the more than human realm" (Abram 1996)? How can we be a conduit of inner listening, to receive the wisdom rising up from the dreaming of the Earth?

Awakening to the Collective Body

My own experiences of Authentic Movement have gradually led me to experience it as a spiritual practice, opening me to a sense of the collective body. My own experience of the collective body has ranged from experiences of group processes in retreat environments, as well as experiences of widening out to include a sense of the Earth and wider planetary life. It is these latter experiences that I will explore further now. I am curious about how

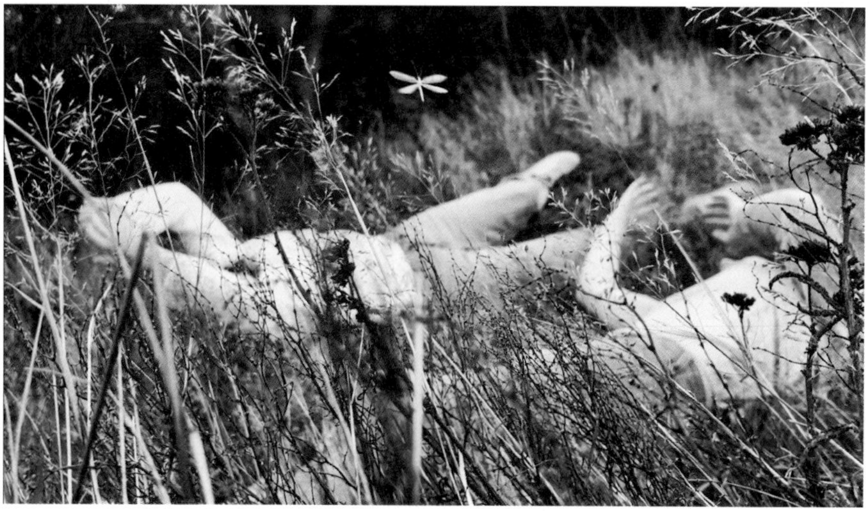

Dancers: Gaelin Little and Cat Westwood. Photographer: Mari Joyce

the practice of Authentic Movement can open us to an embodied connection with the Earth body, and the wisdom such engagement might bring through at this time. I resonate deeply with the words of Native American ecopsychologist Jeanette Armstrong, in "Keepers of the Earth." She writes:

We survive within our skin inside the rest of our vast selves … Okanagans teach that the body is the Earth itself. They say that our flesh, blood, and bones are Earthbody; in all cycles in which the Earth moves, so does our body … Our word for body literally means "the land-dreaming capacity."

(Armstrong 1995: 320)

Environmental activist Marna Hauk explored this possibility of our Earth-dreaming capacity through a piece of embodied spiritual research in which 24 women were invited to "incubate" Earth-healing dreams in a "virtual Hygeian dream temple." I love the reflections that emerged for Hauk in these explorations about where the dreams arise from, whether "the individual women, emergent dreamtime collectives, or planetary supersystem." Whatever the case, she writes:

Earth dreaming practices cultivate reconnection with these larger states of planetary systemic intelligence and wholeness … Through setting intention for incubating earth dreams … we are birthing a renewing world from a dreaming matrix, becoming imaginal, oracular portals and instantiations of the voice(s) of the Earth while re-embodying regenerative and life-giving wholeness.

(Hauk 2018: 186)

My experience of Authentic Movement is that it offers similar tools to open to an expanded awareness that can include a sense of the Earth's voice and our own Earth-dreaming capacities. Adler writes of "the collective body as the energetic consciousness of the earthbody, which includes all living beings" (Adler 1999a: 192). Working with the body, we discover how completely relational we are. We discover that parts that once felt isolated and alone are, in fact, deeply supported by surrounding layers of body systems. Each body system is richly diverse, wild, and dynamic as the ecosystems of our planet, reminding us of our connection to the wider whole.

We begin by listening to the earth, using the resources of the body. As we attend to underlying patterns, we recognize that body is part of earth – inseparable. Each individual is not alone but a participant in local and global bioregions, just as every cell is part of us.

(Olsen 2002: 227)

I would like to share a little personal experience from a group retreat, to reflect on how the collective can emerge, and which speaks to a quality of bodies expressing themselves as "the land-dreaming capacity." On this specific retreat, we gather as an intimate group of four experienced movers, with Linda Hartley in her small studio in Norfolk. Arriving together, we are asked to name what we are bringing. We each speak, and so begin the process of weaving the personal and the collective: "Gratitude and grief … Not knowing … The beauty of the world … Listening to the Earth … ." My description of moving and witnessing here is shared with permission from my fellow movers and I acknowledge that the words are my own perspective on a shared experience.

We work with the ritual practice, a particular form emerging from the Discipline of Authentic Movement, as pioneered by Janet Adler. We come to standing in a circle, creating our container for the practice. Witnessing the empty space, we each take time to feel into whether we will be a mover or witness, then declare ourselves, and make a little eye contact. Witnesses take their place in the witness circle. The bell rings once and movers close their eyes, stepping into the moving circle.

A mover stands, listening attentively
The stillness and presence of the space enter her
As the wind rises up, an extension of her breath.
Another mover sounds, an open channel to the earth
Which rises up and speaks through her now
Her body becoming earth.
Another mover comes to rest on the ground
Heavy with the grief of ancestors
She buries a seed of hope in dark earth.
Another mover stands and pivots slowly, then gathers momentum
The space whirling her being as she surrenders.
We come to stillness together
An open channel here
Body and earth, rising and falling as one
The fullness and emptiness of the space holding us
As we lean into a wider presence.
Threads of connection
Weaving a dance of belonging.

The bell rings again, three times, to mark the end of the moving circle. Gradually, the movers come back to the circle, making eye contact with the witnesses and each other. Time is taken for reflection, to write or draw or simply rest. Some of us step outside, touching the lavender, touching the sage. Slowly, we come back together for the speaking and listening circle, beginning the process of finding words for our experience. In giving language to bodily experience, we deepen a process of weaving personal and collective threads. It is in the sharing of our individual experiences that we affirm our place in the collective, and we witness synchronicities that point to a greater connectedness, and a depth of presence in the space that speaks of collective consciousness.

The moving and witnessing circle acts a container for the ground of experience, which we can observe as continually arising and falling away, each mover a cell within the body, making up the whole but also complete unto herself. Attending to experiences of moving as well as witnessing, I notice a quality of fullness and emptiness all at once, as experiences arise and fall away. Questions emerge: Who is having this experience? What is it that moves us? From what do these experiences seemingly arise and fall away? These are not questions I wish to seek immediate answers to, but rather to keep living, and feed my continuing commitment to the practice.

We make of ourselves an open channel in this work, and in doing so allow something other than ourselves to move us. In this way the Discipline offers glimpses … of luminous presence … stillness in the depths … inner and outer layers weaving together, to create the whole that is each moment … Opening to the collective body necessarily widens us out to these transpersonal dimensions, beyond limiting perceptions of ourselves as isolated beings. We are not alone here, and instead are offered the possibility of feeling our place in the wider dance of creation and connection. Hartley describes this process: "Our personal stories, unfolding through movement and sound, interact and evolve in ways that support each person's developing consciousness and healing, whilst also embodying a greater story in which we all play a special part" (Hartley 2004: 67). We need each other in this work and discover that, whatever we are doing, we are doing it together.

Hope in the Dark

Authentic Movement offers powerful tools to bring us home to the individual and collective body, to

Authentic Movement as a Path to Wholeness

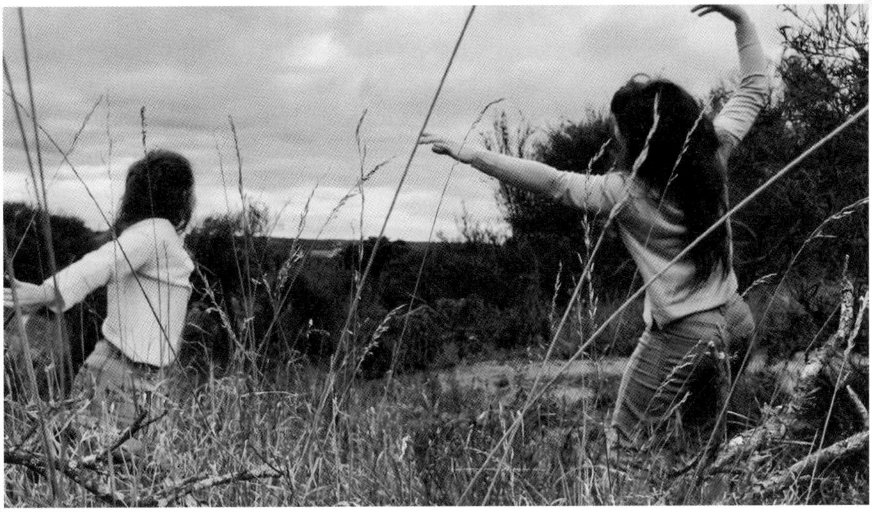

Dancers: Gaelin Little and Cat Westwood. Photographer: Mari Joyce

engage our hearts and minds in order to feel our place as part of the whole. Hartley describes what is unfolding at this time as the archetypal process of Collective Initiation (Hartley 2020). I sense this as a process of being called to a collective awakening. At times, it feels as though the Earth is speaking through dream signals which are becoming less and less subtle, as if having to shout increasingly loud to be heard. We can see the emergence of the coronavirus pandemic in this way too, hearing how environmental scientists have declared that the virus emerged as a direct result of the acute damage and destruction of vital ecosystems and habitats (Carrington 2020).

Environmental activist and Buddhist scholar Joanna Macy has written for many years about the call to awaken to our deep connection to the Earth as our home and an extension of ourselves. We cannot harm the Earth without also harming ourselves. She goes further, describing a quality of consciousness in the Earth itself, also participating in this collective awakening:

It is my experience that the world itself has a role to play in our liberation. Its very pressures, pains, and risks can wake us up – release us from the bonds of ego and guide us home to our vast, true nature.
(Macy 2007: 23)

The longing for wholeness speaks of the spiritual desire for awakening and open-hearted, clear seeing. Such desire connects to the Buddhist vision of the Bodhicitta, which translates as "heartmind of awakening," and depicts a vision of cultivating an equality of self and other: "Those desiring speedily to be a refuge for themselves and others should make the interchange of 'I' and 'other,' and thus embrace a sacred mystery" (Shantideva 1997: VIII, 120). This underpins the foundation of the Buddhist practice of "Metta Bhavana," or "Cultivation of Loving Kindness," in which we allow ourselves to open out into the deeper reality of our interconnection with others and all life. I find such spiritual dimensions deeply nourishing and sustaining, and support a growing capacity to open to the collective.

Transpersonal dimensions feel of great importance at this time, and for me at least help to orient to a sense of a bigger unfolding process. We have only to observe patterns in nature to witness essential life cycles of birth, death, and rebirth. Seen in this light, we might be curious not only about what we are releasing and letting go of at this time, but about what we are birthing into. These are questions for which there cannot be immediate answers, but rather "to live," as the poet Rilke writes, in *Letters to a Young Poet:*

Be patient toward all that is unsolved in your heart and to try to love the questions themselves like locked rooms and like books that are written in a very foreign tongue. Do not now seek the answers, which cannot be given to you because you would not be able to live them. And the point is, to live everything. Live the questions now. Perhaps you will then gradually, without noticing it, live along some distant day into the answer.

(Rilke 2004)

Authentic Movement offers the powerful resource of inner listening, to hear what we do not yet know and navigate ways forward through unknown terrain. I love the capacity within Authentic Movement practice to be an open conduit, to participate in what David Whyte calls the "conversational nature of reality." It reminds me of the following words from a poem by Antonio Machado:

Path maker, there is no path.

You make the path by walking.

(Antonio Machado,
"Caminante, No Hay Camino")

I am deeply grateful to this practice, to my teacher Linda Hartley, and to my fellow movement practitioners with whom I practice Authentic Movement. I am curious about how this work will continue to unfold, especially as we traverse such unprecedented times. Personally, I feel a deep relief in our capacity to drop into our depths of feeling and sensing, and to open to a deeper wisdom from this place – to step forward, knowing that we do not know, but committed to listening and acting with care towards those we encounter. I hope this practice can support us to develop the ability to sit with difference and build our capacity to go beyond polarization and opposition. May we trust in the unfolding of the body's process, as it reveals new possibilities to us in each moment. Every breath, an arrival. Every step upon the earth, a homecoming.

Video link
Dancers: Gaelin Little
and Cat Westwood

Pelvic Bowls – Digging/Drilling/Exploitation: A Performance

Raima Drąsutytė

4

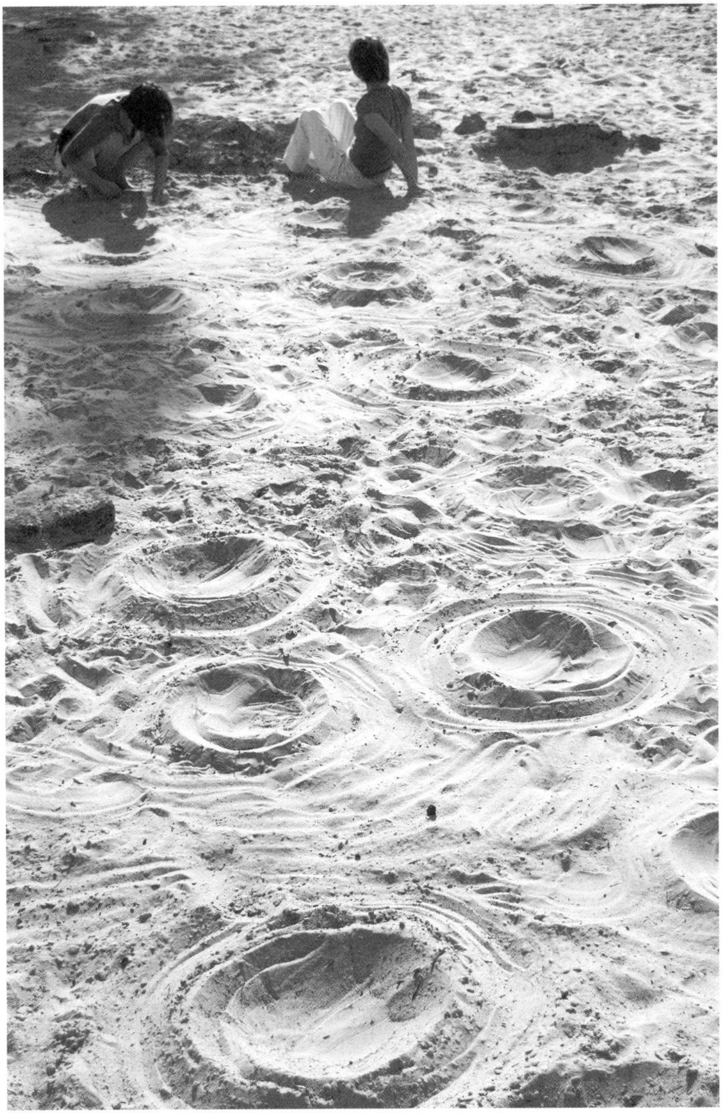

Chapter 4

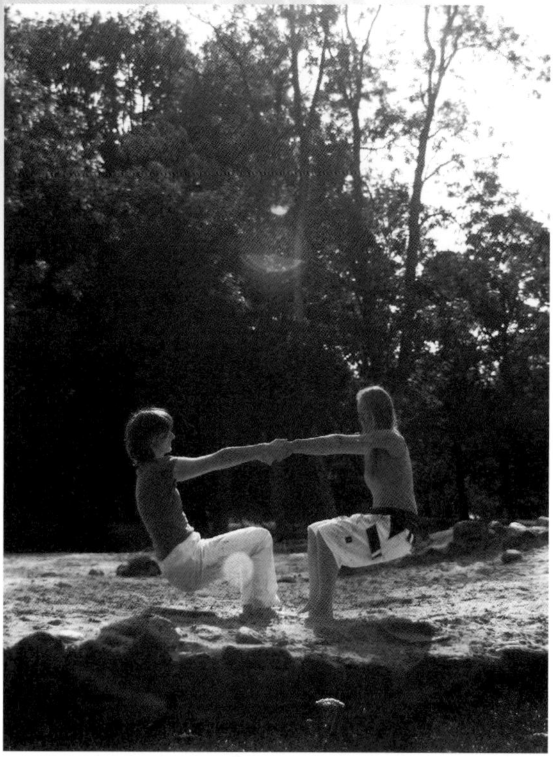

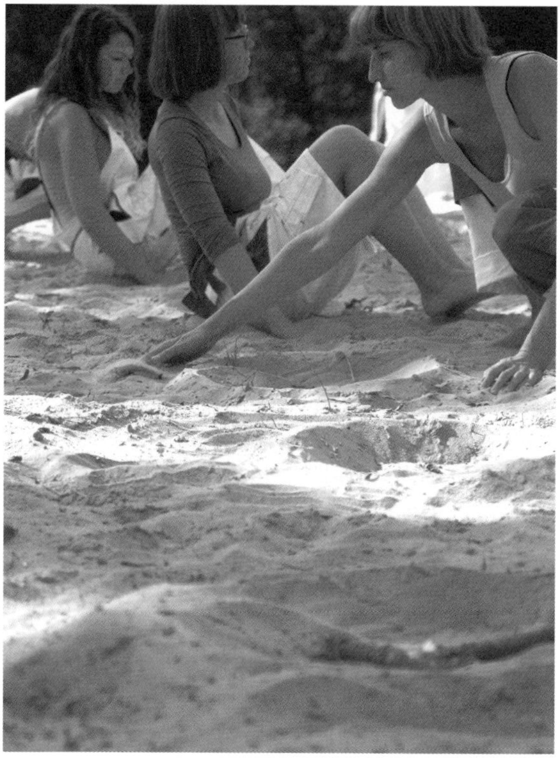

A group of women perform a ritualized action of repeatedly sitting down on the ground and spinning on their pelvic bones. Helping each other to sit down and stand up, the women move rhythmically across a large field of sand, their bodies leaving bowl-shaped holes in the ground. These actions of focusing on the pelvic bowl allow the women both to respond to the massive exploitation that results from commercial excavation and drilling practices and to re-establish their own, embodied connections to the Earth.

Pelvic Bowls – Digging/Drilling/Exploitation

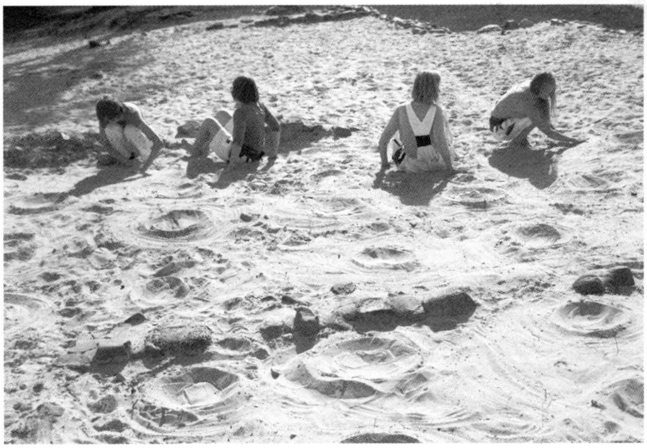

The excavator draws a map in the sand
Water flows through a drilled/embossed furrow
My pelvic bowl of waterways speaks
With the Bowl of Earth.

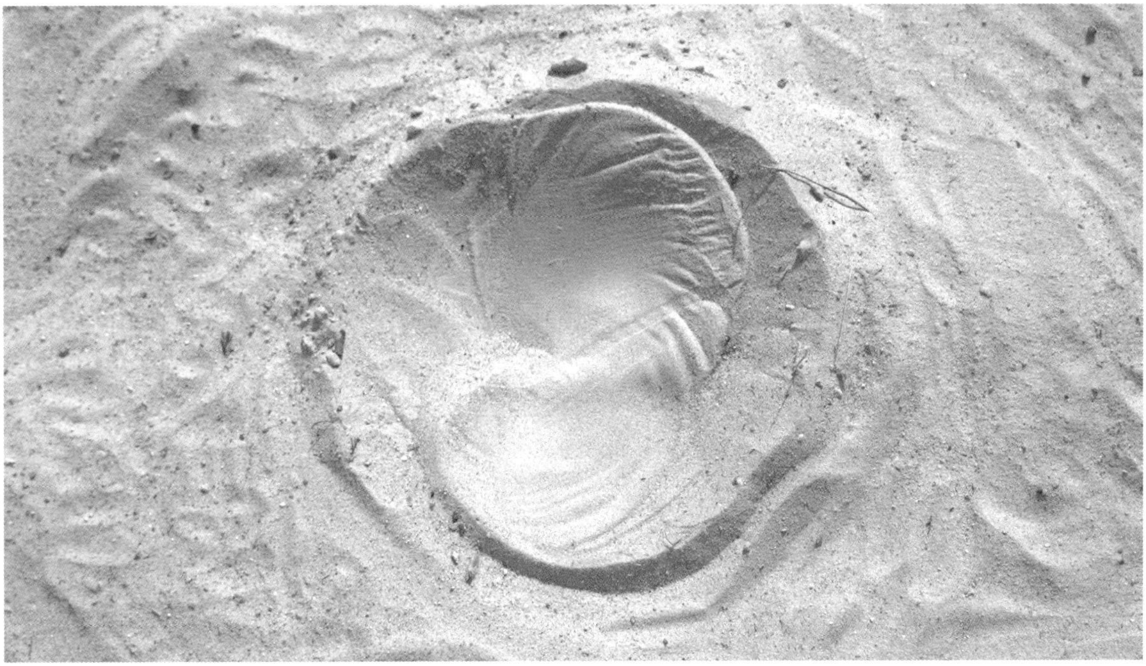

Chapter 4

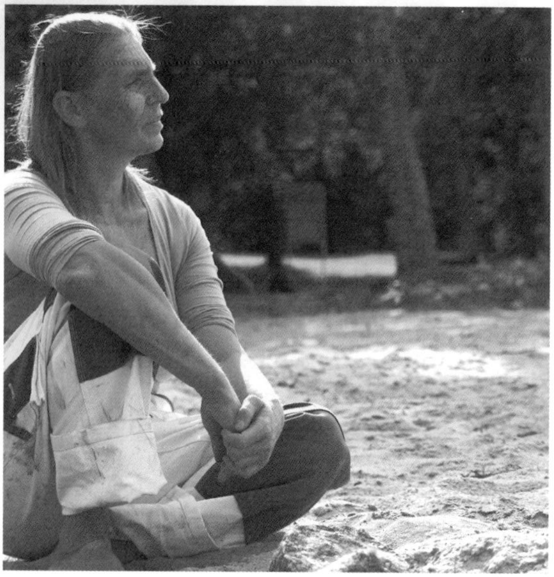

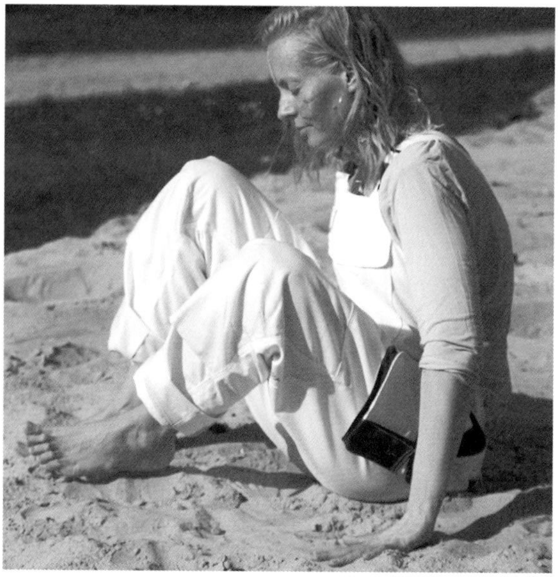

Pelvic Bowls – Digging/Drilling/Exploitation

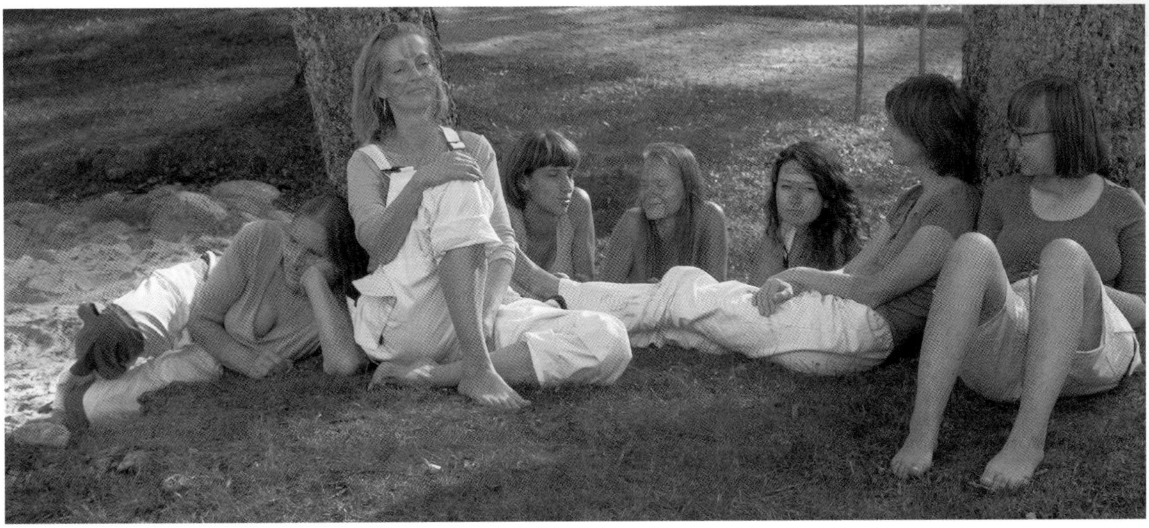

Performance conceived by Raima Drąsutytė and Kristina Skaldina-Moška.

Performers: Raima Drąsutytė, Kristina Skaldina-Moška, Akvilė Mo, Sibilė Marija Brazauskaitė, Sigita Butkutė-Mackevičienė, Aistė Kriukelytė, Julija Šredersaitė.

Poem: Sibilė Marija Brazauskaitė

Photos: Matas Sergijus Šatūnas

The performance took place at the 15th International Land and Environmental Art Festival 2019, Vilnius University Botanical Garden, Kairėnai, Lithuania

Video link
Video: Nojus Drąsutis, Tadas Šlajus

Part 2

Moving into Life 1: Embryological Beginnings

Sailing Backwards Single-Handedly

Beverley Nolan

5

We shall not cease from exploration
And the end of all our exploring
Will be to arrive where we started
And know the place for the first time.
T. S. Eliot, from "Little Gidding"

The possibility that a somatic exploration of early embryological development might intersect with the spiritual enquiry of yoga and the fields of acoustic science was not obvious at the outset. Several years of professional study in Integrative Bodywork and Movement Therapy (IBMT) and even more years in personal practice provided a breadcrumb trail marking the evolution of development from fetus to child in a series of overlapping primitive reflexes and basic neurological patterns. This pathway out of the unknown, through the body I had grown, was providing simultaneously the pathway back to something that beckoned as perhaps the first gesture of a life that was mine. This return journey came with the promise that, as Eliot assures, we will "arrive where we started and know the place for the first time." This sense of coming within reach of an original event suddenly became redolent with the enquiry into the nature of self that accompanies the physical practices of yoga movement and breathing.

Selected extracts from personal journal entries and records of group practices are compiled hereafter to track the experiential unwinding of the journey where key concepts of yogic thought and practice converge with embryological milestones and the pre-echo of discoveries in cymatics and sonocytology. Navigating this pathway turned out not to be a linear journey, a simple retracing of steps backwards through time, but rather like traveling the surface of a Möbius curve, where up is down and down is up, and science is philosophy and philosophy is science.

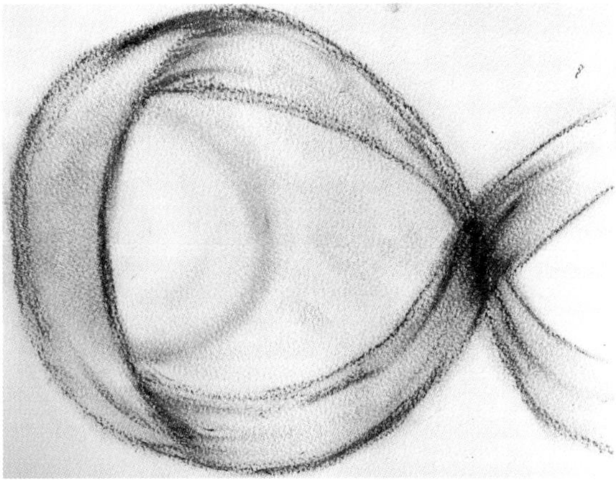

Möbius loop. Artist: Beverley Nolan

The Journey

Setting off

As on many return journeys, the territory and the route seem already known, and what is asked of us is merely a question of reorienting our feet or vehicle to face the way we have come. And so it is with the first stage of my journey through the developmental movement patterns, reversing the known sequence in order to transition from standing to crawling, to creeping, to discovering limbs and the ground, to seeking out sensory and physical nourishment, to resting, to finding a sense of self in those first moments of relationship with another, to awakening my senses to a new world. The way back from toddler to babe-in-arms is clear in my felt experience. Each shape and the way each informs another I know well in my body and there is an ease

Chapter 5

that brings me to the first terminus, here, lying on the ground where the stopping is felt as a sense of taking stock before embarking on the next stage of the journey: birth. Various images arise. I am at the shore of a wide lake, the bank of rushing rapids, the edge of an ocean. There is a sense that the overland part of the journey is done and that it will continue over water. Each image is accompanied by the feeling of something seemingly insurmountable about to be overcome. I must now up-anchor and start sailing against the prevailing winds and currents.

From earth to sea

The inherent challenge in the second stage of the journey is the uncomfortable prospect of unwinding my birth spiral in such a way that my body is able to recalibrate at a body-memory level the sudden transformation from being suited to air, gravity, and a big wide world to being at home in the *in utero* containment of fluids and buoyancy.

I allow the stillness to play out and notice a field of nervous system activity that I interpret to be inspecting the map and the route and making pre-departure checks. These impressions appear as a set of micro-movement sensations of pre-organization in various tissues. Then, an impulse of readiness arises: a sense that this is the best moment, that this is the best shape I can be in to set my course and unfurl the sails.

I am quickly in the squall of it. From a gathering compression of my limbs towards the center of my body, an intensity of focus accumulates over an unmeasured time. Yielding deeply into this shape continues like the coiling of a spring until a swift spiraling outward rushes through all tissues and, equally swiftly, recoils to the small fetal shape I imagined it would. The transition is over in a few seconds. My spine and limbs are now organized more loosely around my center, a center that extends outward as I recognize somewhere close by yet distant: my placenta and my space. The precipitous and dynamic shape changes enacted at speed have been replaced with a profound timelessness. I am quietly refound.

Finding harbor

Stage three of the journey assumes an unhurried pace along a course that is lit by the milestones of my ungrowing body. It is an uncurling and unfolding, the making of space and the filling, each process reversing successfully, safe in the knowledge of knowing itself, until I find myself at a second terminus: an implanted embryo fully nested in the wall of the uterus.

This process of nesting (nidation or implantation) was the result of an intense dialogue with the maternal body. Ordinarily, the immune system holds a memory of its biological identity and will reject an implantation of genetically differing material. A treaty of sorts was therefore agreed, such that my alien nature, resulting from bearing a different set of genes, would be received into the nesting site. To reverse this part of the journey feels like the prospect of another birth, and I notice feelings of reticence to surrender this hard-won harbor in the oceanic womb.

If you are planning to sail around the world backwards, single-handedly, I am guessing that there are going to be moments when you might want to stop, stay in safe waters, enjoy the view, get to know the local cuisine, maybe invest in a harborside property. The nidation site feels just like this. I am wanting to hang out here, sometimes moving, sometimes resting, leaning back in my boat, feeling the lap of the ocean, eyes lowered from the horizon until, that is, the call of the journey starts to beckon and, as with all good travelers, preparations must begin for the next stage.

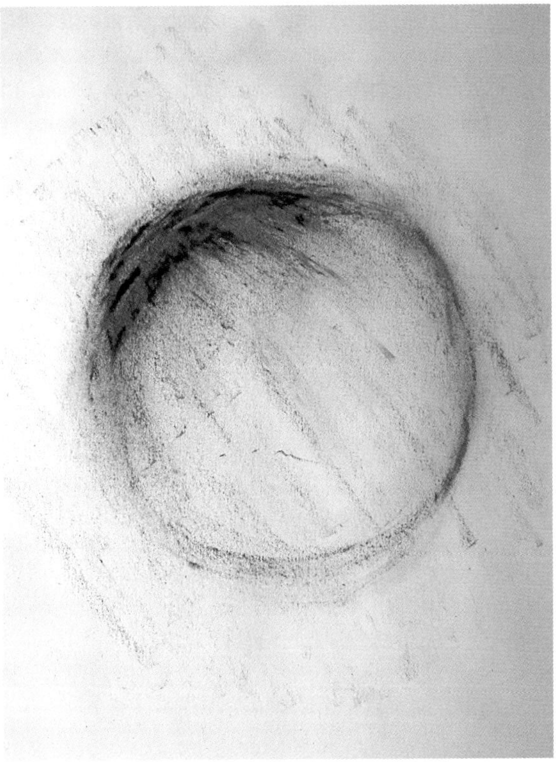

Nidation. Artist: Beverley Nolan

The prevailing winds will be the unhelpful kind and, exiting this harbor, I will be navigating against the currents that want to keep me in place. What focus is required! What clarity of intention! My spherical body shudders, my inner cell mass rotates, and, somehow, I am capsizing and submerging to arrive in calm waters.

Falling upwards

Drifting now on warm currents, I appear to have no means of locomotion, although there is a sense of seeing in all directions as if I might be rotating around multiple axes. This part of the journey is effortless, filled with the sense of falling upwards, coursing across the uterine space and into the fallopian tubes. A feeling of being at one with my body and my environment evokes an intersection with the non-dual yoga philosophy of *Advaita Vedanta*. My body as a spherical ball of cells feels perfect and I notice a great sense of contentment as I am drifting onward along this tube-like structure, even as I am aware that cells are undividing into a smaller and smaller group.

Arrival

From 16, to 8, to 4, to 2: this is the measure of cells inside my original ovum. This moment in the journey is only 30 hours float time away from the moment of discharge from the ovary. A lot happened on that early part of the journey. Some 12–24 hours before the potential for me became a possibility, two very different cells came together to create a one. Accompanying this embryological event lies a second intersection with yoga philosophy and an opportunity to explore the concept of *dvandva*, the play of opposites, this time in embodying the individual nature of both the ovum and the sperm cell and acknowledging that I know them both as my own original experience.

The ovum embodies a singularity. Its discharge towards fertilization is a solo affair and each discharge follows a lunar cycle of an average of 28 days. Its spherical form, unlike that of any other cell in the body, suggests a solitary nature, not requiring of itself to form a collective tissue. It is a form that allows itself to hold the maximum of space with the least amount of contact with its external environment, and it is a form that does not appear to initiate its own way of locomotion but rather is moved by currents. It is large. Dutch embryologist and phenomenologist Jaap van der Wal would ascribe the gesture of "largeness" to the ovum, gesture as a way of describing "the underlying motion that is being expressed in the form" (2003). In my

Chapter 5

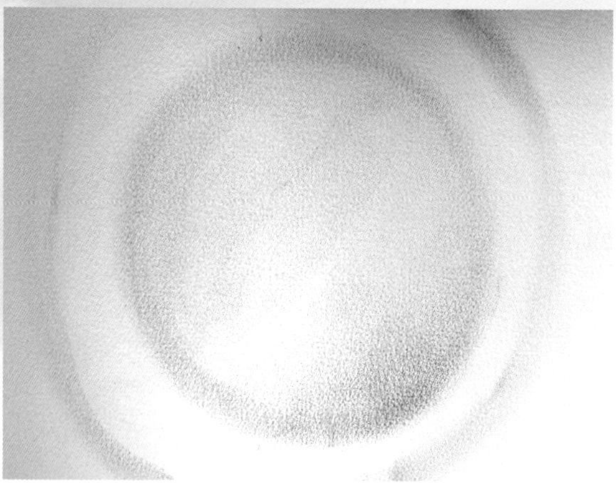

Ovum. Artist: Beverley Nolan

own experiential enquiries, I am drawn to taking up as much space as I can but without effort and to reach in all directions. There is a sense of volume and lightness, and I desire to find a sound from the vibration of its underlying motion: a sound that accompanies the gesture.

By contrast, the sperm cell embodies numerousness. It is small, elongated, and narrow, and its discharge towards fertilization is frequent and random, and in the company of millions of companion cells. It has its own method of propulsion, creating its own current. It is designed for speed, for working in a team and towards a definitive goal. Van der Wal would attribute to it the gesture of "smallness," and in my own movement enquiry into the embodiment of the sperm cell, I am drawn to moving fast and in a clear direction, sustaining focus and speed. I am curious again to use my voice to find a sound that would arise from the gesture of the sperm cell.

Here, in the assignation of the ovum and the sperm, two quite separate gestures vibrate together in the push-and-pull dance of chromosomal organization and the task of locating the first two centers of the first two sister cells. We are in suspense. The ovum will not show visible signs of successful fertilization for up to 16 hours, and we are in suspense again until around 24 hours, when the first cell division occurs. This pattern of experiences evokes the sense of *kumbhaka*, the pause between breaths that is explored in yoga breathing techniques.

And of course, while the vibratory activity of the ovum during its first day has yet to be made audible with acoustic technologies, it is possible to infer that in those beginning moments of the life there would be a primal sound that I could call my own.

The Convergence of IBMT, Acoustic Phenomena, and Yoga Philosophy

There is a point on a journey when cultures meet or collide. It may be in the big cities at the cusp of continents; it may be in the big trading centers and transport hubs. In these places, ideas mix, some coexisting like oil and water, others like oil and pigment. Here, at the terminus of this journey, at the point of conception, there is a convergence of a certain not-knowing that seems tantalizingly close to becoming known.

It is common practice in IBMT to invite sounding from different body systems, structures, and tissues, a sound that seems to emanate from an experiential attunement with the tissues. The practice allows a non-verbal expression of the experience of the tissue type or cell type providing further somatic material for enquiry. The scientific ability to listen to cells was recorded for the first time in the USA in 2002, when Scottish Professor James Gimzewski and his American colleague, Dr Andrew Pelling, discovered that cellular vibration created by the metabolic function of cells could be recorded and played back audibly to the human ear. They named this new aspect of cell biology "sonocytology," and published a debut report in the August 2004 issue of *Science* magazine. They modified an instrument called a Bioscope atomic force microscope to detect the vibrations of the cell wall of a living cell. Once amplified using computer software, the sounds were made audible (Wikipedia 2021).

In the context of the experiential journey described above, there is not yet a scientific rendering of the sound of the ovum or sperm cell.

Other researchers have experimented with acoustic phenomena. Experiments carried out on water by author Masuru Emoto during the late 20th century are widely known, as a result of his 2004 *New York Times* bestselling book (2005); Emoto's work does not withstand scientific scrutiny, though, and he is criticized for not being willing to publish his methodology and data sets for peer review. The findings of German musician and physicist Ernst Chladni in the 18th century, however, who himself was furthering the work of 17th-century scientists Galileo Galilei and Robert Hooke, are consistent with known mathematical properties. Chladni observed that vibration applied to a metal plate with a surface layer of fine dust would result in the dust particles accumulating in different places on the plate, forming geometric patterns and shapes; these are known as nodal point patterns or Chladni figures.

Swiss physician and anthroposophist Hans Jenny repeated Chladni's experiments during the 1960s, coining the name "cymatics" for this field of study. Exploring vibration on different materials, Jenny was struck by the appearance of the mandala-like shapes and geometric patterns already found in nature. He went on to conduct multiple experiments, including one looking into the vibrations arising from the AUM chant, which resulted in a nodal point dust pattern of a circle with a dot at its center, and published *Kymatic* in 1967. While Jenny's anthroposophical beliefs mark him as a pseudoscientist by the measure of many contemporary researchers, his findings are again consistent with known mathematical properties.

There appears, then, at this embryological convergence point of science, philosophy, and embodiment practices, to be at least a common interest. What is happening inside the ovum in those few hours between conception and the first cell division? What sound might be made audible from the vibration of the push-and-pull of chromosomes? Does each gesture of new life potential emit its own "big bang"?

Advaita Vedanta: *non-dual*

Advaita can be rendered from the Sanskrit as non-dual (Sanskrit Dictionary n.d.). The essential teaching from this school of Indian thought is that, despite appearances to the contrary, all things are expressions of a universal consciousness. Every wave on the ocean is never separate from the ocean; every ripple on the lake is never separate from the lake. The invitation is to come to a recognition of this innate oneness by stepping from the foreground of sensory content into abiding and undivided presence.

In the journey of embryological development, as the first sister cells are dividing, they appear within the space of the one fertilized cell (that, in and of itself, is the union of two). They are simultaneously appearances in and of themselves, as well as inseparable from the ground substance of the original cell. During these first 3–4 days of cell division, the sisters create a solid ball of cells, the morula, which continues to have no experience of differentiation, and this singular numerousness floats through the fallopian tube, buoyed by the current of extracellular fluid in which it exists. There is no sense of otherness in this phase.

Chapter 5

It is not until about a day later that the cells start to reorganize themselves to create a space inside the ball (at this point it is renamed as the blastocyst) and to acquire a sense of identity: for example, some may later become neural tissue, some bone or muscle.

Dvandva – *play of opposites*

Another concept encountered in Indian schools of thought is the play of opposites that may be rendered as *dvandva* in Sanskrit (Sanskrit Dictionary n.d.). The proposition is that the sensory world of contrasts consumes our attention and obstructs our ability to understand the true nature of being. Seeing through the oscillations of our everyday life or lifting ourselves up from them is described in some Indian texts as the essential struggle at the heart of yoga as a spiritual enquiry.

As we follow the embryological narrative, we see this most obviously embodied in the original union of the multiple complementary characteristics (that we might call opposites) of the ovum and the sperm. When we remember that we are both ovum and sperm, not only do we retain the possibility of embodying either set of qualities, but we also have a sense of our personhood.

To explore this in another way, a triangulation process can be helpful. For example, I might simply attend to the front of my body and then switch my attention to attend solely to the back of my body, and in so doing gather two discrete sensory experiences. If I then attempt to hold both distinct experiences of front and back simultaneously in my attention, what may arise, after a certain amount of oscillation, merges into a single sensory experience unbounded by the definition of front and back; maybe I name it a whole body. It is quite different to front and to back and arises when the sense of front and back dissolves into the whole. Furthermore, it may become clear that these experiences are the content of something that I am calling my attention to and I may turn towards this, possibly to glimpse the clear and timeless presence suggested by *Advaita Vedanta.*

Kumbhaka – *full pot, empty pot*

Each cycle of breath has four component parts: the movement that we call inhalation, a pause, the movement we call exhalation, and another pause. Yoga *pranayama* practices involve breathing techniques, some of which explore the relationship between these four component parts. This might be done by equalizing the duration of each component part: for example, inhaling to a count of four, holding breath in for four, exhaling for four, and holding breath out for four.

The retention of the breath in or out is a *kumbhaka*, which can be rendered from the Sanskrit simply as a pot (Sanskrit Dictionary n.d.). The pot of the body is filled with breath on an inhalation and, following a suspension in the swing of the breath, the pot of the body is emptied on the exhalation. The practice of *kumbhaka* invites a sealing of the pot (using techniques called *bandhas*), either to suspend the breath inside the body or to suspend the breath outside the body. Whatever action is happening, whichever sensation is being attended to, the body is both full and empty at one time.

The image of the empty pot submerged in a body of water, therefore at the same time full, appears in various yoga texts. At the point on the embryological journey in the post-fertilization phase, in those hours before the first cell division, we experience a type of *kumbhaka*: suspense. At this time, the container of the ovum is full of potential and processes, yet empty of the first cells. It has taken a first great breath in and, retaining this fullness, it will not be for some hours that its cellular outbreath fills the first two sister cells.

IBMT and Yoga Practicum 1: Sounding, the Rise and Fall of Voice

Everyone is arriving quietly, although the door closing behind them is making a prolonged motion of closure that completes with a clang, surprising each one into a guilty glance and a softly spoken apology. They are settling their belongings, retrieving cushions and blankets, and placing them; each begins to create a circle around the wooden floor that warms the space and gifts a few hidden hotspots. An unspoken agreement is apparent that, after finding a comfortable way of sitting, each will add their own silence to the gathering. There seems no intention to the mystical; rather, a respect for the process of coming together, making a beginning out of a collective silence that accumulates.

The agreement is to begin the gathering in a non-verbal way. Once seated, each will simply attend to their breath and wait together in a collective invitation for sound to arise, and if it should arise, to allow it to continue until the sound falls back of its own volition into silence. A timer has been set to ring in 30 minutes' time, after which each person will move, write, and draw for a further 15 minutes before finding a partner to begin the process of speaking and listening.

I sit in my place, arranging my cushion and blanket in my best effort to sustain comfort in my knees, hips, and spine. I am cross-legged. I sway from side to side and forward and back in search of a center where all things are self-supporting and extraneous effort falls away. Eyes are closing. Exhaling audibly. Dropping attention into the movement of breathing. I hear the quiet wave of in and out breath. SO HAM. SO HAM. I notice the non-movements between. I hear someone shifting their cushions. I hear another cough. I hear a big yawn and a few audible exhalations like a sighing, and in one moment I hear a long, hissing sound.

Another sort of silence arises, as if unwrapped by the previous moments of settling. It has a fullness of its own. I am attending to the quality of it when I hear a sound from across the circle, a quiet hum. My listening reaches out through my right ear, through my left ear, triangulating to the sound as it is transmitted across space and time. The sound repeats without need of being heard and then another sound arises, perhaps in response.

In the hearing of the repeated and overlaid humming sounds, I am activated. I notice a longing to find a sound, but my breath is quiet ... and then I feel, just before a particular exhalation, a small contraction in my throat, and a quiet, brief, wavering hum begins and ends. Short. Uncertain. It cracks into the vestibule of my mouth and vibrates for just a few moments. I feel a relief, a small sense of happiness, to have found a voice and I am encouraged. I am encouraged in the etymological sense, emboldened to draw a deeper breath and soften vocal cords to sound more audibly, smoothly, clearly. These sounds seem personal, just for my hearing. I have forgotten the group around me and yet, as I notice again that I am not alone, I hear that other voices are sounding, some with lips closed to hum, others allowing their lips and tongues to make shapes so that vowels and consonants form.

My voice grows desirous to make participatory sounds in this choir of vowels and consonants. No words. No melody. An organic layering of tones and overtones.

At times, the voices crescendo and occupy the containing silence; at times it feels as if an ending is approaching, and then not yet as the tones shift

Chapter 5

and blend again. However, a moment arises where each has come to a natural ending, sound empties away under the doors, and the silent container holds only the SO HAM of each breath. I sit with the silent japa [the silent, internal repetition of a sacred mantra or divine name; Sanskrit Dictionary n.d.] of the soundings resonating in my inner hearing.

We are all waiting now for the bell to ring, and when it does, we lean forward to press our palms to the floor in a gesture of completion and slide our bodies into movement that decompresses joints, and we loosen the focus of our attention. We reach for paper and crayons, notebooks, and pens, and disperse through the space, blankets wrapped around shoulders – a quiet intensity.

A bell rings 15 minutes later, as agreed; eyes look around to find the gaze of another and all manner of shuffling and sliding brings each into a partnership. Smiles break the way into muffled conversations, which continue until the final bell sounds; each partnership finds a way to end their sharing and another round of shuffling and sliding occurs to bring each back to the circle.

Another kind of silence arises, one that expects to be broken through speaking. Someone leans forward and presses their palms to the floor as a signal that they will begin.

IBMT and Yoga Practicum 2: The Anatomy of AUM

Om is the sound of the universe symbolizing absolute reality. It is heard all around us in the movement of the leaves, the waves of the ocean and the stillness of the moon. Chanting Aum connects us with the universe and through our breath, awareness, and consciousness we find divinity.

B. K. S. Iyengar, founder of the eponymous style of yoga practiced worldwide

Another circle of practitioners meets to explore the mouthing pattern. Linda Hartley's work (1995) points out the significance of the mouth to the infant before, during, and post birth, and describes the referred movement of the moving jaw onto the rocking of the skull, a movement that sequences through the length of the spine and back again. The mouthing action plays a role in finding nourishment, as well as offering support for vocal and movement development.

The group examines anatomical images to understand the nature of the relationship of the bones of the jaw, between the mandible (lower jaw) and maxilla (upper jaw), noting the shaping of the bones inside the temporomandibular joint (TMJ) space and the nature of the space itself. We see the possibilities of movement and, after tracing our own bones with fingertips, we begin to experiment with the movement possibilities from the jaw. The mandible dropping seems familiar, creating a space inside the mouth; the maxilla lifting feels less familiar, a little awkward as we note the sensation of the cranium rotating up and back. We exaggerate the opening movement created by both bones with the support of an AH sound that seems to be located towards the back of the mouth. We notice a spontaneous MM sound when we close the jaw, bringing the lips together, and the original AH sound comes to a silence. As we are yoga practitioners, the two syllables are not lost on us, and we note them as constituent parts of the sacred chant AUM.

As we each repeat the process as an exploration of movement inside the TMJ, tracking the movements of the bones in the joint spaces, we notice that the opening movement and the AH sound have a particular connection to the soft palate, and that we are able to find an axial alignment via the soft palate. Further, we note the location as a reference point for the infant sucking reflex, as well as to the *khechari mudra* (seal/contact point) described in many yoga and Tantric texts as being a significant practice for yogins over the centuries. The term comes from *Khechari* (moving into space) and *Mudra* (seal), typically practiced by folding back the tongue to touch the soft palate, said variously either to stimulate the descent of *amrita* (nectar, ambrosia) from inside the head or to stem its flow.

We continue the exploration and experiment with allowing the sound to travel with the changing shape of the mouth from open to closed, from the soft palate forward to the place behind the teeth. In this way, we find that we formulate a representation of all three syllables of the AUM in continuous succession, both as a result of the full movement of the TMJ and also as a way of initiating and supporting the movement, from AH at the back of the mouth to UU as the jaw forms an arc of closure, to the final MM sound, the latter creating a sustained vibration in the bones that form the base of the cranium, until it too falls into silence again.

After a few minutes, we take time to note our personal experiences before coming together to share. We reflect on our received understanding of the AUM as an original sound that has many significances in Indian culture and yoga practices.

Knowing the Place for the First Time

The assignation of Shakti and Shiva as representations of the divine feminine (active, manifesting, changing) and the divine masculine (static, latent, unchanging), respectively, forms an essential image for the union of coexisting opposites. Resuming the journey, the great Shiva Shakti moment is undone. The chemical processes unwind. The surface of the ovum reopens and the sperm retreats and rejoins its tail. The membrane of the ovum reconstitutes and sperm cells, tails spinning, are disappearing from view. All seems to become quiet in the manner of the silence that follows the great AUM. Whatever this place is, it is a convergence, where the somatic understanding of embryological development, philosophical enquiry, and developing scientific enquiry in the field of acoustic phenomena intersect.

I may know myself through the embodiment of the journey that brought me to this place with its abundant somatic experiences and associations, and here I can continue the pursuit of knowledge of the earliest gesture of myself. Maybe I glimpse the clearest form of consciousness that arises before and after the AUM, and I might yet know myself through the song of my cells if I listen closely enough.

And, to circle back to Eliot:

What we call the beginning is often the end
And to make an end is to make a beginning.
The end is where we start from.

T. S. Eliot, from "Little Gidding"

Chapter 5

Glossary

Anthroposophy: a human-oriented spiritual philosophy that reflects and speaks to the basic deep spiritual questions of humanity, to our basic artistic needs, to the need to relate to the world out of a scientific attitude of mind, and to the need to develop a relation to the world in complete freedom and based on completely individual judgments and decisions (https://waldorfanswers.org, accessed October 21, 2021).

Cymatics: the study of wave phenomena, especially sound, and their visual representations (*Collins English Dictionary*).

Sonocytology: from the field of biophysics, the study of audible sound arising from cellular vibration.

Navel Radiation: The Development of the Internal Fascial Network

6

Anna Titova

We are Mind, Motion and Matter.

The body developed out of us, not we from it.

We made the body, cell by cell we made it.

Rūmī 1997: 25

What precedes physical movement? What supports a person's physical movement in space? What makes the movement and perception whole, coherent? These are the questions that travel with me through my personal practice, therapeutic experience, client stories, and teaching. Human experience consists of the manifested and the unmanifested, the visible and the invisible, the subtle spiritual and the dense physical – this is how connections reveal themselves.

"Movement is the language, and the body is the instrument through which it speaks" (Bainbridge Cohen 2018: v, from foreword by her husband, Leonard Cohen). It is through movement that we learn about and explore the space around us; the sense of the inner and the outer space is formed. While studying somatic movement in the Integrative Bodywork and Movement Therapy (IBMT) approach, I had a very deep experience of understanding that a person and their development begin long before birth. We begin as an embryo, as the very first cell – a fertilized egg. While researching embryonic somatic movement, we moved with early images of the egg, sperm, placenta, and umbilical cord, and many others. I became interested in the organic nature of these images and the stages of embryonic development. I found that, according to the osteopath Serge Paoletti, the membrane of the first cell has a fascial nature (Paoletti and Startseva 2012). The formation of the placenta and umbilical cord during the prenatal period is associated with the movement and activity of the fascial tissues. My somatic research from the first days of the IBMT program, then, led me to study the very beginning of movement and connective tissue, or fascia.

What Is Fascia?

Fascia is an amazing tissue of our body, to which scientists previously paid little attention. Even now, in most anatomy textbooks you will find much more information about bones and muscles than about fascia. However, bones are also a kind of fascial tissue, and many muscles are wrapped and packed in the thinnest fascia layers. Fascial tissue is our ligaments, tendons, muscle sheaths, and muscle fibers, the living space around internal organs, as well as bones, cartilage, and fat tissue.

Fascial tissue is associated with our deep sense of self, the sense of our gut and the center of the body. The fascia is an organ of the body that contains about 20 million nerve endings (this is more than in the eyes and skin). Nerve endings located in the subcutaneous fascial layer, in the fascial space around organs and vessels, create a continuous flow of information – a unique sense of self from moment to moment. If our fascia is tensed, the nerve impulses pass more slowly and we feel less well or may not feel some areas of the body at all. The tension can be caused by injuries, strong emotions and stress, overextension, stagnation, or a sedentary lifestyle.

The important properties of the fascial tissue are its integrity and unity. The fascia or connective tissue forms a continuous three-dimensional matrix that permeates the entire body and performs an organizing function for organs, muscles,

Chapter 6

joints, bones, and nerves. The multi-dimensional arrangement of the fascia and the diverse orientation of the fascial meridians or lines allow us to move in different directions (Myers 2001, Huijing 2007, Stecco et al. 2007). The term "fascial meridians" was introduced by Thomas Myers to refer to a whole complex of chains, connections, and lines (based on traditional Western anatomy) that carry tension and movement through the skeleton and through the body's myofascia (Myers 2001: 5).

In the womb, the first movement takes place and our body is formed. In the first years of human life, development and movement first occur in the watery environment of the mother's womb, and then, after birth, on land – in the gravity field of the Earth. For many hours, days, and months, movement integration and body capabilities are clarified. Our cells and tissues remember this time. In the embryonic period, the movement of fluids, cells, and tissues changes the body from simple to complex, from chaos to order. Everything in nature develops through patterns (Bainbridge Cohen 2018: 1). In its movement development the body goes through certain stages or motor series, which Bonnie Bainbridge Cohen called neurocellular patterns. The formation and movement of the connective tissue of the human body are laid down in the embryonic period and can be considered in the context of embryonic neurocellular patterns.

In the embryonic period, during the second week of development, three embryonic layers are laid down:

1. Endoderm and yolk sac – from which the internal organs and digestive system will develop.
2. Mesoderm or middle embryonic layer – which forms everything that will become the "flesh" of the human body: bones, muscles, connective tissue, blood, lymph, and the fascia itself.
3. Ectoderm and amniotic cavity – which will later form the nervous system and skin.

From this moment on, the mesoderm, as the most active tissue, begins its amazing dance. Multiplication, expansion, migration of cells, alternation of folding and unfolding lead to the absorption (invagination) of both the yolk sac and the amnion. This is how our internal organs, nervous system, and skin find their places in the body.

Pattern of Navel Radiation and its Application in Somatic Therapeutic Practice

The first movement in the watery environment of the mother's womb is associated with a sense of space in the human body – proprioception. In our natural unfolding, the first movement occurs with the manifestation of the Navel Radiation pattern (Bainbridge Cohen 2018: 71), as well as the formation of the umbilical cord and placenta, derivatives of the fascial system.

Navel Radiation is a pattern of radial movement of the limbs passing through the center. The image of this pattern is a six-pointed starfish with a mouth in the center. The human body has six limbs: two upper limbs, two lower limbs, a head, and a tail (tailbone). Movement can be initiated from the center or from the periphery of any limb. It is important for movement to be transmitted and to pass freely in all directions through the center.

The Navel Radiation pattern lives and manifests in the human body throughout life. However, due to various complex events, emotions, injuries, and stress, there may be disruptions in the whole body image and then people come to somatic therapy. In my therapeutic practice, some common symptoms of those disruptions are:

- One of the extremities of the body is less warm than the rest.
- Attention does not pass through the limb to the end (for example, it becomes stuck in one of the joints).
- Often, immobile tips of the fingers.
- The head seems to be disconnected from the whole body and does not have a clear relationship with the center.
- There is no movement/respiration/sensitivity in the abdominal area and internal organs.

To work with clients with such symptoms, I use practices focused on the Navel Radiation pattern and fascia of the body. In order for this pattern to be organized in the body, in terms of the Body-Mind Centering® approach and neurocellular patterns, we need to create support through the earlier movement patterns (Bainbridge Cohen 2018). In therapeutic work, I do this through touch, movement, breathing, and the quality of presence. Movement patterns can manifest simultaneously, existing at different levels: from micro-movement to macro-movement, from local areas and tissues to the body as a whole, movement patterns can be more or less manifested. Some of the patterns and qualities of movement associated with fascial tissue that I use in my therapeutic practice are:

- Vibration and flow (amorphous and liquid phase of the fascia, which conducts vibration waves through itself and supports cell respiration).
- Breathing of the fascial cells and layers in any area of the body.
- Movement and transport of complex molecules (proteins, fibers, and immune cells) within the intercellular substance of the fascial tissue.
- Sliding of the fascial layers against each other.
- Compression and extension (fascial layers, ligament and tendons).
- Twisting and untwisting.
- Movement of the spiral, or non-linear movement (the fascial sheath around muscles and ligaments).
- Movement from the center to the periphery.

Somatic practices related to fascia, fascial movement, and the Navel Radiation pattern are often used in work with clients through movement and bodywork. This approach was used in the work with client N, who complained about limited mobility in the joints, chronic pain, and insensitivity in the center of the body and internal organs. While we were working with him, the Navel Radiation pattern helped him to find the necessary integration and to ground his attention in the center of the body.

In its quality, the fascia is similar to a sponge. About two-thirds of fascial tissue is water. Moisture and mobility of the fascial layers are the main conditions for its health. A sedentary lifestyle, unexpressed emotions, and stress can cause redistribution of the fluid within the fascial system and its pathological adhesion. In the case of client N, then, we were able to regain mobility by enhancing familiarity with the fascia through bodywork and the practice of fascial micro-movements, as well as through the state of consciousness and working with attention in somatic practice. In my therapeutic practice, the practice of breathing and movement with the Navel Radiation pattern had a very positive response.

Another important step in working with client N was to create familiarity with the fact that, at the

Chapter 6

level of the whole body, the movement of fascial tissue is non-linear – three-dimensional. Client N's vision and sense of the body map were fragmented and flat. Understanding and practicing movement with the principle of tensegrity helped him to connect with a detailed sense of himself and with a large body volume. The main idea of the principle of *tensegrity* is that the denser areas move in relation to each other in space, due to the mutual tension of more flexible and elastic elements. Moreover, both denser and more elastic elements are represented by different types of fascial tissue. For example, a bone (dense fascial tissue) moves in relation to another bone in the joint, due to the elasticity of the ligaments (flexible and elastic fascial tissue). The movement is associated with the sliding of some layers of collagen fibers inside the tissue against others. In the case of client N, working with the sliding helped both to improve the overall physical condition of the body and to connect the periphery of the body and the center due to the fascial chains/meridians.

An important part of human life in the womb is interaction with the placenta and the umbilical cord. We breathe, receive food, and communicate with the world through them. Embryonic respiration, nutrition and communication with the world are realized in the image of the Navel Radiation. The placenta and umbilical cord protect us on the levels of immune barriers, hemo-barriers, and metabolism. In classes during the IBMT program, we also looked at images of the placenta and the umbilical cord as elements of essential support and connection. They are an important part of the body that a person loses during development. The placenta and umbilical cord are an organic extension of the body and the Navel Radiation pattern. In the case of client N, the final integrating practice was to work at the level of the general process of perception of nutrition and communication with the world through the placenta and umbilical cord and the Navel Radiation pattern.

I invite you to feel your connection to the umbilical cord and placenta with this *somatic practice*:

Focus all your attention on your breathing, on how your ribs and stomach are moving. Think how they expand on the inhale and contract on the exhale.

Imagine that you are an embryo floating in warm amniotic waters and there are membranes around you that protect and embrace your body. These structures are an extension of your body. Find harmony and rest inside the membranes.

Imagine that the navel is a channel connecting your body to the placenta. It is the entrance of the umbilical cord to the body.

Try to feel the flow of power moving through your navel, in and out. You do not need to do or create anything for this; just let the flow go through you. This flow is like a tidal force moving in and out.

Expand your attention to the placenta. This is your center of communication with the world around you. Trust in its wisdom and greatness. Feel your body as a trinity of the embryonic body – the umbilical cord – the placenta.

Allow the breathing and movement of oxygen-rich blood from the placenta to every cell in your body to take place. Watch as each cell receives and lets in nourishment and care.

Observe as the cells of your body exhale and release carbon dioxide and all waste substances into the bloodstream at the same time. Everything that is not needed is collected again at the navel and passes along the umbilical cord to your placenta.

Navel Radiation and the Internal Fascial Network

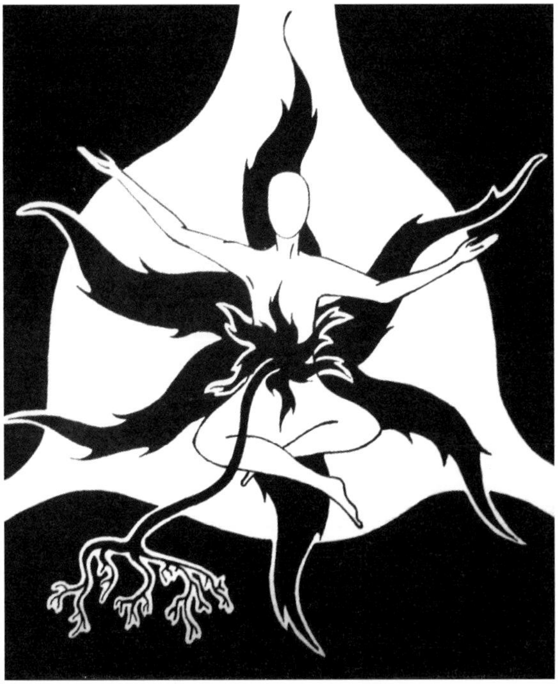

Fascial dance in navel radiation. Artist: Anna Begunskaya

Allow yourself to move in this flow, the flow of fluids, and rest. Thank your placenta for its invaluable work, wisdom, and support.

Gradually, return to the feeling of your body in the present moment. Complete the embryonic movement experience.

Placenta and Navel Radiation Pattern in the Philosophy and Traditions of Different Nations

From the first year and throughout life, connective tissue plays a crucial role in human breathing, movement, and energy. The connection between the center and the periphery is one that is associated with life-supporting functions of the body. A human is a combination of body, consciousness, and spirit. According to A. T. Still, the fascia is the vessel of the soul (Still 1899). We will turn our vision of, and perspective on, the connection between the center and the periphery not only to anatomy, physiology, developmental patterns, and movement, but also to the world of myths, rituals, archetypes, and images. In somatic client work, the level of myths and images helps to connect dense physical movement and the world of subtle sensations and images of clients. Throughout life, a person maintains a connection with his placenta and umbilical cord, a connection with the whole universe. This connection is reflected in the beliefs of our ancestors and opens us to broad meanings and knowledge about the nature and essence of phenomena.

Modern philosopher, physiologist, anatomist, and embryologist Jaap van der Wal writes about the fascia, a derivative of the middle embryonic layer: "Between Mind and Matter the interface is Life itself with Motion as functional manifestation, with the Middle as organisational principle and with Meso as the morphological representation of this quality!" (van der Wal 2015). The fascia itself contains the essence of being and manifestation of life.

At all levels, fascia manifests itself as a connecting and forming space.

> *In that case, fascia becomes the "organ" of Meso manifesting itself morphologically in the architecture of the connective tissues (including muscle, cartilage, bone), physiologically in the principle of motion, in connecting and shaping space on all kinds of levels, in rhythm and breathing and, last but not least, psychologically and mentally in the domain and function of "soul."*
>
> (van der Wal 2015)

Meso layers in general, and fascia in particular, enable innerness; the fascia therefore is the organ of

Chapter 6

innerness, being the domain that Still meant when he said: "The soul of man with all the streams of pure living water seems to dwell in the fascia of his body" (Still 1899).

In many traditional cultures, the placenta was considered important as the vault of the soul. In our time, among indigenous peoples – for example, on the island of Bali – there are still beliefs and rituals associated with the placenta. Balinese people bury their placenta in the ground at a specific location near their home and often come there to ask for support and strength. Ancient rituals reveal to us the value of the placenta and the umbilical cord as an information and energy channel in spiritual terms. The placenta is the place where the human soul is believed to live.

Parents of newborns in the Navajo tribe traditionally buried the umbilical cords and placentas in a specific place that represented their dreams about the future of the baby. The Hopi, like many North American peoples, believe that the first man emerged from the womb of Mother Earth, along with the placenta and umbilical cord. The placenta of Mother Earth was like a tribe feeding its own children (Leavitt 1986).

The ancient inhabitants of Hawaii had a different tradition: the father hid the placenta in volcanic rocks on the shore and then the waves washed it into the ocean – home to the primeval mother.

In Ancient Egypt, the placenta of the Pharaoh was a symbol of the magical, spiritual power and superiority of the ruler. It carried the divine properties that preceded his physical incarnation. The dried placenta was attached high on a pole and carried at the beginning of a solemn procession. Poor people buried their children's placentas or threw them into the sacred River Nile.

On the border of Colombia and Peru, the Kuna Indians believed that the placenta spirit was like a watchdog that accompanied the child and helped to guide the soul boat through the amniotic waters, through the labyrinths of the birth canal to Earth life.

The tradition of the Maya had deep religious roots. Their culture was based on respect for their native land. They buried the placenta of the newborn in the ground and believed that this place would have a symbolic meaning for the growing person. Here, he symbolically "grew" roots to his personality as part of the Mayan people. Thus, according to Mayan beliefs, a person became a part of society, nature, and the cosmos (Lim 2017).

In Cambodia, a prickly plant was planted at the placenta burial site to ward off evil spirits and protect it from animals. Asians believe that the placenta is "a ball – the origin of the soul." In Nepal, the placenta is called the baby's friend, "bucha-co-satthi" (Holt 2016: 48).

In the Indian tradition, one of the energy chakras called "Apara" is located in the placenta. It is a conductor of very subtle energy that maintains a connection with the whole, with the universe and the cosmos. It is associated with such categories as origin, epiphany, divinity, and hormonal cradle. It is responsible for the bridge between soul and matter. Its colors are red, indigo, purple, and crystal; emotionally, it is associated with unity/separation, and its matrix is the mother/child.

Conclusion

The fascia is an organ of form and space – the flesh of the body. Understanding connective tissue and fascia is our access to understanding the space and shape of the body, the processes that organize the body and movement. The study of the organization of the fascial space reveals non-linear connections, multi-levelness, and three-dimensionality. Connections built inside the body and connections with the outside are the essence of a single whole.

The fascia, as a multi-dimensional body organ and binding tissue, has multi-level qualities of movement. We can study it as a mechanical tissue that provides movement in the joints – compression, contraction, and expansion of ligaments. We can refer to the deep fascia between the organs, rich in amorphous substance, hyaluronic acid, and water – the area of gliding and breathing. We can consider the fascial tissue as a connecting web between the subtle worlds of the spirit and the denser material ones.

The fascial tissue opens up the space of the moving body. This is the tissue that begins the first movement of the body in space, the one that meets the internal and external. Being enclosed within the body, it becomes our inner infinite ocean. The pattern of movement of the fascial tissue is the vibration that fills the ocean of life, breathing and flowing, sliding, contracting, and expanding. The pattern of Navel Radiation is an important stage on the path of human movement development and a spiritual bridge between the earthly and embryonic stages of human life, as well as between the material and spiritual.

IBMT and Dance: "Re-Membrane"

Frauke Burchards

7

In this chapter I would like to describe how I use and apply experiences and knowledge from Integrative Bodywork and Movement Therapy (IBMT) and embryology in connection with dance, and what develops from this.

Our body is more than a collection of organs and bones inside a covering of skin. It is a perfect masterpiece of about 70 trillion cells that makes us feel, laugh, move, speak, and dance.

Our innate state of being is movement. From the perspective of our cells, we are in a constant flow of evolution. Every part of us is in constant growth and change. After dance and IBMT training, I continue to research movement. I am interested in simple form, natural movement, lightness and flow, and connection on all levels.

In addition, I am fortunate to have the opportunity to get to know and appreciate Authentic Movement and embryology. In both forms I am impressed and fascinated by how sinking into the body brings movement, feeling, expression, and memory to the surface, and how these can be experienced on the outside: form and movement emerge, rhythm and stillness, flow and continuity.

In experiential embryology, I immerse myself in the choreography of folding and unfolding, taking in and taking out, moving from inside to outside, from outside to inside. I reach deep layers of my being. In Authentic Movement I am with movement and contact and spirituality. My heart is touched.

Embryology

Our history of evolution begins in water. In liquid surroundings, in the depths of the female body, new life is created. From a fertilized egg cell, which is about the size of a pinhead, a complex organism of about 3 cm (1¼ in) in length develops.

"The heart is the first organ to take up its definitive function. It begins to beat in humans around the twenty-first day of development" (Männer 2013: 29). Männer is the head of the human embryology collection in Göttingen, the Blechschmidt Collection, which offers a visual and spatial impression of embryonic and fetal development. Behind these simple sentences lies the unbelievably fascinating embryonic development of the human being. In particular, the first 8 weeks, in which our "Gestalt development" takes place, are highly complex. Our first appearance is as a fertilized egg cell, which represents a whole organism: it is the whole. Rather than joining together part by part in an additive way, it develops and differentiates from within. It divides, reorganizes, reshapes, and transforms. It grows and spreads into space. It is an ever-repeating process of folding and unfolding, bending and stretching. "The embryo continuously changes its apparent shape in a steady metamorphosis of its form" (van der Wal 2005: 3).

Jaap van der Wal describes embryology as a life-long process. The embryonic dynamics do not cease.

> *The embryo is not a past or only a temporary stage. "The embryo within us" is a fundamental principle that still works in body and soul. Embryo is something actual in us. There is an embryo in us, which is apparently the primary fundamental thing in our body and in our mind.*
>
> (van der Wal 2020)

Chapter 7

My teachers, Linda Hartley and Bonnie Bainbridge Cohen, understand embryology as:

- transition from flow into form
- creativity of our being, connected and full of feeling
- the greatest moment of change.

Inside I am resonating with "transition from flow into form" and "greatest moment of change."

This touches me and awakens the impulse to learn more about it and to make it more visible.

From the beginning of our lives, we are with movement, flow, form, and change.

Flow

> *Flow manifests as fluid motion spiraling through the body, connecting each cell to all other cells. It is the fluid field in which the cells breathe and move. Well-being is a deep sense of ease, comfort and inner restfulness ... It comes when we balance the liquidity of our free flowing movement with a deep sense of form.*
>
> (Bainbridge Cohen 2016)

Form

> *Our form or structure is more than our external shell. It is our body and mind and all the many aspects that we think of as being "me." We hold our form through intellectual concepts, emotional patterns, physical compensations and physiological imbalances.*
>
> (Bainbridge Cohen 2016)

To understand the form means going back to embryology.

Dance

In dance we are looking for a way to make visible the invisible, inner movement and images. The movement, the expression, the form is created from the inside out. In embryology, the direction of movement is from the outside to the inside.

Isabelle Schad writes about experienced embryology and is very impressed by how "the formation of the human body as a biological process is connected with the outside, i.e. the visible form; how it determines the direction of movement. This process resembles a choreographic process" (Schad 2019). And van der Wal (2020) has this to say about embryology: "[T]he design of the embryo is a performance, an achievement in due time."

Although the embryonic structures no longer exist in physical form, I can feel the relative place and form in the body that they once occupied as an inherent material/structure, as a lived experience. To bring the sensed into form, into dance, to follow the choreographic process of embryology, this is the idea that leads to our dance performance.

Together with my dance friend, Bettina Löns, I developed the duet "Re-Membrane," based on the experienceable embryology and embodied cellular consciousness. Authentic Movement, Contact Improvisation, movement, touch, breath, and silence accompany us and give us new impulses again and again. Our treasure is our body with all its perceptions, feelings, and subtleties, and an inherent knowledge within us. All this knowledge, all these experiences flow into our choreography.

How Our Dance Piece Is Created

There is an idea. Inspired by two workshops in embryology with Hartley and Bainbridge Cohen, the desire and the need to work and research more intensively with this material arises. We dive into the emergence and not-knowingness, and start to explore directions and polarities: front–back, up–down, inside–outside, outside–inside.

IBMT and Dance: "Re-Membrane"

At the beginning, nothing is visible: no form, no structure. Only the encounter with our being and with the movement allows the form to come more clearly to the fore, rising from the depth of our bodies.

We follow what is created, often with the questions: What are we doing? Do we need a concept? There seems to be an inherent plan that we follow with our bodies, trusting in what appears and unfolds. We let our bodies find forms, flow from form to form, change, and redesign. It is in not-knowing that movement arises.

Everything is there – we follow the flow.

Now, as I write, I become even more aware that, similar to the embryonic tissues and cells, in the creation of the piece we follow a path that is unknown. It cannot be followed cognitively and finds its form only by following the flow of movement.

Using photos from the performance, I will show excerpts from our dance piece "Re-Membrane," created out of movement, flow, lightness, and learning and researching about experiential embryology, Authentic Movement, and craniosacral biodynamics.

Beginning

I lie in the child's pose and let my weight sink to the ground, it is dark.

We start with hands-on work.

I perceive hands on my skin, tender touch, like hands on the surface of water, my cells feel the contact on my back, I feel warmth and the light pressure of hands, calmness rises, my cells relax, my outer shell becomes softer, I sink deeper and am aware of my inner skin, which is connected to my outer skin by fluid. I am connected to the outside and inside, and feel the rhythm of expanding and contracting.

After some time, I feel my heartbeat. I listen to the rhythm of my heart and perceive it deep inside me.

I feel my skin, my outer limits, I breathe, I am. Arrived. In the right place.

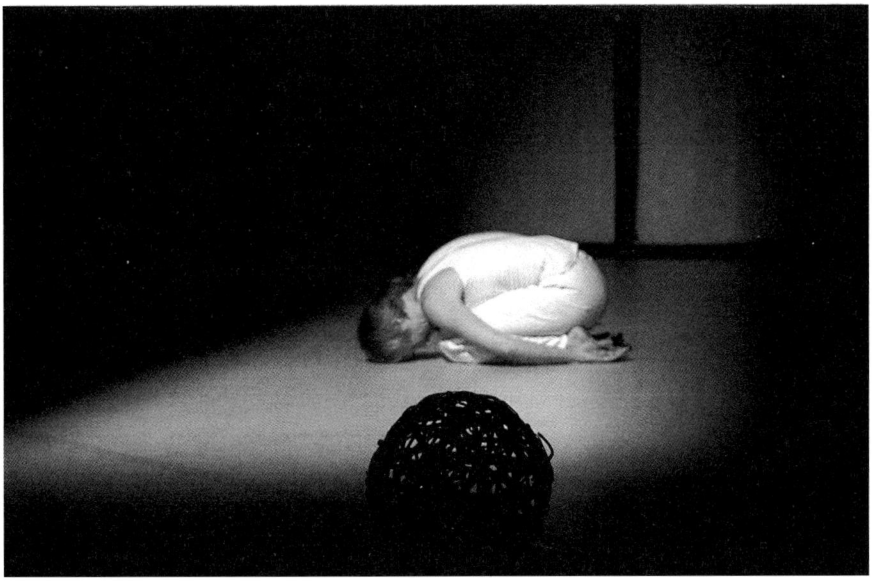

"Re-Membrane." Dancers: Frauke Burchards and Bettina Löns. Photographer: Ralph Hormes

Chapter 7

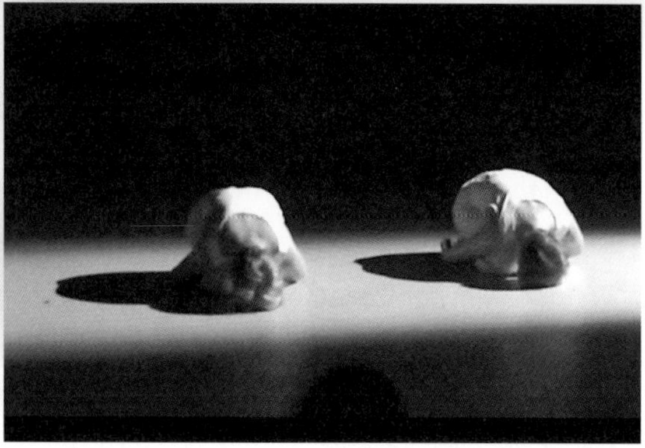

"Re-Membrane." Dancers: Frauke Burchards and Bettina Löns. Photographer: Ralph Hormes

Each cellular membrane has an outer layer of molecules facing towards the outside and an inner layer facing towards the inside. A layer of fluid lies between them and connects them.

In the beginning we are two who are one, says Bainbridge Cohen, and this delights me: "[T]o begin, the egg and sperm unite." We are thinking that from the union of the egg and the sperm we "have a primary cell, that divides and duplicates. But it turns out that the first cell is two cells" ("After a process of 12–24 hours, the instant the genetic material from the sperm and the egg (one half each) determines the unique genetic code for the new individual, two cells are formed. The first cell of the new person is two, from which all other cells and tissues will form" (Bainbridge Cohen 2012: 164).

Front – back

Now the fertilized cell begins to divide: one cell becomes four, eight, sixteen ... until this one cell has become a sphere of many individual cells. More and more cells continue to grow until some of them differentiate.

One part of the sphere of cells becomes a developing embryo (embryoblast); the other part becomes a cell membrane (and later placenta) – a container filled with liquid.

The embryoblast also differentiates into two layers of different tissue types: namely, the endoderm

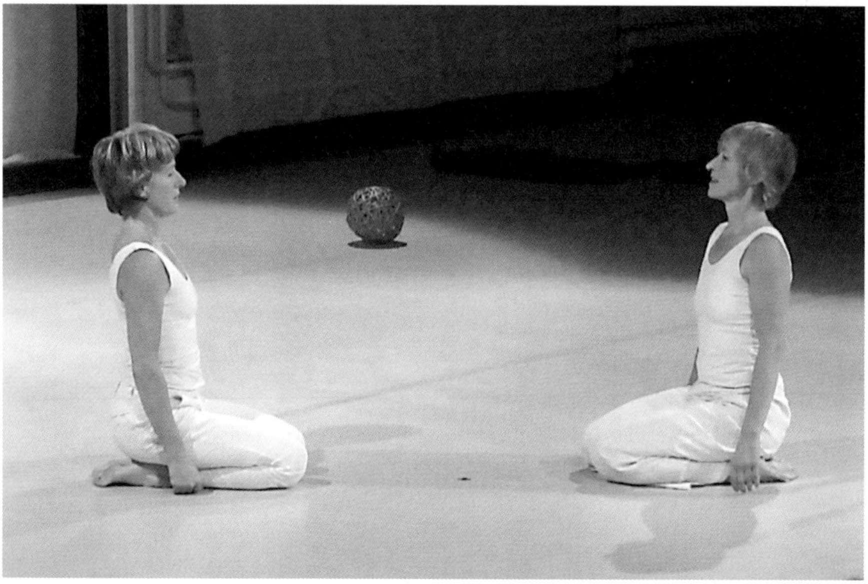

"Re-Membrane." Dancers: Frauke Burchards and Bettina Löns. Photographer: Ralph Hormes

and ectoderm. (Later, a third cell layer is added – the mesoderm.) The embryoblast is now a kind of intermediate layer, a disc, between two fluid-filled cavities (yolk sac and amniotic cavity).

For a while we have a front and a back, and the first spatial direction is not the axis between top and bottom, between head and rump, but the axis between back and front. This is due to the fact that the embryo now forms a flat disc.

I stand, my hands pluck and stroke delicately over my front, touching my face, breastbone, stomach, pelvis, legs, following the shape, the curves.
We are "in front" with our attention and move through the room. How does "the front" (where the organs grow) and "the back" (from where the nervous system and skin grow) feel? How does it feel when I am in relationship? Who am I in relationship? We lean with our backs against each other and feel our backs.

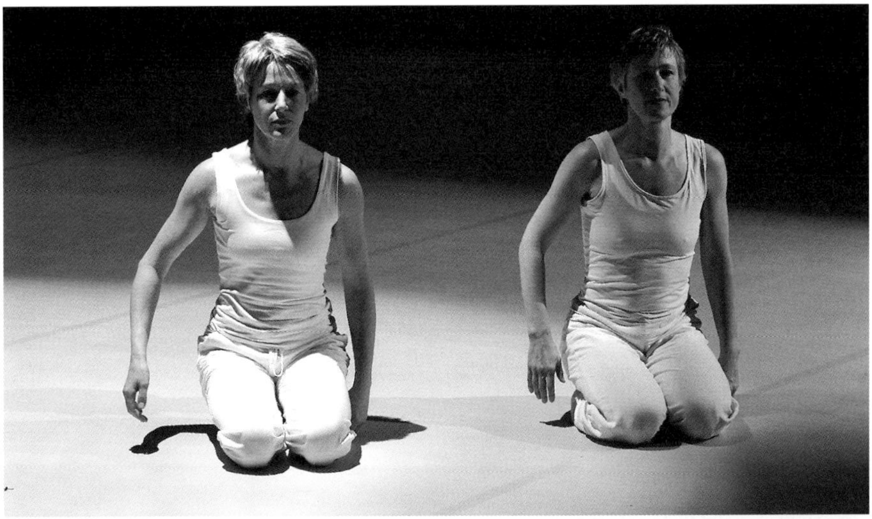

"Re-Membrane." Dancers: Frauke Burchards and Bettina Löns. Photographer: Ralph Hormes

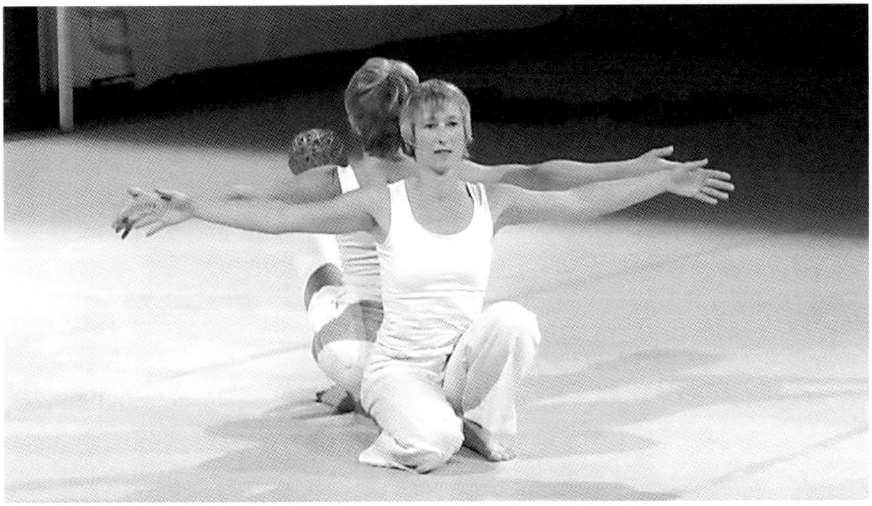

"Re-Membrane." Dancers: Frauke Burchards and Bettina Löns. Photographer: Ralph Hormes

Chapter 7

Flow of fluid – rhythms

"If we now imagine a two-week-old embryo, we find the endoderm with the yolk sac at the front of the two-layer embryonic disc and the ectoderm with the amniotic fluid at the back" (van der Wal 2016: 92). We imagine two balloons filled with liquid: one at the front and one at the back. What is exciting is that, during a certain period of embryonic development, there is a connection between these two balloons: at this time there is "a subtle flow of fluid between them that causes a rhythmic movement of opening and closing, extension and flexion" (Hartley 2014: 20).

We are researching how the liquid is distributed forwards and backwards:

I stand, lean my body forwards, lean it backwards – forwards – backwards, I feel the inner movement. Fluid shifts: forwards, backwards, slightly, slowly, flowing. I bend forward and feel yielding, condensing of the front side; fluid flows forward and gives support to my front side. I stretch back; a slow flow backwards begins, my back widens, expands. I lean backwards and am supported, my arms are spreading out, reaching out into space, wonderfully light to the wrists, to the fingertips, connected, like water, flowing through. Again bending forward, and I feel the alternating flow of fluid from the front part to the back part, slow, steady, calm, safe, infinite.

This flowing movement, the alternation between flexion and extension, folding and unfolding, rounding and expanding, accompanies us in our further research work and development of the piece. We are in contact and yet each with herself; we feel ourselves through the rhythm that is within us, which connects us and our form with flow and rhythm. This rhythm connects us; no words are necessary. We dive and trust, into the developing form, and follow the flow.

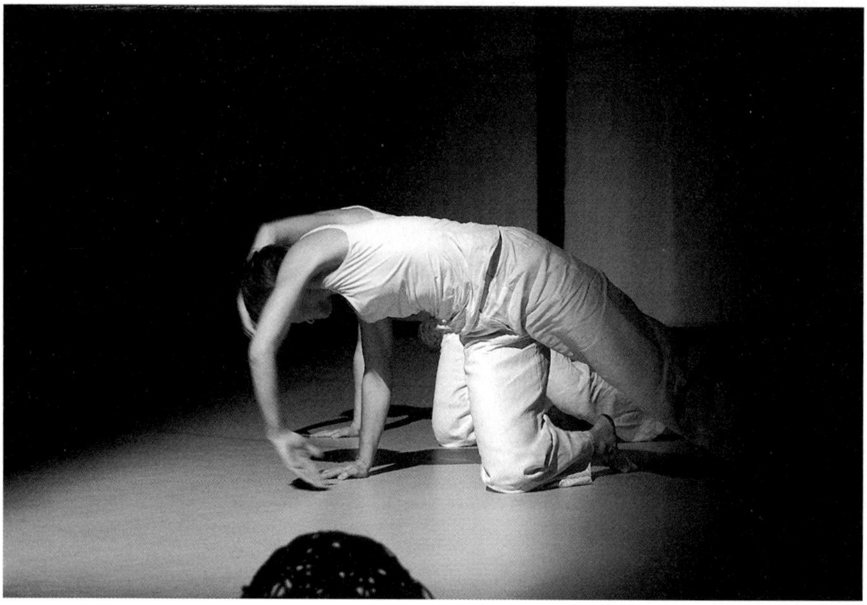

"Re-Membrane." Dancers: Frauke Burchards and Bettina Löns. Photographer: Ralph Hormes

IBMT and Dance: "Re-Membrane"

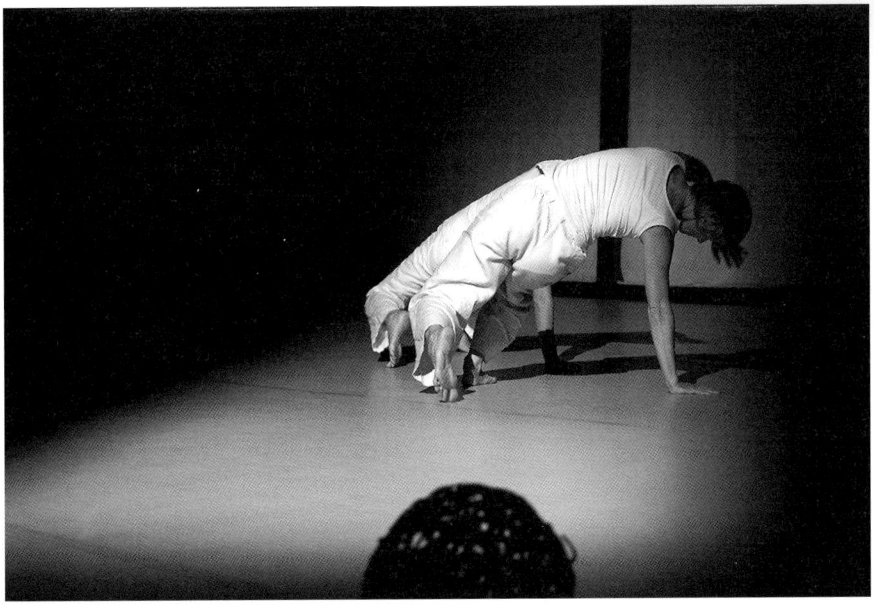

"Re-Membrane."
Dancers: Frauke
Burchards and Bettina
Löns. Photographer:
Ralph Hormes

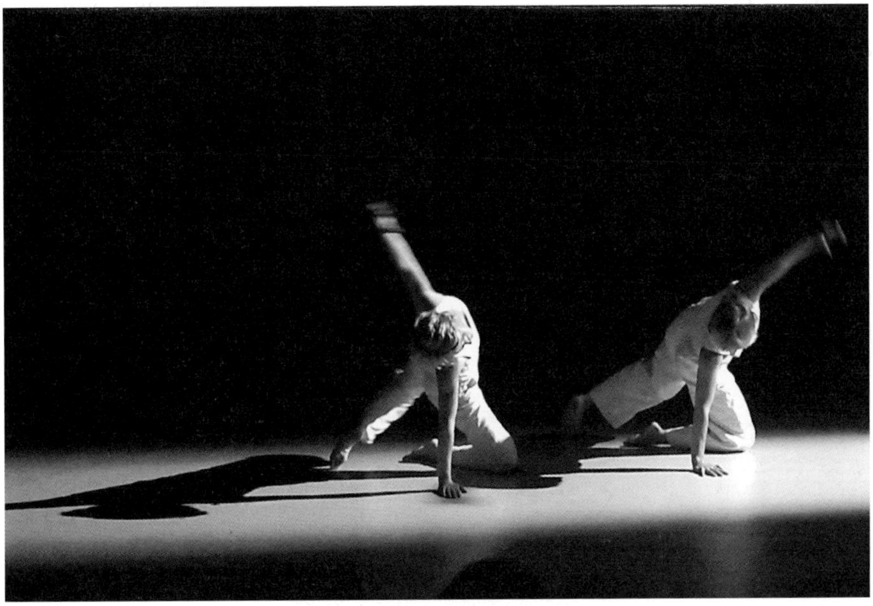

"Re-Membrane."
Dancers: Frauke
Burchards and Bettina
Löns. Photographer:
Ralph Hormes

Chapter 7

Outside – inside

We continue to follow the process of development and meet a moment that moves us very much: upper and lower end of the embryo round and bend towards each other, the embryo folding into a deep C-curve. To do this, however, it first has to lose the uprightness it achieved in the second week, only to regain it later in a new and fuller state. The yolk sac, the front balloon filled with liquid, flows inwards and creates the digestive tract. The outside is brought to the inside. Interior is created. At the same time, the rear, liquid-filled balloon stretches around and envelops the whole embryo.

We are looking for the movement of inflow, our arms form the front yolk sac, I am aware of my mouth and my tail/anus, I feel my tail stretching and allow the distance between head and tail to increase. At the same time, I am with rounding, with bending of head and tail, and also my yolk sac becomes smaller; the fluid of the yolk sac begins to flow inwards from the periphery. At the level of the solar plexus, I imagine the taking in, flowing inside, taking it in, bringing it completely inwards, slow, soft, fluid. I hear it gurgling inside me, flowing up and down, spreading out. My back continues to round itself, expands, and I let the fluids envelop me and feel safe. The fluid inside me is flowing and streaming: a long journey in which caves and spaces are formed. I know that there is room inside me for my organs. I am happy and feel softness inside me. I am so touched that what was outside is now deeply inside me.

Inside space and heart

Now, a third layer of cells has formed. The embryo is no longer the two-layered disc of the second week and has developed into a three-layered form. This layer is the mesoderm, from which, among other

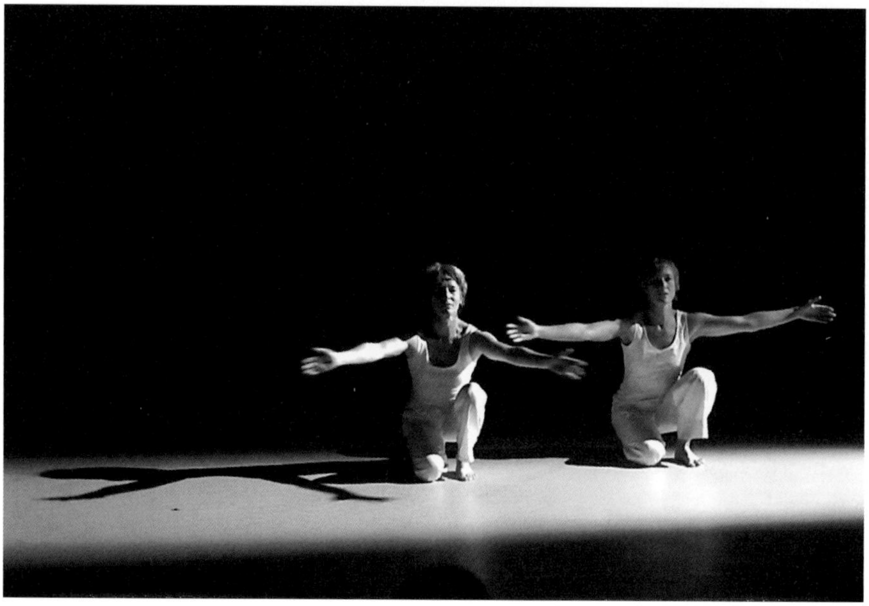

"Re-Membrane." Dancers: Frauke Burchards and Bettina Löns. Photographer: Ralph Hormes

IBMT and Dance: "Re-Membrane"

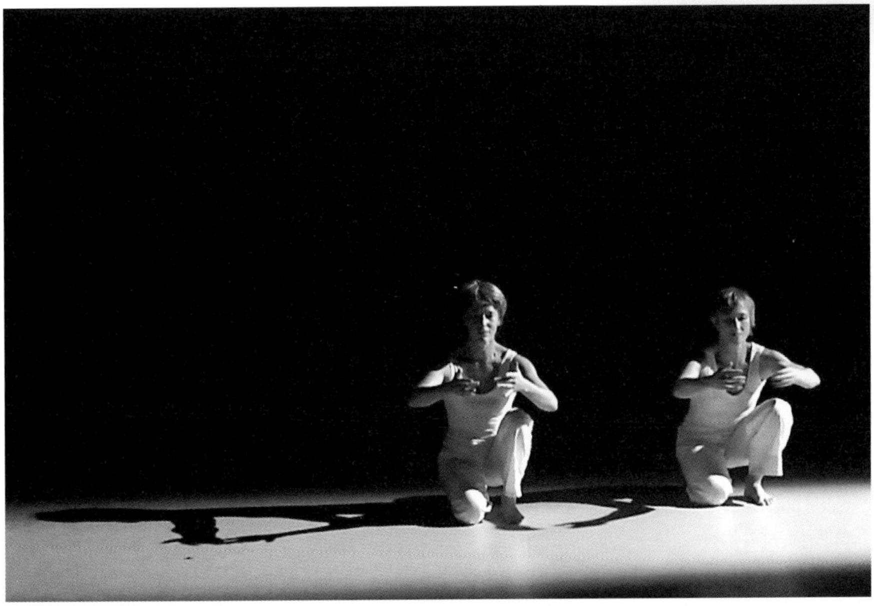

"Re-Membrane." Dancers: Frauke Burchards and Bettina Löns. Photographer: Ralph Hormes

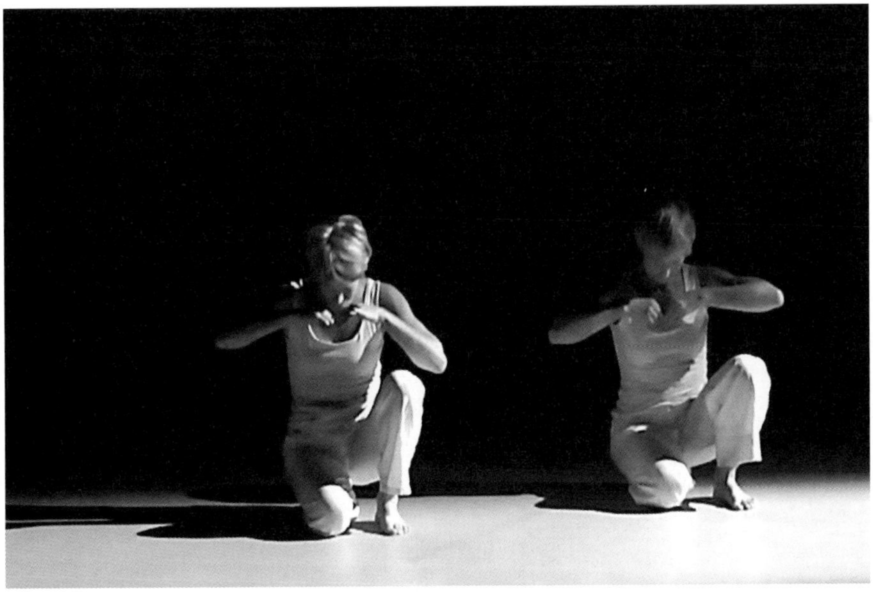

"Re-Membrane." Dancers: Frauke Burchards and Bettina Löns. Photographer: Ralph Hormes

things, the bones, muscles, heart, vessels, blood, kidneys, and gonads develop.

The first blood vessels appear. The blood vessels that grow in the mesoderm are tiny. They are capillaries that emerge and, with them, "primitive," primary blood is formed: "When blood vessels first start to form, the heart does not yet exist … early blood flow stimulates the development of the heart" (Talbott 2013).

Chapter 7

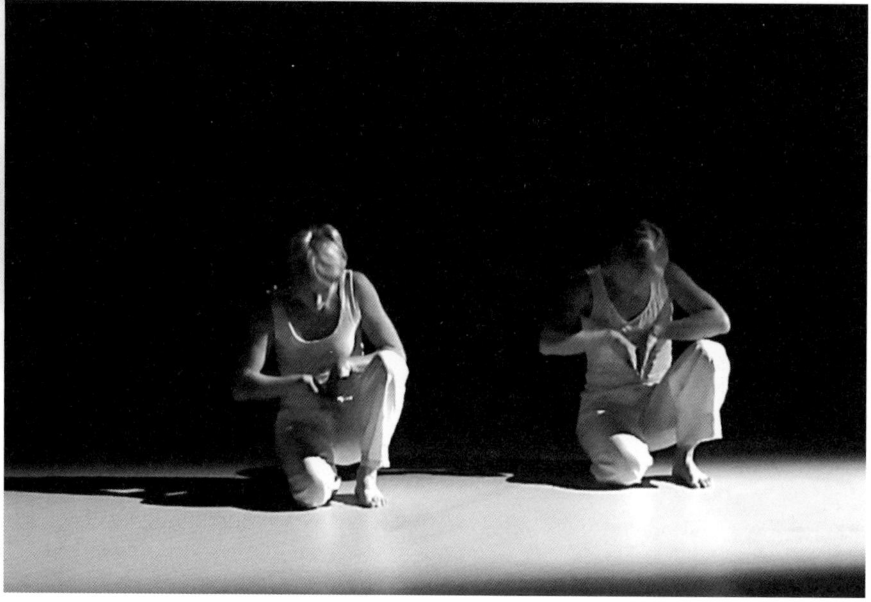

"Re-Membrane." Dancers: Frauke Burchards and Bettina Löns. Photographer: Ralph Hormes

Heart

The very first form that the embryonic heart takes is a simple tubular structure, and is located at the very top of the embryo, sitting as if on the forehead. Only a membrane separates it from the embryonic brain. During the second week, the heart folds into the centre of the body; from its outward and upward facing position it now becomes deeply embedded within the body.

(Hartley 2014: 20)

Before the heart has developed walls (septa) separating the four chambers from each other, the blood already flows in two distinct "currents" through the heart. The [blood currents] in the right and left sides of the heart do not mix, but stream and loop by each other, just as two currents in a body of water. Thus the movement of the blood gives the parameters for the inner differentiation of the heart, just as the looping heart redirects the flow of blood.

(Talbott 2013)

The heart is excited and beats: close the mouth and bring it inside to the heart; I lay my hands on my heart: the left hand lays over the right hand, the right hand embraces the heart and the left hand lies on it. I feel my heartbeat.

Again, we seek the movement of inflow and connect with the inflowing fluid of the yolk sac up and down, and imagine the tissue of the two tubes that become our heart, spiraling and curling around each other; the right tube of the heart shifts a little to the right and curls into the left half of the heart, my lungs envelop the heart. Our heads bend and follow, sink into the heart. When we straighten up again, we keep the connection to our heart.

Closure

During the next few weeks of development, the embryo continues to change its shape through a constant metamorphosis of its form. The change of shape is movement, created by the consequences of

IBMT and Dance: "Re-Membrane"

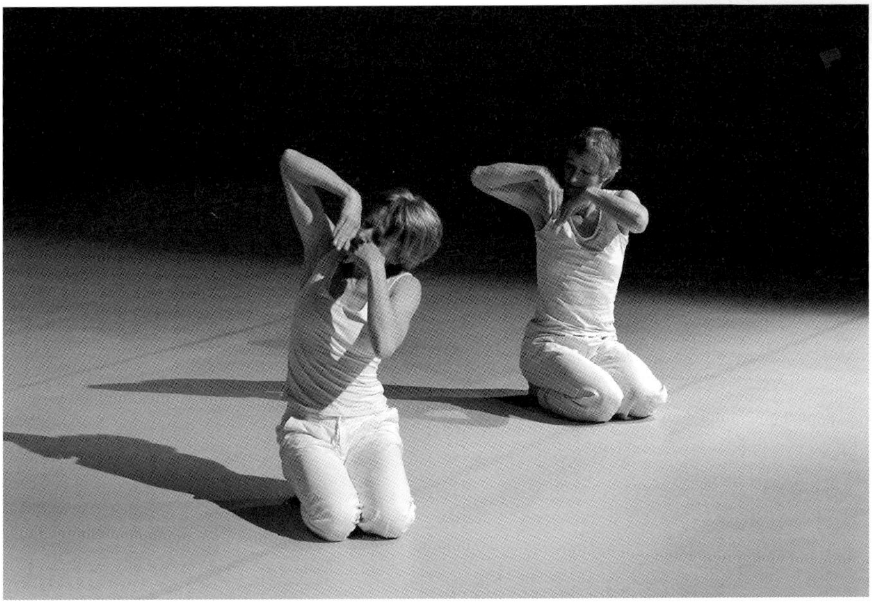

"Re-Membrane." Dancers: Frauke Burchards and Bettina Löns. Photographer: Ralph Hormes

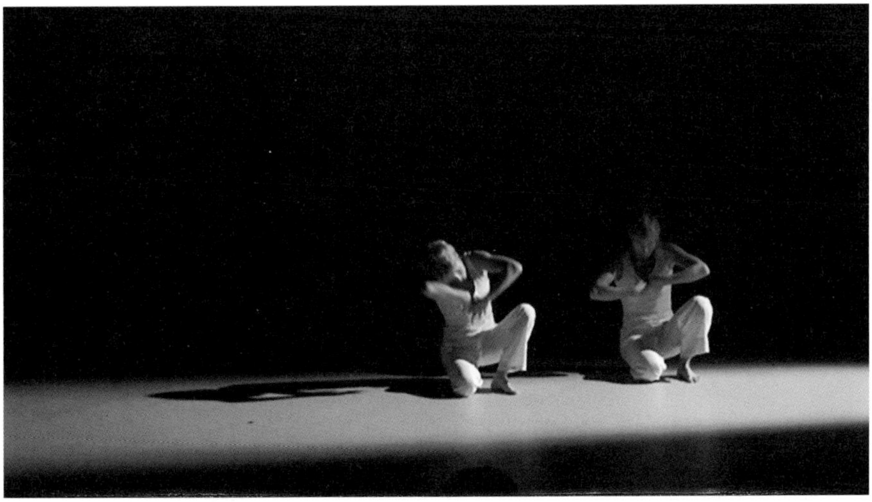

"Re-Membrane." Dancers: Frauke Burchards and Bettina Löns. Photographer: Ralph Hormes

a current, by the interaction of pressure and pull, by rotation and compression. The form comes out of movement.

[The] cells from all three layers engage in a stunningly complex way as they endlessly differentiate, flow and stream into their own specific locations to form the different tissues of the body. This miracle of shape-shifting organization continues until all the organs and tissues of the embryo have formed and is completed after about eight weeks.

(Hartley 2014: 20)

Chapter 7

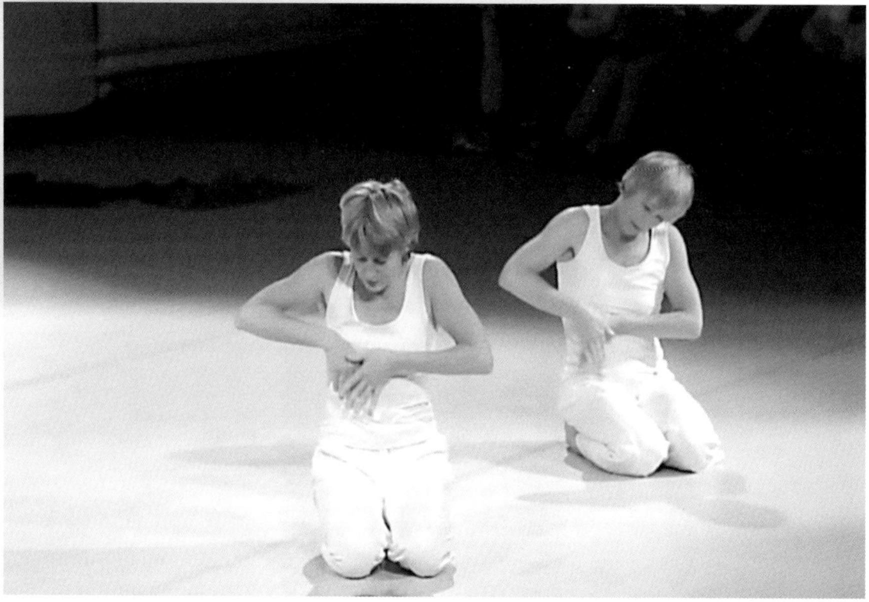

"Re-Membrane." Dancers: Frauke Burchards and Bettina Löns. Photographer: Ralph Hormes

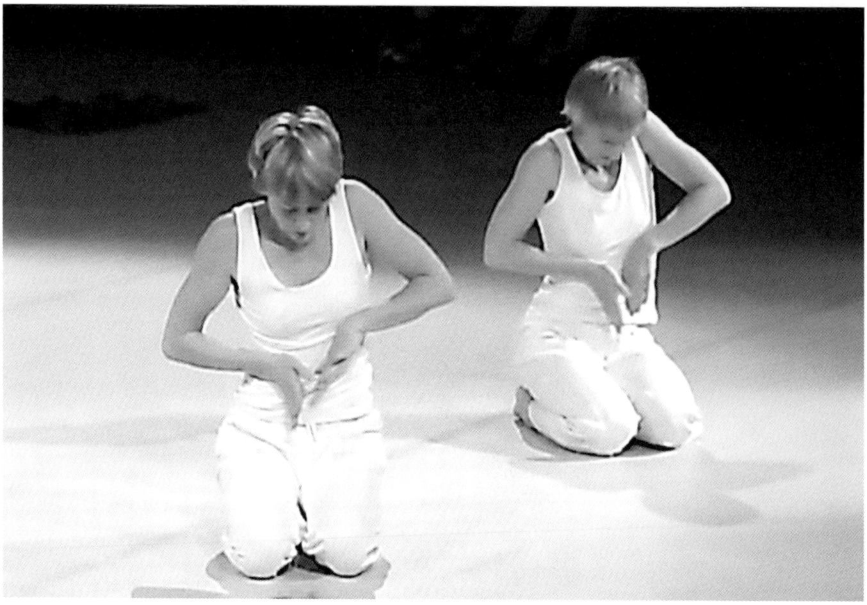

"Re-Membrane." Dancers: Frauke Burchards and Bettina Löns. Photographer: Ralph Hormes

IBMT and Dance: "Re-Membrane"

We roll on the floor, I roll my heart with me, with me across the floor, enveloped, and I feel a streaming and flowing, all cells are permeated, flowed through by liquid. We spread out and dive in and follow the currents, spirals, and rotations of our bodies.

We dance with ease, feel the flow, follow the form, and change it again and again. We create an atmosphere of togetherness.

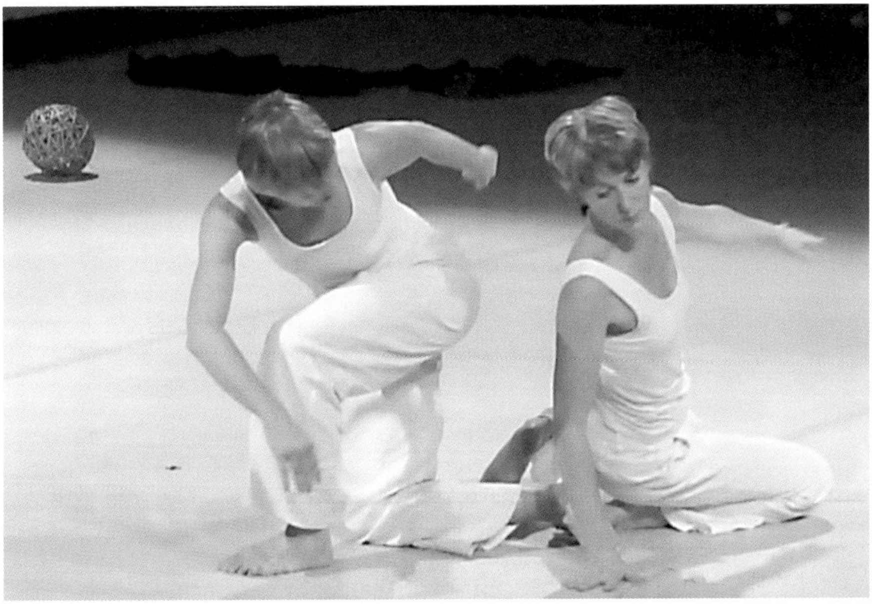

"Re-Membrane." Dancers: Frauke Burchards and Bettina Löns. Photographer: Ralph Hormes

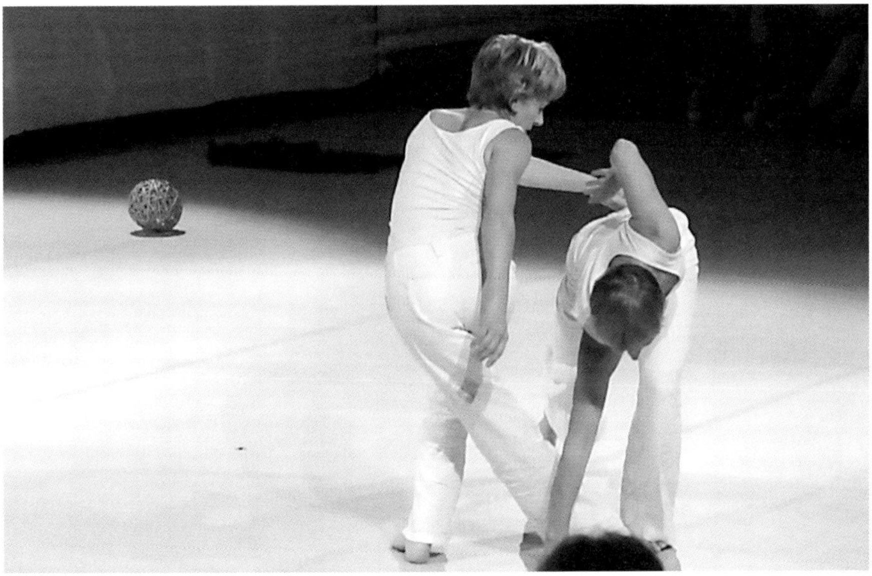

"Re-Membrane." Dancers: Frauke Burchards and Bettina Löns. Photographer: Ralph Hormes

Chapter 7

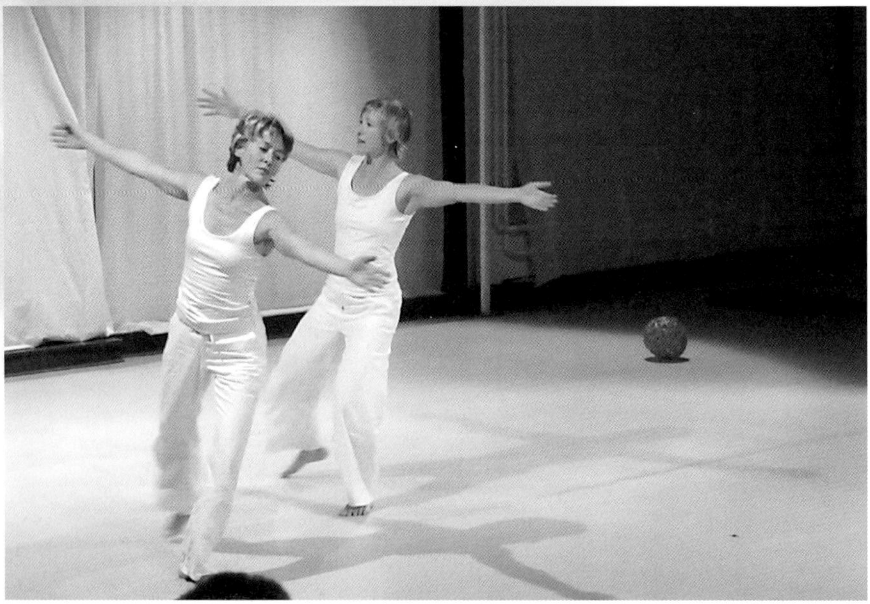

"Re-Membrane." Dancers: Frauke Burchards and Bettina Löns. Photographer: Ralph Hormes

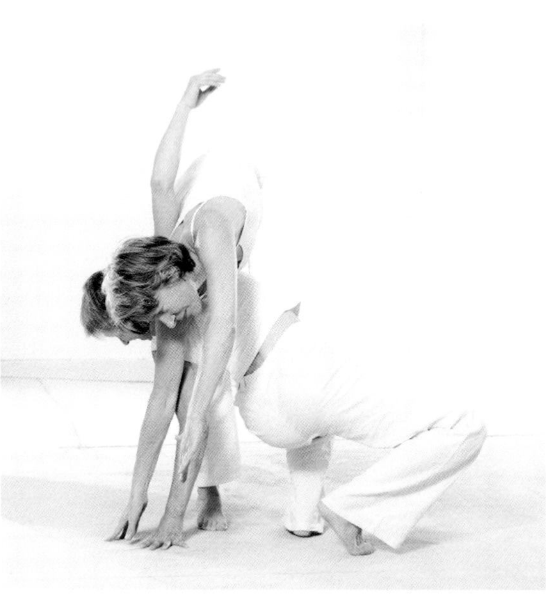

"Re-Membrane." Dancers: Frauke Burchards and Bettina Löns. Photographer: Mirko Plha

The more I write about the performance in retrospect, the more fascinated I am about what is (present) in us and what unfolds in space and form.

There is joy in me about what has been created:

"Re-Membrane":

A dance piece, which

reminds us of our beginning and our completeness.

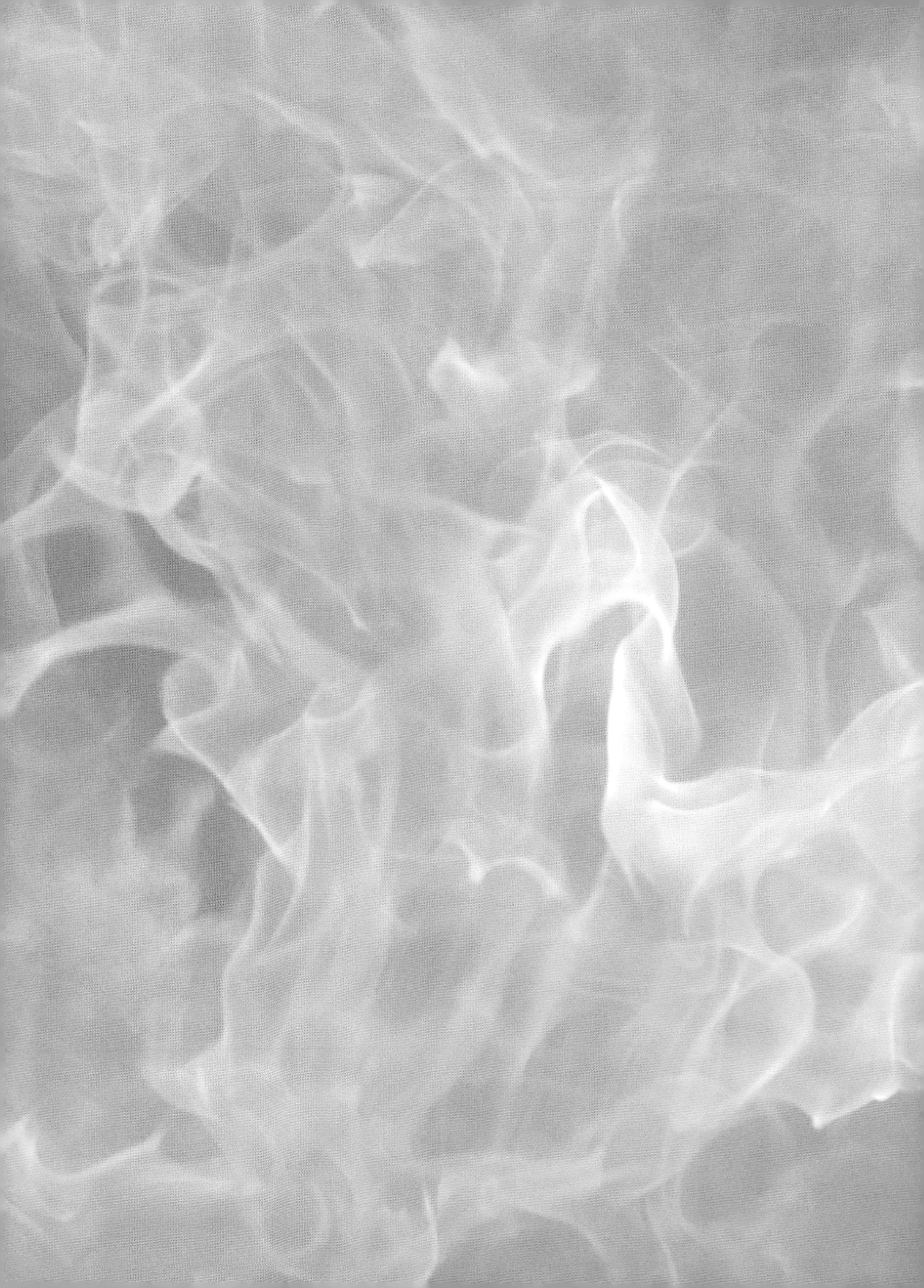

Part 3

Moving into Life 2: Birth and Beyond – Supporting Development

Support on the Path of Motherhood

Anna Feoktistova

8

To my mother

And her mother

And all the mothers of the world.

How long will it hurt?

From now on – always.

I hear these words from my yoga teacher as I sit on the yoga mat. It is the beginning of the class and our teacher is talking about some cases from her experience as a doula and answering some questions. She is giving support to our emotional state – anxiety, confusion, longing for some information, and an opportunity to relax.

I hear her saying: *"From now – always."* I am shivering inside just a little bit and put my hand on my belly. I am pregnant. There are 10 pregnant women and a yoga teacher in the room with dimmed lights.

"How long will it hurt?" It is a question from the story the teacher was telling us, from the birth process and the moment when labor begins. At this moment the pelvic bones are moving further away from each other, the ligaments are stretching, the muscles of the pelvic floor should be as relaxed as possible, but relaxing them means a new level of pain.

"From now – always." This answer relates to the birth process, the period after it, and the whole of life following. It means that nothing will be the same again.

"But the pain will be changing." The child will be born and the sensations will change. Then he or she will grow up day by day, step by step, year by year. The physical pain will calm down but pain in the heart will do a lot of different work. It will bulldoze the space inside the heart, inside the mother's soul – the space for love, acceptance, self-devotion, and the capacity for letting go. The pain in the heart will clear out the space inside for all the qualities necessary for being a mother – to a newborn, to a toddler, to a pre-schooler, to a schoolchild, to a teenager, to an adult.

There are many texts about babies: about how they develop during pregnancy and after birth; about what they need; about what parents should or should not do and have to provide – gymnastics, doctors, education, and so on. There is so much information about babies! But I want to devote this text to mothers: to those who are around the baby, to those whose bodies and minds do such great and subtle work, for so long.

How to Use This Text

In this chapter I write about different stages on the path of motherhood: pregnancy, labor, and recovery after birth. I invite you to read the chapter and do the practices sequentially, one by one, even if you are not pregnant at the moment and your interest lies in the recovery after birth. Please start with the sections "Asking, Listening, Hearing, and Answering" and "Pregnancy"; there you will find the main embodied ideas and skills that will penetrate all the other practices and periods to come. Step by step, we string the rings of skills and practices on the pyramid, and each ring finds its basis, the Earth, in the previous one.

Asking, Listening, Hearing, and Answering

I adore mothers all over the world. I suggest that we direct our attention to the mothers and that

Chapter 8

they do the same – turn towards themselves. I am sure that the first skill that should be developed by a pregnant woman is that of listening to herself, to her needs and individual qualities. The skill will become a habit of paying attention to her own sensations and feelings, thoughts, and desires.

When I was pregnant with my second son, I was a student of Integrative Bodywork and Movement Therapy (IBMT). Everything we were doing in class was exactly what my body, emotional state, and mind needed. IBMT teaches us to be patient and attentive to ourselves. We are looking for a cellular breathing mind in our bodies; we are listening to the organs, bones, muscles, and nerve tissues. We are finding movement patterns which live in our bodies and give support to our adult movement. Through all this anatomical and physiological work, we are learning how to recognize our needs on all the levels of our being: body, feelings, and mind. We begin to hear our inner voice and treat it with deep respect.

One of the main IBMT disciplines, which serves all other skills and therapeutic presence, is Authentic Movement. The ideas presented below do not describe the form that the discipline is practiced in, but they are based on the skills used in it. Authentic Movement taught me how to turn my attention to myself through the body's impulses and its movement, how to be a patient witness to myself, showing me great benefits that appear later on.

Asking

Within the broader skill that I call Listening, we can distinguish four different stages: asking, listening, hearing, and answering. Each stage is significant and supports all the others.

What do I feel right now?

What do I need right now?

Where is my attention?

Who am I now?

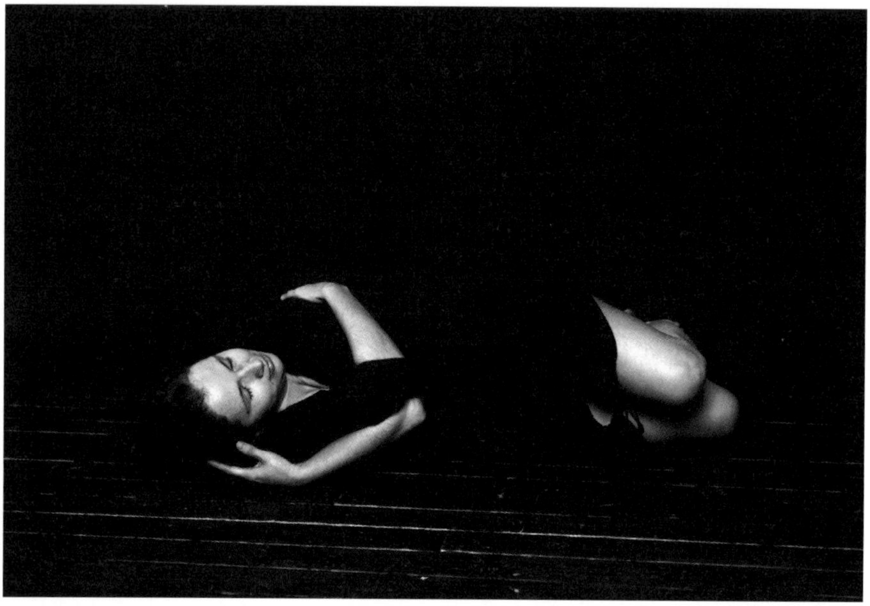

Asking, listening, hearing, and answering – listening. Mover: Anna Feoktistova. Photographer: Daria Yarkova

Asking these questions can be a regular ritual that helps you to return to yourself, to find your center and vector of movement, to create a quiet moment that will give support to the mother as well as the baby.

Sometimes, especially after giving birth, a woman can be frustrated. All her attention is with the baby but she is still stressed. The attunement is obstructed. The old knowledge that the woman had about herself can seem irrelevant. It can really be a challenge for her to begin to recognize her own needs and reactions again.

At first, questions may be as simple as: *"What is my feeling of warmth now? Is it warm enough for me? Maybe I need more clothes?"*

Listening and hearing

After asking a question, we need to be calm for a while; we need to open our awareness to the body, inviting it to speak. It takes time to build a relationship with our body based on trust.

It may be helpful to put your hand on the heart area or on your belly, to take a few deep inhalations and exhalations, to feel how your feet are placed on the floor.

An answer can come in different ways. It can be a clear understanding – some words in your mind. It can be a silence which allows you to recognize a small compression in the chest area or a facial grimace that will become a key to understanding. Or it can just be a big exhalation. Any movement, any image, any sound can be an answer. Please hear it.

Answering

After you ask, listen, and hear a reply, you have a beautiful moment – to make an answer. This answer can be an expression of your support, love, and care. It can be the safest and most reliable hug into which you just yield. It is about giving patience and acceptance to yourself and satisfying your own needs in the best way possible. You can talk to yourself, dance, make different sounds, lie down, and rest – all of that while being tuned in to your needs.

Please say to yourself, to a place from where the answer comes to you:

I see you,

I hear you,

I feel what you need,

And I'll take care of you in the best way.

And listen once more. Your body will answer again by expressing emotion, creating sensation, breathing, by movement and stillness, the heart beating. All body languages are so different! It is such a beautiful time when you learn about how your own body speaks.

If your understanding of your needs is clear – can you satisfy them right now?

If not now, can you choose a time and make a promise to yourself to do it? And then really do it?

Or – if this is impossible – can your awareness become a place where you shed your tears, dwelling in futility about it?

You can be a good mother for yourself. You can take care of your health, feelings, needs. You can learn this art now. Your inner little girl can be met, seen, heard, and hugged by your inner adult.

But what about the babies? Maybe, while listening to herself, a woman will do something wrong that will hurt her baby? Or she will not be attentive enough towards the baby and it will cause trauma? My answer is: NO. I am deeply convinced that if a woman knows her real needs, if she creates a safe and nurturing space for herself, if she is tuned in to herself, her connection with the baby will work in the best way automatically:

I hear you, I feel what you need – because I feel myself.

When I am in a strong connection with myself, it is the best base for my connection with others, including my children, parents, and friends.

Listening and hearing are the basic skills necessary for making different choices and doing various practices and exercises.

Feelings and states we meet unexpectedly

There is another issue I want to mention. Very often, the experience of pregnancy, labor, and being with a little baby brings us back to the time when we were babies ourselves. This experience is pre-verbal; it is a subconscious layer that can unexpectedly manifest itself when we become mothers. We can meet with really deep feelings that return us to the time when we were so small and helpless, and to the experience of our own mothers.

It is an important time that can show us many places we can heal and use as a support. My strong recommendations here are:

1 Be prepared and create support for yourself in these places, rather than falling into the emotional pits unexpectedly, finding yourself in a hopeless position.

2 Find time and help to meet with those feelings and traumas, to be in kind hands and a strong therapeutic container.

Most of all, it is important to accept: now this is what it is like. Here is a pit. I need to be conscious of this place, build a temporary bridge for now, and work deeper for the future.

Pregnancy

I am pregnant. And it is magic. I am breathing with my hand on my belly. I sense a pulse and movement there. My body is creating a new body. There are two souls inside me.

I'm abandoning tormenting thoughts. I'm breathing. Being grateful. The changes in the horizontal are aligning. Life is breathing and the heart is pumping. The vertical will resist.

(Excerpt from my diary, March 2014)

During the fourth month of my second pregnancy, I started to feel a strong pressure on the pelvic floor area. I had a feeling that my organs were falling out through the perineum. My gynecologist diagnosed me with vaginal prolapse. During the remaining months of the pregnancy, I learned how to treat my body in a kinder way and not to overload it. This problem became a new door for me. I went through it and found myself in a big, unexplored space, so important for the health and life quality of each pregnant woman and each mother. I began to learn more about it, and 2 years after my labor, I created a somatic course for pregnant women based on IBMT practices.

Pregnancy brings a lot of changes to a woman's body, mind, and emotional state. It happens without mind control or conscious choice. The previous world is crumbling; changes happen rapidly and are out of control. Through the IBMT approach, we find the way to our bodies as our homes. We learn how to listen to the body using our attention (to the sensations, to the breathing), imagination, and movement. We begin to allow

Support on the Path of Motherhood

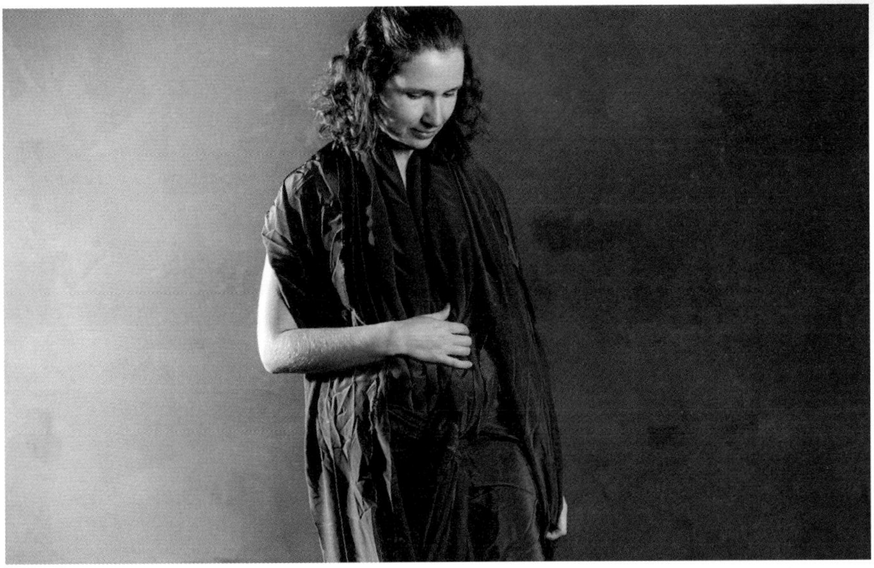

Pregnancy. Mover: Anna Feoktistova. Photographer: Daria Yarkova

this inner wisdom to lead us through investigation of our changing needs. We yield to the earth and the power of breathing, releasing the blocked zones and finding the core of our inner power and support.

Changes During Pregnancy

Body level

During pregnancy, the body tissues, especially ligaments, become more elastic. The hormonal balance changes. The breasts prepare for feeding. The weight gained in the belly influences bone structure. Common problems caused by this process are flattening of the feet and hemorrhoids.

Organs change their position, form, volume, and structure quite considerably:

- The uterus grows a few times larger (by delivery, its volume can be 520–550 times bigger), the amount of muscle fiber increases, the ligaments grow longer.
- Ovaries, heart, and lungs enlarge too, to create special hormones which support the new cycle of placental blood flow and nourish it with oxygen.
- Intestine, stomach, bladder, and liver are moved and squeezed, subject to pressure (Argamakova n.d.).

Psyche level

There is a saying that, during the 9 months of pregnancy, the soul of the mother goes down to the meeting point between two worlds: the world of the living and the world of the dead. It moves there to meet a new soul. The birth process, then, when the door between the two worlds opens, is full of mysticism and can be unpredictable. Later, 9 months after at the birth, two souls move up – back to the world of the living.

Over the course of a pregnancy, a woman's attention changes. It is directed inside, towards the inner

Chapter 8

world. This period can be experienced through different states and with different feelings: it can be calm and harmonious, or full of worries and panic. It brings a woman to another level of being and, of course, she now needs some new knowledge and support.

Practices During Pregnancy

These practices have three main goals:

- To give support to the changing bodymind, to find new comfort in the body and life for the period of pregnancy.
- To prepare a woman for the stressful birth process.
- To find and establish new ways for a woman to communicate with herself, with kind witnessing and support. In the period of life to come, after the birth, these ways will become the basis for communication with the baby as well.

Below I describe the four main necessities I discovered for myself and other women in a pregnant state, and practices related to them. I found IBMT-based practices very helpful for achieving these goals, and have also added some others that I applied in a somatic way.

Silence, deep rest, supporting space

Any pregnant woman needs to be in a place where she can meet with herself in silence and acceptance. She needs to take a deep rest and hear herself. She also needs to meet other women who will understand her and share their experiences. And, as usual, there is not much time for this!

Cellular breathing is the first aid for coming out of a stressful state. It helps us to take a deep rest over a short time, to find support on a fundamental level. It also helps to tune in with the baby in a basic place connected to the wisdom of the body.

You can have a taste of this practice within 10–15 minutes, creating a time when you will not be disturbed. Start by sitting down in a comfortable way, with the sit bones placed higher than the knees. Take a few inhalations and exhalations in the silence of your heart; allow all your attention to turn inwards. Feel your connection to the Earth, allowing it to support each cell in your body, each thought in your mind, and each emotion moving through your presence. Allow yourself to yield into the palms of the Earth. Take these minutes when time changes its speed; let it be slowed down.

Put your hand on the chest area or on the belly, observing how the breathing changes the shape of your body. Inhalations expand it, and exhalations make it shrink. You can notice it. The next step is to imagine that there are millions of cells, making up the body, right under your palm. Each cell is breathing as our lungs do – expanding and contracting, filling up and emptying.

Cellular breathing has a different speed and amplitude than the breathing of the lungs. Just imagine this small movement in your body and open your awareness to the sensations. Maybe you will feel a tiny vibration inside, perhaps warming up or cooling down. Maybe a deep sound like a hum will emerge. Please be open to this experience, listening to the whispering of your cells. This time of witnessing the inner mystery creates a magical opportunity for all bodymind systems to reset and to tune to your health, your strength, your needs.

Be here for a few minutes; rest and yield in the cells, listen to them. Then bring your attention back to the bigger breathing of the lungs, feel the movement under your palms again. Notice the sensations on your skin; open your sense organs to the sounds, smells, light, and colors. Caress your body with pleasure. And switch to your next duties, allowing the connectedness to your sensations and feelings to support you.

Our need for **touch** is so strong! In somatic practices you learn how to feel and to satisfy this need, at first – by yourself. An opportunity to give touch to yourself can be exactly what you need in a particular moment. It helps to regulate the nervous system, creates the feeling of safety, and switches the bodymind system from a stress state to a state of rest and recovery. Touch is our way of connecting to the world, and by changing the quality of it we can regulate it and tune to our needs.

First of all, take a look at your hands, acknowledging them. You can meet yourself in your hands, palms, fingers, their lines, skin, hair ... You can move them in the space, witnessing their dance, flexion and extension, reaching out. Make your hands and your gaze alive. Touch one hand with another; feel their meeting, letting them investigate each other. You can rub and push them against each other, feeling the circle going from one hand to another through the heart. Feel how the blood and warmth are activated (Olsen and McHose 2004).

Feel which place in your body asks for touch or more attention. Put your hands on it, allowing this touching to be open to listening. Feel what quality of touching your body needs now – lighter or heavier, pressing and pushing, or just giving a slight sensation of presence. Let all of your body respond to it through moving, stretching, yawning, and making sounds. Allow yourself to be touched and respond to it. Allow your hands to change the place of the touch. Follow the sensation of pleasure – our bodies respond to touch like cats. Kind and safe touch helps to build the trust between body and mind.

New ways of breathing and making sound

During pregnancy, the fetus becomes bigger and bigger in the uterus and the belly area rises. The lungs and heart grow too. Movement of the diaphragm therefore becomes more difficult, as there is more pressure from above and below. It becomes necessary to find new space and freedom for breathing.

The chest (thoracic) diaphragm is not alone in this, being part of a whole system of diaphragms. It is supported by the pelvic and throat (vocal) diaphragms, which move in sync with the lungs. The thoracic and pelvic diaphragms move together in one direction and the vocal diaphragm in the opposite direction. The main purpose of this movement is to give more space for the lungs to inhale and to help them to shrink on the exhale.

For this moving with breathing practice, put your hands on the sides of the ribs. Witness what tone there is here at this particular moment, what sensations, and maybe what emotions. You can use cellular touch to bring more relaxation to this area.

Then witness the movement of breathing that lives here right now. How are the ribs moving, to the sides, to the front, to the back? Be attentive and curious about all the directions of movement that are possible. With patience, invite your ribs and diaphragm to move in directions that may be less familiar. You can help by applying some pressure on the sides of the ribs, on their upper lobes, inviting attention and movement to these places. Let all your body participate in this movement. Allow your pelvic diaphragm and throat ligaments to move as well, providing more space for the lungs. You can move as you like or rest in any position that feels right. Open your mouth, make facial expressions, allow sounds

to be released. Let your body show you the best way to move, to make sounds, to breathe. Stretch in any direction, roll on the floor, rock your extremities from side to side. You can also play music you like, if it helps you to move and rest, to be attentive to yourself.

Accompanied by this free movement and sound, the body tissues are renewed. The inner fluids activate and fill cells and organs with the necessary nutrients and oxygen. They help carbon dioxide, any waste, and excess fluids to find their way out of the body. Such movement activates the lymphatic flow and assists the body in coping with edema as well.

Making **sounds** can be useful during pregnancy and serves as a guide during the birth process. It helps the body to open for labor, allowing the baby to travel to the outer world in synergy with the mother.

Explore the sound that lives in your body. What is it like: louder, quieter, deeper, lower? What changes in you – in your body sensations, in your emotional state – when you sound like this? And like that? Let the sound out. Launch the sound vibration inside the body tissues. Play, research, and rest, while making sounds in different ways. Let your body follow your needs, with sounds and breathing. Be curious, not serious, open to the unexpected ways that the body will choose to heal you and to show you the best qualities for pregnancy and giving birth.

One of the techniques that I tried during pregnancy was valuable in the birth process. It was in a class for pregnant couples; pregnant women and their partners were howling long and loud, making sounds like wolves. The men were hugging the women from behind, giving more support. The women were leaning back on to them, opening their chest and neck and letting the upper jaw open freely. The teacher told us: "Wolves never howl at the Moon alone. It is not about wistfulness and loneliness. Wolves howl in pairs; their sound is a song of love." I do not know if this is true or if it is a fairytale, but from that moment I loved to sound loud like a she-wolf who is in love.

In the eighth month of pregnancy, I came across **Taoist Female Practices** that helped me to **tune in with the pelvic floor**. These practices work with the pelvic diaphragm and perineum through the thoracic diaphragm and the connection between them.

Lie down in a position that is comfortable for you. It is better to lie on your back but if the baby is already big, or you feel strong pressure, feel free to find a better position on your side. Take a breath; observe how your chest is moving, following the inhalations and exhalations. Let your attention stay with this process, yielding into your breathing, becoming softer. Put one hand on your chest and the other on the lower belly. Sense the movement that happens there synchronistically. Feel how all the organs in the belly go down on the inhale and then come back up on the exhale. Each breath massages all the inner organs. Just stay tuned in to this process. Let your pelvic floor release on the inhalation, giving more space to the lungs and organs of the belly. Notice the moments when the pelvic floor draws in. Make these moments a little bit slower, letting the release happen. You can feel your neck and jaw responding to the release of this tension. Be free to move your neck and head, to pull faces, to yawn, and make any sounds if they come.

Calming the worries and panic

Authentic Movement is a practice that teaches us how to be a patient witness for the movement that lives in the body, for emotions, feelings, and the stream of thoughts. We learn to listen to our inner impulses, to give them space and body for manifestation, and to observe this process. We put aside criticisms, assessments, and judgments. Our goal in this process is to be open to the present moment as it is. Authentic Movement gives us a gift – the opportunity to witness without needing to do something. It calms down the panic and worries, clearing the space for free e-motion. This is the place where the opportunity to interact with the baby from a conscious, loving, and peaceful state is established.

Reclaiming the area of the genitals, opening the natural sexuality

Another practice to prepare me for giving birth was **perineum and vagina massage**, which helped to release tension and stretch out the tissues. During the first delivery – 2 years before the second one – my body had a strong negative experience connected with a breakdown of the perineal tissue. I came to the second delivery with more awareness and care towards the perineum area, and massage helped release tension around the vagina, approximately 1–2 cm (½ to 1 in) inside the entrance. Psychologically, it was also easier to inhabit this area of the body – alive, sexual, and intimate.

In the process of these massages (I was taught how to do them by a doula and later on was able to do them myself), I became aware of how closed this part of the body was for me. It had to do with my childhood and education, with assumptions passed on to me by my parents and teachers in the process of growing up. From this moment on, sexuality and sexual energy started to open up for me and I realized that I was only just starting to get to know and embody them.

Giving Birth

We are naked, raw, a little naive, emptied of what is unnecessary. In this state of openness there is room for something new to enter.

Hartley 1995: xxxvi

In my experience, delivery creates a new body. Each delivery does that. During labor, the pregnant woman disappears and dies, and two new people are born – a mother and a child. These are two new bodies, and so the term "recovery after delivery" does not entirely appeal to me. For me, it is a process of embodiment, inhabiting a new body, exploring, collecting, and aligning, together with building a new life in a new family.

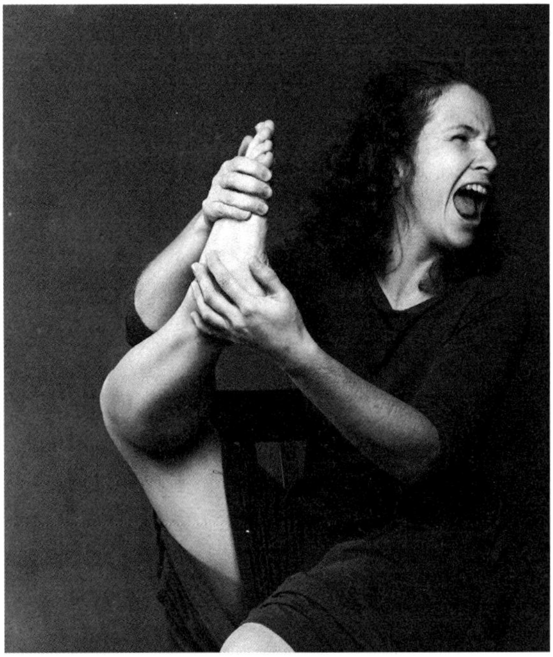

Giving birth. Mover: Anna Feoktistova.
Photographer: Daria Yarkova

Chapter 8

I have two sons. In both cases the labor was fast (3½ and 3 hours). Here is what supported me during the birth process.

Connectedness to my body sensations, free movement and sound, breathing

At the beginning of the birth process, an abundant cocktail of hormones is injected into the bloodstream. The neocortex is switched off as far as possible and the reptilian brain is activated. There is no chance – and no need – to remember all that you have been keeping in mind about the labor: how to breathe, what the periodicity of the contractions means, what you need to do. The memory and the skills in your body arise and become the leader in this huge stream of birth power.

You can move, make sounds, ask your helpers for touch – being tuned with yourself. During birth, it is impossible not to hear yourself. It is a time of truth and trying to get out of its path may cause much more pain. But if you are honest with yourself, if you trust that the birth-river will bring you out on the right shore and you can yield into its waters, the journey becomes smoother, the pain eases, and you feel it within these powerful and intense sensations.

As you now see, it is important to prepare your bodymind system during pregnancy: to build the skill of listening to your needs on a bodily level and to try different movements, sounds, poses, and kinds of touch. All of this becomes memory in the body, the body's encyclopedia that can be opened without conscious impulse, by inner choice.

Navel radiation pattern

The strongest sensations during the birth process are collected around the belly and the pelvis. It was refreshing for me, and helped the process, not to be too concentrated on these areas. During contractions, I found that stretching my limbs away from my belly started to expand the tight lump of sensations from the center further out, in rays, making it more diffuse and tolerable. I directed the contractions in diagonals – to the left hand and right leg, to the head and tail (coccyx). I asked someone to press on my sacrum so the force could pass through. An image of a sea star helped me, and I felt that all I was doing was spreading the force of each new group of very intense sensations from the belly throughout the rest of my body using my limbs.

My body knew this movement from the Navel Radiation pattern that we studied on the IBMT program. It comes from the embryonic period, when nutrition, breathing, and movement are organized around the umbilical cord. The navel is the center of life and connectedness to the mother and the world. Through the navel, the connections between developing limbs are created.

Opening the chest area and lower jaw

As I noticed during the work with breathing and diaphragms, the pelvic floor has a strong connection with the neck and lower jaw. Opening the mouth wider, releasing my lower jaw and grinning, I felt how the process of the labor went further. I found that the chest – the space of breathing, feelings, love, and future nutrition – should be widened as well. As I made an inhale towards all the sides of the lungs, spreading the ribs and opening the sternum, I felt how my pelvis responded, widening and opening the birth path for my baby. Opening the chest area and lower jaw helped the pelvic area to widen, to open, to let the baby come out. Now, as I am writing these words, I am thinking about the connection between the possibilities of becoming a mother and letting go, to expand love more and more on each contraction, in each labor, each new stage of your child's life after birth.

Support on the Path of Motherhood

After Birth

I am lying on my back,
My chest and opened arms
Are holding a huge translucent sphere.
It is like a milky fog, a light
That pours on me from heaven ...
I am lying on my back
And the light rains in me –
And inside of me becomes milk.
I'm feeding my dark-haired son
With this milk from heaven.
I feel how deep in me
The door of the chest cage is not closed any more
And coolly warmed air easily coming deep inside.
I'm the one who carries the milk in myself.

I see black soil
A huge field with grass ...
I am lying on this ground – white, naked.
I am sensing with all of me –
I was born from the Earth
And full of milk.
Steam is coming out from the opened womb,
I am embraced and warmed
by the One, who's supporting the Sky.

(My first Authentic Movement practice after giving birth, August 2014)

The birth process is over. There is no pregnant woman and no fetus any more. There is a mother and a baby, two newborns, two separate people who will be connected by an invisible umbilical cord for the rest of their lives.

I will now describe some important points and practices that helped me during the ambiguous period after giving birth.

"My body is filled with power and love" – these are the words I wrote after my *swaddling*. This is an ancient ritual, which aims to bring a woman's energy back, to help the organism regain its strength and tone. In essence, it helps a woman to recollect

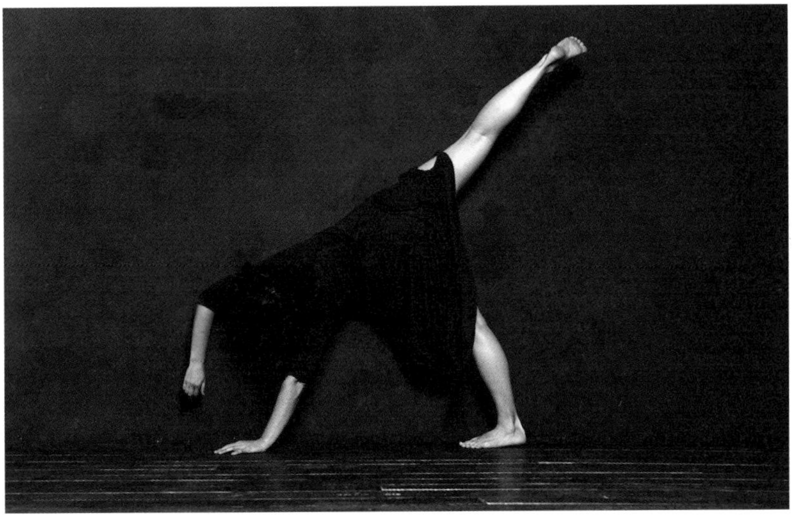

After birth – recovery.
Mover: Anna Feoktistova.
Photographer: Daria Yarkova

Chapter 8

herself after delivery – her body, psyche, emotions; it releases the mind and helps her to shift from a state of pregnancy to a state of motherhood, to redirect her attention to a child outside, to re-establish a family.

The ritual lasts about 5 hours and is done by one or two women. It consists of several phases. While it lasts, a woman has time to relax deeply. She sweats and warms up from the inside with the help of special herbal drinks, massage with ethereal and warm oils, a hot bath (or sauna), swaddling, and finally a ritual of *swaying* (or delivery closure, sometimes called the technique of seven locks).

IBMT work with the organs as a whole helps organs to "dare" to spread out inside the body. It creates awareness of a new space, released from the expanded uterus. I had the feeling of a space between the organs. I had an image of a bud that started to blossom and I could see each petal separately. I felt how the bones of the pelvis moved closer to each other, the lower back feeling supported by the organs.

You may practice this by yourself or with a helper. Lying on your side, release your belly. Let your weight fall down to the center of the Earth. You can say to yourself: "I am secure now. It is safe for me to relax, to rest, to be soft, to move from within." Put your hand on your belly, noticing the movement of breathing there.

Connect with the sensation of your organs. Take time to sense and feel. It would be wonderful if someone could give a supportive touch to your organs but you can also do it by yourself. Lift the belly and organs with your hand a little, let them hang. The belly is soft; continue to exhale in this position. Let your organs and all your body and mind rest. You can sway the organs, activating the inner fluids.

Then roll slowly to your other side and take your time to rest here. Make rolling movements and pauses, allowing the silent listening to grow into movement. Move just as you need, as you feel, as you want, being connected with the force of the inner organs.

Upside-down positions gave me real insight and support. At the beginning, I started to notice that my body tried to go to upside-down positions and stay there for a while during warm-up and Authentic Movement sessions. After being in those positions, I always felt good – I was full of energy and toned, my legs felt lighter, my upper body was lifted. An upside-down position is any position where the pelvis is higher than the head. Because of gravity, the abdominal organs move from the pelvic floor towards the diaphragm, up towards the chest organs. It helps to ease the muscle work of the pelvic floor, activates the diaphragm, and brings relief to the legs and their venous blood flow.

To practice upside-down positions, open your curiosity, be playful, and stay in touch with your body sensations. At first, just move as you like, tuning to the music of movement that lives in your bodymind in the moment. You can stretch and roll with pleasure, yawn, spread your limbs into the space, or gather in compact, baby-like positions. Let your movement be pleasant and free. Invite your body to try to lift the pelvis higher than the head. You can use the shoulders, head, and hands as a support, pushing from your feet or lifting the legs and feet higher as well. Play like a baby who knows the potentiality of three-dimensional movement, where any position is possible. Stay in such poses for a while, breathe there, feel how your diaphragms are moving. Find rest with your pelvis higher than your head. This can also bring us back to the experience of being in the mother's womb, where we can recharge with the energy of peace, finding availability and readiness for a new phase in movement and life.

Support on the Path of Motherhood

Work with the pelvic floor muscles and strengthening of the vaginal walls was an important area of research for me. Here I mention a few of my discoveries:

- There is a thorough description of all the muscles and exercises for them in a book called *The Female Pelvis: Anatomy and Exercises* by Blandine Calais-Germain (2003). There are exercises to differentiate all the muscles and to strengthen the pelvic floor muscles, and practices for the small organs of the pelvis (bladder, vagina, uterus, intestine, and anus).
- Taoist female practices include exercises based on the synchronized movement of all the diaphragms in the body, using special eggs to tone and reanimate the vaginal walls.
- Special post-natal yoga sequences work with the pelvic muscles and diastases.

I enter all of these practices and exercises with the sensitivity, trust, and respect for the body and its wisdom that I have gained through IBMT practice. During recovery from the delivery, I had times of calmness and inner concentration, but also periods of despair, frustration, and anger. I found myself weak, with a desire to restore everything back to how it was before I had children in my life. I went through many different states and emotions. Everything I had discovered before and during pregnancy – the quality of inner witnessing, tuning in to my needs and places of pleasure, connectedness to the power of breathing and cellular breathing mind, and so on – helped me to stay true to myself in all these states, and not to throw myself away, not to run away, not to freeze, while waiting for better times. I was with myself – my body, my inner child, my heart – playing, talking, hugging, crying, waiting, holding hands. And things changed with time.

I'm a woman,

I was born by Nature,

I am Nature,

I'm free in the play of Elements in me,

I know how to conceive,

I know how to carry,

I know how to give birth,

I am body with psyche inside

Hear my call,

Join it.

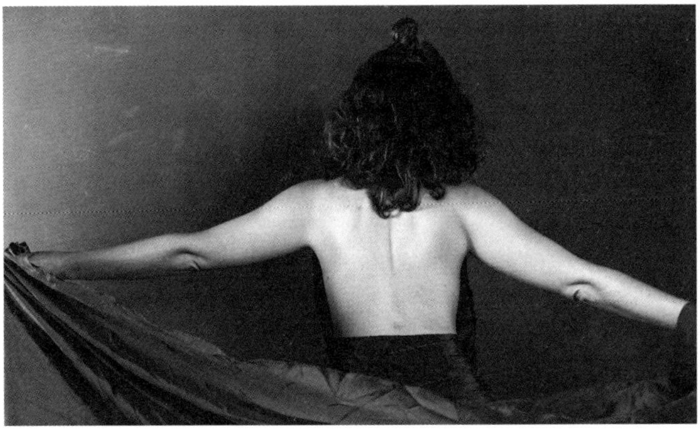

After birth – when your child is not a little baby any more. Mover: Anna Feoktistova. Photographer: Daria Yarkova

Mother Witness: Revisiting Rupture at Birth Through Somatic Movement Practice

Penny Collinson

9

This is a story that acknowledges the lived experience of a birth, is a return to birthing, and describes the journey afterwards. It is about connection and speaks of what happened and what did not happen, and the importance of that for mother and baby.

The chapter begins in **the studio**. It will recount a process which took place during my training in 2009, focusing awareness on my uterus through a hands-on partner exploration. I had had my second baby 4 months earlier and was aware that this exploration could reveal body memories, and that emotions, feelings, and associations held within my tissues might be brought to consciousness (Hartley 1995: 106). What makes this a remarkable event is that it unexpectedly involved the participation of my daughter, Stella (who has given me permission to use her real name); her spontaneous responses throughout played a profound part in what unfolded. In verbally tracking back with my partner what had emerged through this hands-on process, I reflected on Stella's actual birth.

The chapter continues with **the birth**, where I recall my experience.

The studio and **the birth** are historical reflections and are mainly written in the past tense. They include passages from my study notes, and reflective writing from my journals.

While preparing to write this chapter, I cried every time I thought of the birth, and speaking about it was very difficult, so I decided to ask my body how she feels, what she knows. This became a 4-week creative process that involved a stilling–sensing–moving–touching–imaginative dialogue with my womb, a process of embodied imagination (Hayes 2013; Pallaro 1999, 2007; Tufnell 2017), and journaling in response. Journal entries included both recalling and tracking **back** to bodily experience, and to a **forward** emergence where I invited what is present now to come on to paper.

The creative process tracks a 4-week enquiry and is the embodied renderings of the "story" as they live in me now, out of which the themes of body, birthing, and relationship emerged.

All journal passages are in italics and indented, and are generally written in the present tense. The nature of piecing together bodily perception has at times involved disrupting their chronology.

Furthermore, arranged around the journal passages are insights, reflections, and thoughts on practice, as they were emerging throughout the creative process. These signposts carry forward insights from one passage to another. They are not indented or in italics, and are written in the past tense.

Following this are **the reflections**, in which I consider overarching insights from the creative enquiry. I reflect both on how the process brought personal healing, and on how it has impacted on me as a practitioner in my work with clients and graduate students. I share how the 2009 encounter in the studio revealed the nature of embodied imagination within a co-creative practice and how the relationship between the three of us was dynamic and live, as each of us was present to the others through sensation, image, touch, and movement. It has reinforced a sense of trust in my body towards the unseen felt expression accessible through a widening field of attention, in which we (all human beings) are interconnected. Attention to my sensory-perceptual experience not only brought a material connection to my body but also re-enlivened a felt visceral sense of holism

Chapter 9

and connection to the transpersonal (Williamson 2010; Hayes 2007, 2013). Throughout this and the final section I turn to writers such as Linda Hartley, Stanislav Grof, Jill Hayes, Steve Haines, and Shaun McNiff, whose theories illuminate my practice.

The chapter closes with **the conclusions**. Here, I reflect on the power of our birth stories and see that if my ground is firmer around the start of Stella's life, it can have an effect on her and on our relationship. This process comes at a point when another individuation is taking place, where she has stepped into a new chapter of her life which takes her away from home to secondary school. However, as the chapter reveals, we are both understanding more of the possible impact of her birth story on her life now. This is bringing healing in ways that continue to surprise us.

The Studio

This is a story of co-creation, connection, and disconnection.

It started in the studio and involved myself, a practitioner, and my 4-month-old baby. The teaching that weekend had focused on the experiential anatomy of the uterus and reproductive organs.

All the usual protocols and preparations were observed: my partner and I had taken time to find a comfortable and supportive space on the ground and sensed the presence of our own and each other's bodies. Hartley observes, "[r]elationship encompasses a mysterious world of energetic exchanges" (2004: 221). With this in mind, our focus went to our non-verbal communication: posture, gestures, movements, and sounds emerging. We widened our attention to sensory and affective responses, to sounds, and to any images and memories which arose. The bodily presence and touch my partner offered supported my own presence to my womb.

While we were settling, someone volunteered to take Stella so that my partner and I would not have to attend to her. The entire weekend, Stella seemed to want to be close to me and, as she was taken, I intuited that she should be staying. Sure enough, within moments she was crying and shrieking and was returned. I laid her on my chest to breastfeed and she was quietly settled. Once again, we became three. The exploration began.

My partner moves her hand to the area of my womb; we both breathe and settle our focus here. She says to Stella, "This is your first home." In that instance, Stella responds with short breaths and sighs and squeals. She's talking to us. Over the coming minutes, her sound and movements escalate in volume and size. They are relentless. I try to soothe her through feeding, holding her closer; I move her to the other breast. She sucks and gulps, throwing back her head, kicking legs, and squeezing hands.

I am lying back ... I feel your warm hand on my uterus. Just stay there, no words please, just there. But where am I? You invite me to consider other organs. No thanks, I can't, just here is enough.

I'm calm and curiously I have very little sensation around my uterus. I'm not picking much up physically or emotionally.

Stella's responses are ferocious: she can't find any satisfaction. She whimpers and cries and is never still. Nothing seems to console her, and she becomes more and more troubled, sucking for sustenance from my breasts, as though her life depended on it.

Suddenly, I feel overwhelmed. I'm hot, distracted, anxious that something is really wrong, longing for Stella to quieten and relax. My legs are tight and heavy, my head is whizzing, my chest is congested, and I want to push Stella away. I've had enough. I don't have enough milk and I don't know what else to do.

At that same moment someone lifts and rolls Stella's stomach and legs closer into me above my chest. I clasp around her and pull in further; this is just what I needed. I breathe her in and out, slowing myself, feeling her close. I have a very clear thought that I couldn't have done this myself, I needed that person to help me, I couldn't have done this.

I'm invited to the brain, heart, and uterus connection, and I cry. I am moved, I am in love. I see Stella's commitment to stay with me, to survive, to not stop getting sustenance.

My system is calming, I'm slower again, I can be here and do this now. I can be here now.

We finish and, just as quickly as she had started, Stella quietens and rests. When I sit up later, I cry again. I love Stella. Thank you for fighting for me – not just you – the fight supports me too.

My partner and I spend time writing alone and then verbally track through what emerged together. I saw many connections with Stella's actual birth. It was useful for me to hear what happened for my partner, and I am struck by her witnessing:

My hand has been there for some time ... I see a flash ... a silver line ... an opening ... you both seem to drop in.

The Birth

Having had a previous C-section, I went into hospital as soon as labor began this time. The baby was monitored, and it became evident that its heart rate was consistently dropping, suggesting the baby was distressed and that something was wrong. After further close monitoring, the midwife and consultant agreed there should be an emergency cesarean section.

I am still hopeful I can do something to help the baby's distress, and for a vaginal birth, and so I try to help by changing my position and moving. They tell me, kindly and firmly, it's not anything I can do, it's not about me, it's about the baby.

I am given an epidural and it numbs all sensation between my breasts and pelvis.

I have done this before. I feel relaxed and confident this baby will be okay now, we're excited that this little creature will be with us in a matter of minutes. I focus on breathing, and relaxing. I want to take in all I can of this birth. I'll see their face, hold them in my hands. I have no pain, and soon into the operation, I feel strong pushes inside me. I'm told that some people describe it as though someone is doing the washing up in your belly. I breathe deeper, trusting that my calmness will be felt in the cells of my tissues and the umbilical link to my baby.

I have felt nothing quite like the anticipation in the moments just before seeing my baby, of actually seeing, smelling, and holding this new member of our family. The times in life when I feel so present and alive are rare.

The consultant lifts her into the air and tells us "it's only a girl." I hear one small cry and she is taken away.

I recall my response clearly: it is a collision of surprise (that she was a girl), a pang of guilt (that we "expected" a boy and might she "think" mistakenly that I wanted a boy?), and stunned confusion at the consultant's words. What

Chapter 9

becomes more pressing is that my baby has been taken with no explanation. It's at least 10 minutes before we are reunited on my chest; she has been washed, wrapped, and lies very quietly

Grof reminds us that, in a C-section birth, the child moves from the womb directly to the external world, "where it must face separation, hunger, cold, the need to breathe, and other difficulties" (1985: 254). He observes birth as an attack on the defense system, and its potential for emotion and sensation to be held at the perinatal level.

I'm told later that "it was good we got her out" because my uterus lining had been close to tearing, and had it ruptured, this could have been extremely dangerous for both of us. How did she know there was a problem? *Thank you, clever, clever little angel, for saving our lives.*

It was a few days after Stella's birth that I felt the true assault of the consultant's announcement as she entered the world, something which has distressed me for years since. I felt an anger at the carelessness of his words, which had landed as misogynistic, disrespectful, and degrading to us both. It was not the welcome I had wanted for this tiny creature, who we knew had endured a frightening labor and was at the threshold of her next home.

Returning to the birth story as I did in the studio, my anger had turned to despair, with shame that I had not voiced my feelings to the consultant. His words and actions represented all I did not want to remember about Stella's birth. Furthermore, although I understood that she was taken away to be checked over, I had not anticipated her being washed and the vernix caseosa skin covering being washed off. As she lay on my chest, we reunited. I felt huge relief and joy, and I suppressed my shock and upset.

Tracking the effects of the epidural helped me to understand why I had had very little sensation of my uterus or torso in the studio. The eruption of overwhelming helplessness that I felt as her distress escalated was reinforced as I recalled my anxiety about Stella's wellbeing when she was taken away and my feelings on being reunited.

I am curious that I developed hyperthyroidism 6 months after the birth. Its effects crept up on me - weight loss, stress, palpitations, tiredness. Come four o'clock in the afternoon, I did not think I could cope and would reduce everything down to a minimum just to get through to bedtime. I felt helplessness and inadequacy. Apparently, it can be misdiagnosed as post-natal depression. It was not until my legs started to tremble involuntarily that I realized something was very wrong and sought medical help.

In the years since, I have thought about Stella's birth and noticed a freeze response in myself. It is subtle. As I write, I feel the sensation strongly – a suspension behind my sternum which is quietly creeping upward into my throat and down into my belly. Perhaps the freeze has been protecting that in me which was hurt … **you**, womb … your pain. What is your story?

The Creative Process

An underlying premise of somatic movement practice is that we evolve who we are in relation to where we are (Hartley 1995, 2004). Awakening early each day into an embodied exploration emphasized this premise: how does the world touch me, and I the world? I recognized a deep urgency for self-reflective, imaginal, bodied time, to be intimately held and contained in the presence of a living, soulful world, however that may show itself (Hillman 1979; Hayes 2013). In handing over to my body - to the silent levels of my experience - I opened to this dialogue. I moved to connect to other. I moved to discover who I am. Hayes suggests,

Revisiting Rupture at Birth Through Somatic Movement

Embodied Imagination trusts in sensations, emotions and images which it does not understand, so expands and changes as they expand and change, never knowing where it is going, never understanding, only listening to the emergence of the unknown through new sensations, new emotions, new forms.
(Hayes 2013: 23)

The structure for my practice was simple and took place almost daily over 4 weeks. In a quiet, private space I oriented to my bodily experience and the environment, moving then writing for 1 to 2 hours. This occurred through various methods, using all my tools: sensing breath, weight, the presence of feeling, mood, and emotion in me as I interacted with the space, tracking and following my energy, pace, and capacity for movement.

Between practical sessions I observed what was happening in my outer life, and how and with whom. I journaled spontaneous thoughts, reflections, and dreams. McNiff warns us, when attempting to reveal hidden states of consciousness, not to project our views or overlook what the "artwork" presents and how its expression influences us (2004: 21). With this in mind, I took time to be with the movements, words, metaphors, and images that arose, allowing things to present themselves in their own way.

Extract 1

Yield listen allow

arriving bodily has a particular emphasis towards my lower back, and steady sustained focus of breath. Imagining an old wooden box with stiff hinges blowing off the gritty dust

womb warm

I trace the scar tissue it still has some numbness even after 11 years and a little discomfort to touch.

thank you sweet womb for carrying the girls and holding in to the last

I wonder how long she had felt distress in my womb, could it have started before labor? silent cries I couldn't yet hear through the layers of my flesh. somehow you knew, you sensed danger

You're sounding in the studio in a way I hadn't known before, trying to get as much as you can as quickly as you can, as though your life depended on it. There's not enough "I don't have enough milk." I can't console these cries. Gulping, sucking, wants me, doesn't want me

Breathe in

Breathe in and let out

Reading this later, I see that my sensing and moving located familiar and unfamiliar body experiences. I knew the tightness of the pelvis and lumbar region, and I needed to go steady. I recognized the numbness of scar tissue. But the drop into gratitude was tender and unexpected. I was transported back to the time of labor and the thought of baby in my womb, the imagined cries and real cries in the studio. The body knows no time.

The studio encounter had revealed the extraordinary interconnection between the three of us. Had Stella relived her time in my womb? Had she re-experienced her birth? If we were connecting to the presence of energy, affect, sensation as remembered, as held in the tissues of my uterus, then was my womb recalling her experience during Stella's birth?

Extract 2

I'm drawn to my sacrum and lower lumbar; they feel tight and restricted. My movements release tension but a bend and a dip to the right sends a shoot of pain up into my spine.

Head finds relief through pressure, pressing, massaging, twisting into my scalp, circling into

Chapter 9

the crown. It is unscrewing, igniting a push. Legs support my back and enable head to push. Is this Stella's voice saying, "I need to push but it's too dangerous?" Is it my unfinished process? Does my head need to push? I've been putting my hands on the dense bone of my pelvis and the soft warm hollow tissue of flesh; hands bring comfort, support, love

Tender strokes soothe fingers, palms, wrists, and arms

I must give each movement the space to reveal itself. I feel a commitment to following this path

My body was sore. My head had found relief in slow, steady contact and resistance, reaching me forward into movement. Amidst the tightness I realized there can be gentleness, and I noticed compassion towards myself. Later, a thought was thrown up: What was my own birth like?

Extract 3

I am perfectly contained, back support, knees bent feet firm

and able to push   a dim light in the room

I sense how you still float within the fluids of my own body

we are two in one body, and together our hearts and flesh bond

Throughout the rest of the day, the frame of my body felt strong but I also sensed deep sadness too. Is the umbilical link still so strong between us?

Extract 4

It's a crisp, chilly morning outside, inside I am warm and contained and feel able to do my movement within the ease of central heating. I'm lying on the ground curled up on my side. My mind goes to something I read last night, a cesarean section birth in a war zone with the barest of anesthetization ...

pulling a baby from a uterus is a very bloody job.

cutting through layers of flesh requires care but a lot of firm, direct, and clear-handed actions to pull the tiny creature through a small slit.

There is reciprocity of touch between mother and baby

Shock ... pulled it out within seconds.

I see Stella for a moment, she is held up in the air, like a trophy. All that is known gone

change of pressure, light, sound, temperature, umbilical cord cut all containment gone

but she was frightened in there too ... maybe she didn't want to leave home?

Questions about Stella's experience in my womb keep rising in me for days: why was she distressed? Imagining the speed and handling of her birth goes around and around. The time without her and not knowing how she was kept returning. I felt stuck, deflated, and wretched.

Extract 5

It takes time to draw mind to body and away from sleep,

breath moves life in. Eventually, tenderly I find space

ground   freedom to pour and roll, the river starts to flow again

attention drops to my uterus in the final movements.

You bore two children, two souls

I love you   thank you

I imagine Stella touching over my uterus. She understands

we both longed to be close, to be connected forever

and all I longed for was to hold her, to have her with me, on my skin. To see her, know her, love her, protect her, we longed for each other and a void had opened up, a void of fear and shock

this birthed a gentle companion, she knows what it's like on the peripheries, a place of resistance to kick against and come more reassuringly towards center

The slow arrival into my body had brought deep satisfaction and, with it, liveliness and flow in my movement. Thoughts returned to the birth and to Stella coming out of the womb and not being welcomed. My own welcome to her was unclear: joy, care, awe, yes, but something else too … something hesitant, more fragile, fear, confusion. In those early days and weeks, I had mild anxiety that my baby was not happy and that the world was not receiving her with open arms. I felt frustration and resentment towards everyone. Could they not see she needed to know they really loved her?

I am wondering whose story this is.

Extract 6

I'm pulling up and away from ground support

Fluttering heart, flapping my wings

an hourglass,

the salt

pouring

down

my spine dry vertebra.

It soothes my sore lumbar, as liquid strokes tired bones

and pours through vagina to the ground between my feet

I am empty

I trace blubbery soft gut tissue

it aches, no tone, dull

She's stoic and private about it but I see a furrowed brow and dark eyes in her pale face

I'm floundering in the blur

My practice this morning was in two halves, stopping part-way to support Stella to eat and relax. I am anxious about her and it brings me up in my body and away from my base support. It triggers right into feelings of helplessness and inertia, from the birth. My mind fires off, recalling many years of her tummy-gut pain and I am scared this is continuing.

Extract 7

I looked forward to holding my baby.

I relaxed, stayed calm, prepared myself

The imminent arrival is truly exciting

And then I heard the consultant's words … shock one

Stella was taken away, no sound … shock two

She is returned washed and quiet … shock three

I am starting to understand why my upset,
why my shock

Formed in my womb, I have carried this soul

and the ritual of birth, the emergence of a soul into the world

brings us close to Source

Chapter 9

This is a ceremonious act

we are the gatekeepers.

Yet the hand which pulls forth the child forgets the two are a shared flesh

As I listen to these words from my womb, and the strengthening container of the pelvis, I am seeing the larger picture at play. His words hurt so much because they contained no love, no reverence for this rite of passage. They were empty of awe, no feeling for mother and baby's transition as we both crossed a threshold, leaving behind that which we had known.

Extract 8

> **I move, breathe, stretch to awaken my cells live LIVE feel**
>
> **let go forgive**
>
> **I am transfixed by the sun. Its warmth penetrating my body**
>
> **I soak you in with each breath, you spiral through the pores of my skin**
>
> **I go tenderly, small figures of eight, sways, rocks and gradually more freedom and flow ... suspending reason**
>
> **whisperings to ground enliven the soles of my feet ... here the creature stirs**
>
> **I feel a pulsing in my womb heart racing**
>
> **breathe deeply yield yield and listen**
>
> **I have interpreted her sounds, cries, sucking, kicking as a reliving of her experience in the womb, but it's your pain your agony of disconnection from the Great Mother and the threat of losing connection and separating again**

I sense a turn in the road here, somehow claiming back my own body rather than feeling numb and helpless: a reconnecting to the whole from which I have become separated and adrift.

Extract 9

> **Last night I had two dreams: the first is disturbing, with horrific images of brutality and bullying against a defenseless boy. He has no one to turn to. I seemed to be the observer, looking in**
>
> **Unable to sleep again, and my mood low, I feel discomfort and despair as I try to relax and find ease for tight hips and an achy lower back.**
>
> **The second dream involves making a dance performance: I am with my close friend. I sneak off, and under branches which reveal a large open space beautifully lit by the sky, I run into it with the momentum to launch into a cartwheel. There are others close behind me, and we are all magnetically pulled into the openness of this space to "let go." My friend is sad, and sore, and out of energy. I offer to touch her with strokes, massage, to pour my weight and to hold her ...**

These dreams speak to me of deeply felt emotional polarities: the agonies of physical pain and loneliness, the ecstasy of freedom and abandonment, and the tenderness of care and companionship. Body, movement, and physicality. As I see the open space and rush into it, the presence of my body is visceral, powerful. Yet there is a faint whisper of doubt - doubt in my capacity to really let go - to move my body and feel as I once could. I have aged! Where is spontaneity, joy, and ecstasy?

Extract 10

> **Stella can't go through the school gates today; her anxiety is overwhelming. We head home. Her system eases, my system eases, her feelings flow, mine flow. We park up by the sea, watch the dogs jumping in the puddles, take in the sky, the**

grasses, the sandy beach beyond ... Stella shares all the things she felt in the morning:

Dry throat, gagging sensation "which goes into my tummy and feels really painful," hot, sweaty palms, fear, a feeling of being "paralyzed" and "I can't move through it."

She tells me she likes the school, loves her friends, and doesn't understand why she hates leaving home

and here I am

the gatekeeper. Can I meet her at this threshold and welcome all that she is with all that I am?

I tell her the story of her birth. She listens

something in her seems to know

Breathe in

Breathe in and let out

We are two bodies

Breathe in and let out together

In reading this passage back, I marvel at Stella's willingness to name and share with me these strong, frightening symptoms that she experiences. I wonder if, in sharing my version of the story of her birth, has some non-verbal, pre-conceptual voice in her been heard? Did our sharing together offer her feelings more grounding, some roots? Does this dear young soul remember home and feel its absence?

The Reflections

The creative process has been a significant personal experience. My interactions with the space I moved in (textures, materials, places of resistance or expanse), together with a presence to my womb, have enabled me to discover feelings, movements, and images which have lain fallow in my bodyself. Embodied imagination requires a loosening of control so that things outside my awareness can arise. This dedicated time to go beyond the edges of my consciousness, with openness and resources, has brought new expression.

It was days into my creative process before I sensed the holding and sacredness of the time/space framework. With this came a sense of safety and ease in my body. I was able to notice more detail and stay longer with the emerging sensations and images. This has been emotional, relinquished areas that felt blocked, and increased my psychological wellbeing. For example, there is relief in more clearly perceiving sensations associated with the shock and freeze.

Significantly, I have a more nuanced awareness of the first moment of meeting Stella when she is put on my chest after being taken and washed, and greater self-compassion for the resistance I had carried. I asked my body to show me what happened here, and strong sensations emanated from my heart and womb, an immense flow and flurry of moving energy. The image was a mass of quick, gold, snake-like shoots searching, sniffing out its kind. As an animal will smell and lick her newborn, my (animal) body wanted this too. But the energy was blocked. I am seeing my baby for the first time and my body is a jumble, a confused clash of shock, worry, anger, and love. With shame and discomfort, my process revealed that I felt rejected by Stella. It is clearer now that perhaps, more accurately, my body instincts, which were on full power, had been sharply curtailed by the removal of the vernix caseosa on her skin. Nature's bonding lotion had been washed away. There is more to this moment, of course – Stella's experiences up to that point.

Chapter 9

The studio story has helped shed light on this - her spontaneous surge of energy, which seemed to turn to distress and a ferocious need to be connected to mother for reassurance and sustenance.

Though the loss or absence of bonding might seem a trivial sacrifice for the success of an emergency cesarean section, I began to realize that there was misattunement, misalignment, an anger (of sorts) which subtly caused some disruption to our attachment process. Tracking the details as I have, and giving my uncomfortable emotions space and voice, has been healing. They are easier to be with, the love (revealed as **longing**) has been freed and I sense flow.

The studio and **the birth** convey something of the co-creative interpersonal processes at play. Each story conveyed how our presence interlinks on silent, felt levels where we pulsate, receiving and responding to one another in known and unknown ways. The practice of Authentic Movement invites these unknown qualities to be expressed and become more conscious. For example, in staying with a sensation, movement, or image, we trust that its own logic will unfold. The reflexive process of moving, journaling, and verbal exchange gives us the opportunity to describe what occurred and the insights arising – furthermore, to consider how they serve us personally and collectively. It is a valuable process which honors each person's participation and viewpoint of the experience.

I facilitate embodiment processes for clients, and I teach my graduate students methods of embodied imagination, drawing on the principles and pedagogic values inherent in Authentic Movement and somatic practice. Reflecting on the studio experience with Stella, I have been curious to know if a baby can be part of an experience in such fluid, spontaneous, and affective ways. **Is it that our "training" in perceptual awareness is not so much about learning, but noticing what is blocking or hindering our innate abilities to connect, communicate, and interact?**

Much of my facilitation, then, goes into creating conditions conducive to our needs for safety, structures which support innate and natural healing processes, and means to establish containment and reflexivity consciously around what has arisen. Whether our enquiries are solo or collaborative, attention must be paid to the space with consideration for the temperature, air, light, and materials with which we will interact. Simple movement methods are applied to awaken somatic awareness and loosen intellectual/cerebral control. The sensate or felt sense can be arrived at through methods which are stilling, sensory, and meditative or active and dynamic, and students and clients practice these options so they have choices and can move intuitively and spontaneously to impulses in the present moment.

These activities are vital stages in preparing the body as a container or "vessel" for deeper emergence (Adler 2002; Hartley 2015; McNiff 2004; Stromsted 2015; Williamson 2010). Soul is known through embodied imagination and, given the right conditions, can enter and lead the way. There is no place for control or willfulness, only receptivity, surrender, and compassion. The rewards come in many ways. For me, in this process the gift is in knowing more fully the fluid, impermanent nature of being human, and that change in and outside of my body is always happening. When I stand unafraid at this threshold, I am in touch with Source.

Another area of my teaching is concerned with timeframes and how they are used in methodology, particularly transitions between interaction and emergence, rest and reflection (artistic, written, verbal). Pacing and shifting our consciousness in different ways within the creative process has an important regulatory function of enabling material which arises from our unconscious to integrate, and ultimately to make change in our everyday lives.

The Conclusions

My final thoughts bring me back to the topic of birth. Traditional medical models considered the child in delivery as not aware of the environment and not experiencing pain, to the extent that the child was viewed as "an inanimate object" (Grof 1985: 251). Thankfully, more contemporary neonatal care recognizes newborn babies as sensitive, vulnerable, and conscious sentient beings, in the womb and at birth (Baring 2013: 407). Of interest to me is the impact of birth on the child's emotional and psychological life, and the potential for the experience to determine a child's feelings about existence and their image of the world (Grof 1985: 251). Haines suggests that birth is an early defining story that leaves an imprint outside of conscious awareness and is encoded in our body intelligence (2015). For this reason, it has been important to revisit my experience of Stella's birth by asking my body what is known and listening with compassion to my story.

Birth stories can be healed through love and bonding with parents, but the attachment process is affected and shapes experiences going forward. Stella's birth story is in her body and I see it living out as nausea, pain in her abdomen, sweats, and freezes, all of which are recognizable trauma responses. I have never seen these symptoms and responses so clearly as I do now. For some years, the social/relational process of leaving home, joining groups, or going to school has been difficult for Stella. Now they are more acute. She does not know what frightens her and she wants it to change.

In order to write this chapter, I chose to focus on the first 4 weeks of a creative process. However, this process continues; there is more to discover, and with it the potential to feel support and connection to those I live with, and those with whom I work. I value and trust the wellbeing that comes through being present to my moving body and being perceptive to this depth of relational connection.

Stella's journey is a longer, ongoing process. While our current enforced isolation at home, due to the Covid-19 pandemic, means no school (and no symptoms), creative play and reflective chats are central, whether it be costume make-up, drawing, making a dance on TikTok, or playing with the cat. Stella and I are aware of what a return to school and social activities may bring and, with support from others, we will keep listening, communicating, and developing her resources.

The Development of Movement and the Self

Heike Kuhlmann

10

In this chapter I will share significant aspects of human movement development. These key aspects of Developmental Movement Patterns (DMP) influence brain development and the foundation of self. At the end, I will offer practical applications for working with children and adults, and a way of using Contact Improvisation for children with their caregivers. I view touch and play as vital influencers for wellbeing, nurture, and personal development.

The DMP are sequences of patterns that a baby needs to learn and go through in the first 2 years of life in order to arrive into standing and walking. They follow a genetically laid out pathway, and the outer environment further supports the movement into being. Human development occurs through a dialogue between nature and nurture. The nervous system holds the potential to be stimulated, through inner movement and outer environment, into expression of pre-existing patterns. Examples of stimuli are touch, interaction, light, sound, temperature, and objects. Those stimuli shape the development of the brain.

In the first year, millions of new neurons are created; the neurons myelinate and build numerous synaptic connections with each other. The synapses are created rapidly and randomly, so that children have twice as many synapses as adults by the age of three. Movement and experience form the brain's connectivity and plasticity. Movement and experience are needed throughout our lifespan for the continuous maturation of the brain.

The first dialogues of a baby with its caregivers are through touch interaction and movement expression. A major part of the DMP evolves while the child is still in a non-verbal state of development. Sensations invite movements to unfold. Movement generates more sensations. This dialogue between sensation and movement stimulates further development of the human being. It forms the foundation of our unique perception and, through that, our sense of self; it is through the DMP that one forms the ground and foundations for one's sense of self. As Bonnie Bainbridge Cohen, the founder of Body-Mind Centering®, describes, the understanding of a situation arises out of perception (interpretation) of previous experiences. She says in an interview: "Your understanding depends on the poignant experiences of your own history and pursuits" (Bainbridge Cohen 2018: vii).

A child's sensations and movement are accompanied by the caregiver's glance, touch, and words. Their presence and appreciation are meaningful to the child, as the interpretation of sensation and movement that form the perception happens within the caregiver–child dialogue. The development of verbal expressions arises much later.

Movement by its nature is preverbal. Speaking about it requires translation from movement to verbal. This is a far greater leap than any translation between verbal languages. Yet, when the words arise directly out of experience, there is a recognition of their authenticity.

(Bainbridge Cohen 2018: viii)

The development of language brings the chance to name and create a mutual experience of meaning. It also allows one to distance oneself from the direct experience. "Language causes a split in the experience of the self" (Stern 1985: 163), as language moves the relatedness into the impersonal. This can be different when one is speaking directly out of the movement experience because the direct experience is still resonating in the language.

Chapter 10

I invite you to notice the difference between sensing something and perceiving the information that comes from that sensation. Valuation and judgment are formed after a sensation is perceived. Reflecting on the personal perception of sensations can give new insights. Socialization has been inscribed into the body. It is in the interpretation of sensation and movement that socialization forms the body and movement pattern. This understanding provides tools to be active with the body and movement inscriptions. The first step is to become conscious of those inscriptions. The second step is to make choices about whether or not to continue with the known pathways or to choose a new response. This means actively responding to the socialization acting on us.

I would like to invite you to pause and take a moment for reflection on your own movement history. This reflection can continue through reading this chapter. Please allow your inner witness to perceive your inner sensations and allow yourself to connect to those sensations, the content, and your own history.

Sense of Self

A sense of self – a sense of what and who is me, and what and who is not me – is of importance in development. When a baby is born, it breaches out of the mother's womb, out of a fluid environment into the airy world. Gravity starts to pull on the baby's body. Movement starts to be more difficult. Air needs to be breathed in and out. Where are the nutrients? Before, nutrients and oxygen arrived effortlessly through the umbilical cord. Now the baby needs to move towards the nipple and to suck in order to receive food. Almost everything is different.

In the first 2 months, the world of a baby is full of learning basic elements to survive. This includes sucking, sleeping, feeling hungry, sensing the caregiver's body, listening to the tone of their voice, feeling gravity pulling on its body, moving the body, and experiencing the difficulties of controlling one's own movement. Although those actions appear very natural to us, they are all new for the baby. All these experiences are part of the formation of the baby's inner organization. Therefore, these acts of movement are important not only for survival, but for laying out the foundations of the self. They are also the primary manifestations of vitality.

The Vitality Affects describe the energetic flow within the movement, using words like melting, ephemeral, effortless, or exploding. It is the research of Daniel Stern that has provided evidence of these basic Vitality Affects and how they contribute to the emergence of a sense of self (Stern 1985: 37-68, 2011: 19-28; Hartley 2004: 77).

From 2 months onwards, the infant starts to engage in interpersonal relatedness with its caregivers; it is this relationship between caregivers and baby that allows the baby to bond and attach to them. Through this relationship, the forming of the brain and the sense of self occurs. "Interpersonal experience plays a special organizing role in determining the development of brain structure early in life and the ongoing emergence of brain function throughout the lifespan" (Siegel 2020: 53).

The sense of self emerges while places in the brain, like the hippocampus, are still under construction. Without a functioning hippocampus, conscious memories are not really accessible. Throughout later life, movement can bring to the surface moments of memories of that very early, pre-verbal time. They are stored in the brain as intrinsic memory. Once the core self has emerged, it allows a configuration of the verbal self. With the verbal self, the pre-frontal cortex is more evolved and explicit memory can be stored and remembered. It is the way the baby moves and experiences itself in the world and in relationships that shapes the development of the different brain areas and their interconnectedness. That is why, from a developmental perspective, the brain is fully embodied and relational. "Development is a product of the effects of experience on the unfolding of genetic potential" (Siegel 2020: 50).

Experience has a long-lasting effect on how we learn, on the nature of our genes and their regulation, and how these affect our response to experience. The interrelatedness between experience and gene expression shapes neuron growth and interconnections. This is even more important in the first years of life, when the body is still in development, but that interrelatedness stays alive for our whole life. Allan Schore defines this time as the period in life that makes us human because the foundations of our relational behavior patterns are laid down here.

I want to emphasize the difference between the sense of self and identity. As the word "identity" suggests, I identify with something; the sense of self reflects a deeper connection with oneself, while developing a coherent sense of oneself means that one knows that one is and that the other is somebody else. One can experience very different identities, depending on the circumstances. Life and identity can change completely, yet a sense of self offers a grounding for all identities. It is of importance for people who had more challenging beginnings in life, to support them in generating their sense of self through DMP. Working with a knowledge of the developmental patterns in Body-Mind Centering® and Integrative Bodywork and Movement Therapy (IBMT) supports human beings to develop a sense of self, to create solid foundations and resilience.

Basic Neurocellular Patterns and DMP

Basic Neurocellular Patterns (BNP) and DMP pre-exist in the genetic blueprint. (Over the years Bonnie Bainbrige Cohen has used different names

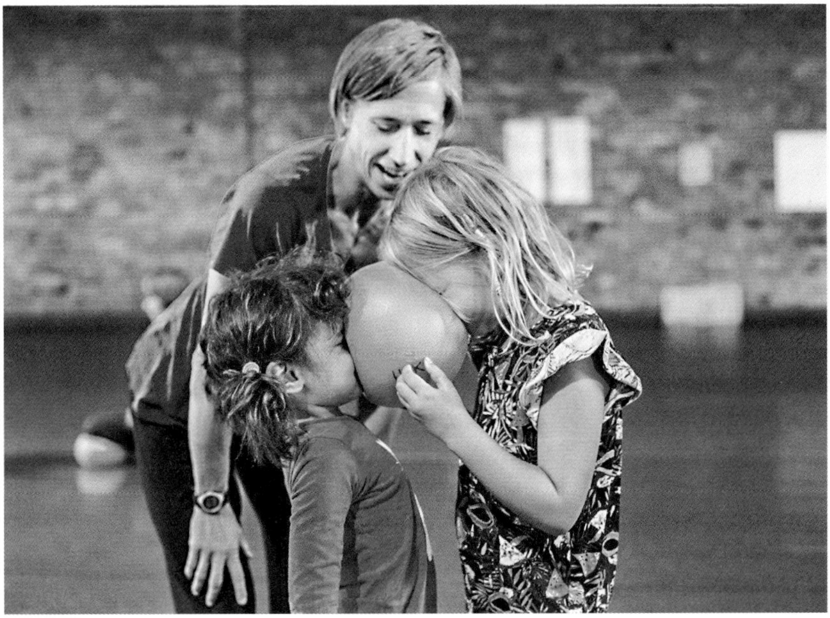

Heike Kuhlmann and workshop participants. Photographer: Jakub Krzyżanowski for Art Stations Foundation by Grażyna Kulczyk

for the series of DMP that a human being unfolds and learns at the beginning of life. Laban–Bartenieff Work had already been influenced by the DMP. Bainbridge Cohen finally arrived at the name Basic Neurocellular Patterns – also the title of her 2018 book. The term describes for me the dialogue of neurological and cellular processes.) Genetic expression occurs in dialogue with the environment and its challenges. The completion of one pattern modifies the following pattern. The progression of the patterns mostly occurs in overlapping waves. Two hundred years ago, the biologist Ernst Haeckel observed that human embryology and infant movement development mirrors phylogenesis, the evolution of species on earth. Phylogenesis began with the one-cell organism and evolved into more complex types. The human being is one of the most complex species on earth.

Human development starts when two cells (the egg and sperm) become one cell. This one cell multiplies until it becomes the morula, a group of many equal cells. From that multitude, differentiation emerges. Becoming different cells with different functions, an embryoblast and a trophoblast emerge. They create the nurturing environment (trophoblast) and a body that has a front and a back (embryoblast). How is it to sense back into that beginning? How is it just to sense having a front and a back body? This simple layer of front body cells will differentiate and form our organs. Out of the back layer, skin and nervous system develop. How is it to sense into the cells of your back body – somatizing that they will become skin and nervous system? If they had been somewhere else in space, they would not have become skin and nervous system. It is an interesting question to ask: How much space and where you are in space influence what you become or what possibilities you have. Space has an influence at the microscopic level of the cells, as well as at the macroscopic level of the globe.

The BNP include movement development from the single cell to the multi-complex human being. They are subclassified into pre-vertebrate and vertebrate patterns. The pre-vertebrate patterns are comparable to the movement patterns of animals without a bony spine. The fluid environment and cellular communication permit the early organization and structuring of the body. The first patterns to emerge are Vibration and Cellular Breathing. Supporting Cellular Breathing in each of the trillions of cells in our body invites each cell to have a known space and surroundings. Sponging and Pulsation can be practiced with images of the sponge and jellyfish. The fluid exchange through the membranes, from inside the cells to the extracellular matrix/interstitial fluid, is of significance for tone modulation.

The emergence of the notochord gives rise to a distinction between upper and lower, right and left. The genesis of the limbs creates a radial symmetry, with the navel as center and the limbs – legs, arms, head, and tail – as the periphery. This radial symmetry pattern can be associated with a sea star (an example of an exercise for the Navel Radiation pattern is included later). The nervous system develops through initiation of the notochord, beginning with a folding of the ectoderm in the back. Almost at the same time, the yolk sac (part of the entoderm in the front) is invaginated and starts to develop into the organ system. The cells develop and differentiate in dialogue with each other and with the environment (the womb of the mother). Already, at this early stage, the cells and tissues can be toned and patterned in a certain way. The nervous system is the registering and regulating system of the body. The autonomic nervous system regulates our stress reactions. The tone and vibration in the cells and in the fluids influence how the autonomic nervous system will function. The developing baby will feel, through the tone and vibration of the fluids, if the outer environment (the mother) is in stress or in a relaxed state.

Birth is initiated by both the child and the mother. The baby's flexion pattern increases through compression of the womb-space. That compression allows the flexion pattern to complete and produce a response to move into the extension pattern that is needed for passing through the birth canal. Over the first year after birth, the development of the extension pattern is predominant in order to calibrate the more developed flexion pattern. One exercise to practice the calibration of the flexor and extensor tone is the movement sequence of total physiological flexion and extension. In side-lying, one moves from a totally flexed position into a fully extended position. Movement into extension and back into flexion is initiated from the soles of the feet.

At around 4 weeks, the baby is able to hold its head up. Coordination of the upper and lower body is starting to appear. Two arms or two legs move together in a Homologous pattern. An example is the swimming or jumping motion that can be seen in a frog. At around 4–6 months, development continues with the emergence of a coordination pattern of body halves, the right and the left body halves, which allows the baby to roll and crawl. This is the Homolateral pattern, and it underlies the most complex pattern, the Contralateral pattern. The Contralateral pattern allows us to walk and run. We can see this pattern in vertebrates; wild cats, like a jaguar, can crawl and run very fast.

Primitive Reflexes are genetically programmed, so they can ensure survival of the newborn and support the appearance of the DMP. Once they have done their job, they should integrate and therefore allow movement choices to be made. If primitive reflexes remain active, they interfere with the child's development and inhibit the freedom of movement choice. Active primitive reflexes can complicate and hinder the learning of reading and writing. Instead of there being a choice, there is a hijack by the active primitive reflex. As a child wants to be part of a group and perform an activity like other children, it either has to use more effort or show resisting behavior.

When teachers have an understanding of DMP and primitive reflexes, they can notice and analyze a child's movement and see how best to support the integration of that active reflex with activities and exercises. A child that has certain tension patterns or an active reflex will try to compensate in order to be like the others. This is how humans develop compensation patterns from early on. The longer a compensatory pattern exists, the stronger its neural pathway, and the longer it can take to find a more functional and efficient pattern.

When adults practice somatic work, they become conscious of their movement patterns, of where a movement is more effortful. Somatic work also includes understanding how to move more efficiently and where to use less effort, and this allows more brain capacity and the freedom to choose a range of movements. Working with DMP can support a repatterning of the foundation of our movement.

We find that this reeducation of underlying developmental patterns not only gives more inner strength, clarity, and aliveness to our movement and perceptual responses, but it also frees more of our energy for creative thought and activity. The sequence of movement patterns will unfold according to its own innate timing; regardless of whether a pattern has been embodied or not, the next pattern will emerge at its appropriate time. If a pattern has been missed, this gap will weaken the support for all subsequent

Chapter 10

movement development. Generally, we learn to compensate for such weaknesses, usually through the creation of rigid holding patterns, from which areas of tensions and immobility in the body ensue. Much energy is used up in maintaining such an inefficient method of support, and that energy ceases to be available for creative work and play.

(Hartley 1995: 92)

Children can be supported in their movement pattern more easily than adults. Most children move and play a lot during the day. Activities and games in which the developmental patterns are included support the building of a solid foundation for movement. Examples of activities are inviting children to move like a snake, to jump like a frog, to crawl smoothly like a cat, and so on. Depending on their age, one could offer children tunnels to creep through or structures to climb over. In these activities I move and play with the children; I do not distance myself from them. I rather become the snake or the crocodile that wants to eat somebody and we play together. I move with them at eye level. By moving with them on the floor, I am the role model, showing them that the floor is our friend and it is fun to roll, crawl, slide, jump, and play on and over it.

In my experience as a somatic dance movement facilitator, I observe and analyze what I see in the children's movement and adjust my class plans accordingly. When I see a child having difficulties with skipping, I offer activities like crawling on the belly for the whole group. I invite them to come back to the floor to practice Homolateral movement patterns, which support skipping. We creep like a salamander, in a Homolateral pattern. The upper and lower body halves on the same side move together. Creeping on the belly can be awkward, many adults having difficulty doing it.

Children love catching games, which are all about running. What if you change the setting and catch while creeping on the floor? I do not mention to a child that it cannot do something. I trust the activity is helpful for everybody and that the child feels included.

The Navel Radiation pattern is a good example to use in class. I use information and pictures or videos of sea stars to introduce the pattern. I offer a movement sequence that gives them the direct experience of moving like a sea star, where all the limbs connect to the center and radiate out of the center. The children experience how it is to move from their center, and how it feels different when the limbs initiate. The Navel Radiation pattern supports traveling through different levels and planes. After having spent time on the floor experiencing that pattern, we move together with partners so that one can support the other with touch or guidance. This practice offers a lot to children and nurtures their movement foundation.

Bonnie Bainbridge Cohen differentiates the learning processes of a child and an adult. A child can learn without thinking consciously about it because the nervous system is waiting for stimulation of that potential to come into existence. "When you are an infant you have that pattern in the Nervous System without thinking about it. As an adult you do it with consciousness" (Bainbridge Cohen 1984: 25). An adult needs to bring consciousness to a non-functional movement pattern in order to change it. This awareness allows the adult to direct the movement pathway away from the commonly known pattern to an unfamiliar new pattern.

If the body is the instrument through which the mind is expressed, then one can just play more kinds of melodies, or different kinds of verse, kinds of timbre. As an adult, one's compensatory patterns are also deeply woven into the emotional and thinking patterns, and need to be acknowledged and validated.

(Bainbridge Cohen 1984: 26)

An uncompleted or weak underlying pattern will then produce a weak upcoming pattern. A weak pattern can be indicated through the use of more effort, or a higher tone, or initiation in a different body part. Coming back to the underlying DMP can support the repatterning of that weak pattern.

All natural phenomena fall into patterns. The nervous system is designed to function by patterns. The nervous system has the potential for innumerable patterns, but the patterns are not accessible to us until they are actually stimulated into existence, until we actually do them. Patterns will fall on a continuum between efficiency and inefficiency.

(Bainbridge Cohen 1984: 25)

On one hand, it is the practical rehearsal of the pattern that forms the pattern. On the other hand, it is the execution of the pattern that educates us about efficiency and inefficiency in that performance. Returning to the underlying pattern is a way to support the next pattern to develop in a functional and efficient way. Human learning occurs through connection. New experiences are connected to known experiences. The interpretation of the new experience through the old experience influences and informs any new learning. In IBMT work, processing different layers of a sensation invites revelations of unconscious aspects of self. As we become more conscious of our movement patterns, we repattern the brain through rewiring neural connections.

Development of the Brain

The DMP stimulate the development of the brain. "Each basic developmental movement pattern is coordinated by a specific area of the brain" (Hartley 1995: 93). Allan Schore and Daniel Siegel researched the relationship of the environment (caregiver, adults, surroundings), DMP, and the inner blueprint of the developing brain (Siegel 2020: 167-80). Their research confirms the rewiring and repatterning of nerve connections through sensation and movement, demonstrating the complexity of the developing brain, which includes genetic potential, type of experience, and gene expression. It is the brain's neuroplasticity that allows us to adapt to many changes and circumstances.

Most areas of the brain evolve in the first three years of life (Siegel and Hartzell 2009: 41). The human brain consists of several parts: brainstem, midbrain, limbic system, bridge, pre-frontal cortex, and left and right cortical hemispheres. The corpus callosum serves as a bridge between the two hemispheres. Both halves of the brain perform different tasks. The right hemisphere is responsible for understanding emotions, concepts, implicit messages, and art. The left hemisphere is responsible for language, logical thinking, and objectivity. Both cortical hemispheres are in constant communication through the corpus callosum.

When a baby is born, only the brainstem is developed, as this coordinates functions like breathing, sleeping, digestion, body sensations, and senses (tasting, smelling, hearing, and seeing). It includes the thalamus, pons, and medulla oblongata. The brainstem is also called the reptilian brain, whose functions are vital for survival. These functions originate from our evolutionary patterns of searching for food, reproduction, and the fight, flight, and freeze response of the nervous system (Bentzen 2016: 18-29).

The midbrain and limbic system are called the mammalian brain because it developed with mammals 250 million years ago (Bentzen 2016: 30-43).

Chapter 10

It sits on top of the thalamus of the brainstem like a bonnet, and consists of various structures like the hippocampus, amygdala, mammillary bodies, and central gray areas. It is viewed as the emotional center. It becomes fully active after 8–10 months of life (Siegel and Hartzell 2009: 44–7). From this time onwards, babies learn to manage as best they can, regulating their needs and feelings depending on the environment their caregivers provide. The attunement between caregiver and child forms the child's emotional foundations.

"The developmental patterns in turn underlie all human movement possibilities, from the positions we adopt while sleeping to the way we hold a pen or perform the most intricate dance movements" (Hartley 1995: 32). This knowledge allows a facilitator to support a child in developing their potential at a later age, or even as an adult. Coming back to the DMP can stimulate certain brain areas. "Areas of the brain and nervous system can be stimulated through the practice of specific movements. It is the actual practicing of the movement patterns that stimulates the developing functions of the brain areas involved" (Hartley 1995: 94).

The right hemisphere develops first. Its development acquires dialogue with a caregiver because the right hemisphere learns in relationship. It supports us in understanding our bodily states and the context in which we exist. It is through interaction with the "good-enough caregiver" that the right hemisphere wires itself. Schore's research shows that the wiring of the right hemisphere happens mainly through non-verbal communication like tone of voice, facial expression, touch, and body language. These build and shape the affect-regulating system in the right hemisphere. "[The] right brain stores the internal working models of the attachment relationship. It processes emotional social information – its functions are as diverse as enabling empathy, humour, and many of the capacities that are fundamental to human subjectivity" (Carroll 2007).

The mapping of the bodily states (visceral, muscular, skin) is fundamental for the processing of emotions. By mapping, I mean sensing into the body in order to perceive and feel little changes like tone or fluidity. The good-enough caregiver, as Schore points out, addresses the child's bodily states and therefore supports the building of the emotional regulating system. Once those foundations are properly established through a well-functioning attachment with a caregiver, a child can adapt with greater resilience to difficult and traumatic situations (Rass 2012: 111–51). This is the reason why Schore and others speak about a paradigm shift. In learning, rather than prioritizing the development of the left hemisphere, the development and wiring of the right hemisphere can be promoted. Bessel van der Kolk's research shows the important role of the right hemisphere in dealing resiliently with traumatic events. Although the left hemisphere reacts at the beginning of a traumatic situation, it is the well-functioning right hemisphere that provides the resilience to come out of it. Once the severity of the situation increases, the left hemisphere switches off and the right hemisphere takes over (Rass 2012: 14, 19, 27, 29, 31).

I must emphasize that the relationship established through movement and touch shapes the development of the brain. Bonding and attachment support the building of a resilient and adaptable brain. The BNP and the DMP develop in relationship with the outer environment. A good enough caregiver provides the emotional base for the child to stimulate its potential into existence. A conscious practice of the DMP in adulthood supports the repatterning of the brain and establishes the recreation of solid foundations for a more resilient life (Hartley 1995: 91).

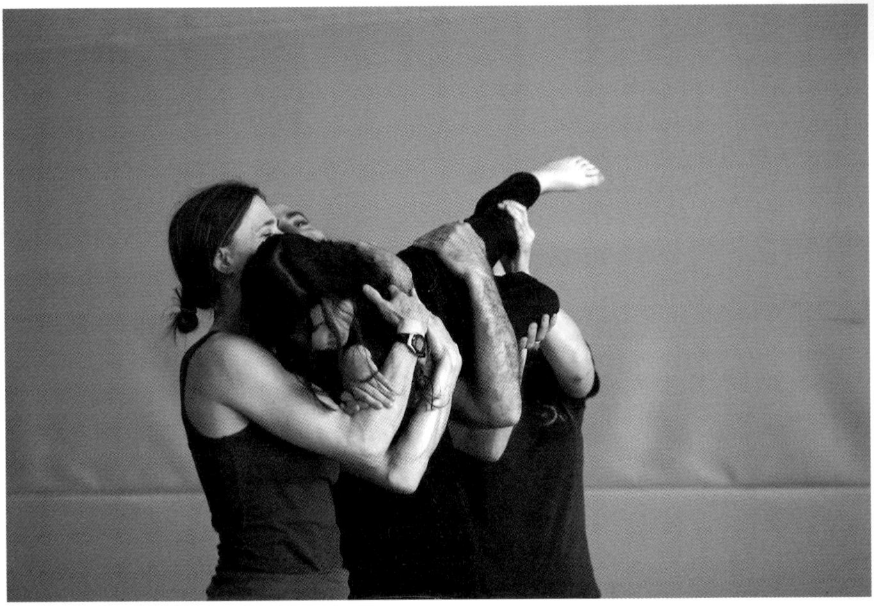

Workshop participants. Photographer: Patrick Beeleart

Practical Aspects of the Work

Above, I underlined the relatedness of movement and touch for the development of self. This means that focusing on the relational aspects of our beings is an important body of work. The knowledge of that Developmental Process has allowed me to value very different movement experiences than I was able to with my dance and physical education background. I began emphasizing the creation of spaces with a playful, creative atmosphere. The relational aspect is that I am with the children. I am clear in my intent to support them to unfold their potential, with the consequence that I tailor the content of my planned class. The work is not just about moving together; it is about creating spaces that invite nurturing, repatterning, and unfolding of potential. The relational aspect in movement and touch is further emphasized when offering workshops of movement and play "for tall and small." (I try to find an open title for the workshops that I offer for caregivers and children, using a distinction that is visual rather than referring to form and content.) These workshops are playgrounds for adults, mainly caregivers, with their children (from 4 to 6 years, and 6 to 10 years). The principles of Contact Improvisation are applied in combination with the body of knowledge described above.

Movement and play for tall and small people

Contact Improvisation is a playful dance form where two or more dancers explore their relationship with gravity while being in physical communication and touch with each other. Touch can have different qualities. The skin is our largest sense organ and has numerous receptors that can listen to touch. If I listen to how I touch another skin, my skin is also being touched while it is touching another body's skin. In Contact Improvisation, each dancer follows the impulses that arise from listening into her/his/their own skin or what she/he/they perceive(s) in the other's body. Thus, a common movement is created. This includes sending impulses to the other and following impulses from the other. This dialogue can lead the dancer through space and in positions where one dancer is moving over the other dancer, finding support in the other body. An experience of being supported and carried, as well as supporting and carrying, is created.

(For more on Contact Improvisation, see https://www.youtube.com/playlist?list=PL32CFE3B0B49F196B. I can recommend watching this video as it shows the beginning of Contact Improvisation, with Steve Paxton's research into how bodies move with and resist gravity.)

Moving together in physical connection can lead the dancer to places where they could not have gone alone. Through being in the moment of connection with the other dancer, one enters the realm of not knowing but trusting the physical connection. Therefore, Contact Improvisation gives an opportunity to get to know your own body in its functions and abilities; it creates a space without planning, and an opportunity to perceive and consciously experience the moment. If I look at the benefits of this dance practice, it can actively promote mutual respect and joint action. It also allows a togetherness without fixed roles. Contact Improvisation and attentive play can therefore enrich parents and children at the same time. The physical dialogue of a Contact Duet is about finding out together where the journey is going. In doing so, it is possible to enter and immerse oneself into an unknown space. This immersion requires an intensive listening on the physical level, in one's own body and in that of the partner. Where should our dialogue go? What do I want? What does the other one show me? Where do we go together?

Contact Improvisation for adults and children differs from the dance practice of adults because of different body proportions and body weight. Experiential and movement knowledge, as well as movement possibilities, might be different. There might also be a different drive for movement in adults and children. Spaces for movement, dance, and play for both adults and children are rare in our society. For smaller children there are activities where caregivers accompany them. In wanting the best for their children, some parents might not be self-aware enough to recognize what they want and need, but rather focus on the child's need. The emphasis in my classes is on reminding the caregivers to feel their movement drives and needs, and from there to meet their child. A dialogue of togetherness is created out of being in contact with oneself. Caregivers provide a safe harbor when they are in contact with themselves. In my experience, that can be a challenge and, when taken, it can be a nurturing place for everybody.

Contact Improvisation for tall and small offers us a space where everyone can learn to feel themselves, to deal with themselves and to encounter the other at "eye level" from that very personal connection. It offers the possibility of a temporary suspension of the normal fixed role distribution for caregivers and children. When caregivers dance Contact Improvisation with children, both sides are allowed to pay attention to their needs and enter into a playful dialogue. The negotiation process can now take place on a physical level. That trains us in the responsibility to listen to our own needs and it offers possibilities for making choices. Bainbridge Cohen points out that, "in the process of exploring movement, what is perceived is informed by our environment, our preconceived expectations, and the choices we make" (Bainbridge Cohen 2018: vii).

To come back to the beginning of this chapter, it can be especially interesting for adult caregivers to realize where there is a difference between the felt sensation and the actual interpretation of that sensation in their perception. It can be valuable to recognize any preconceived expectation that an adult has of a child. The playground of Contact Improvisation for tall and small can create little seeds that then can inform daily life practice. Contact Improvisation creates a learning process that cannot take place in the head but only in the cells; it requires a physical presence, a being at home in the body. If this presence is not yet present, the dance can make it possible to arrive in one's own body; it trains the body's own ability to perceive. Contact Improvisation enables a re-anchoring in the body.

By playing with weight there is a constant relationship with gravity. Through the constant connection of the inner axis with gravity, the cells receive updated kinesthetic information about where we are in space and what tension we need for movement. The sense of balance is finely tuned. Through this awareness of our natural connection with gravity, we feel ourselves clearly and receive confirmation of who we are, and what our limits and challenges are, and it informs us with choices.

To create a space where caregivers can move together with their children in this way is very precious. In offering activities and games, the DMP are smuggled in. I do not talk about repatterning. I just create settings where everybody can go back to explore those early movement patterns.

Having given a short introduction into the underlying somatic knowledge of the DMP and their importance for movement classes for children, adults, and children with their caregivers, I hope you might appreciate the complexity and the relatedness to human development. As social beings we are in relationship. Bringing awareness to those relationships starts with bringing awareness to oneself. We can start, right here and now, to sense and feel our body and its relation to the surroundings and to this written material. What is waking up in your inner needs and nurturing necessities? Would you like to go to the floor, to lie down and feel the floor supporting you? Feel your ground below and your breath moving you? What are you drawn to or what is waking up your curiosity? What would you like to move towards? Notice those needs and give yourself permission to follow them and feel the effect of that. If that means being still or moving very little, follow this. If that means moving fast or big, go for it. I would like to conclude this chapter with two practical examples to try out with somebody (a child or an adult) that you feel comfortable with, which you could try at home:

First partner exercise: Go down on all fours, side by side in a pair like sheep, no matter what the proportions are. Now start to push each other away. You can try to get either under or above the other person. Your partner can support you by making themselves smaller or bigger, and you can change sides and roles. Then rest a little together. How is it if one of you lies down with a body part on the other? If you like to receive weight, you can also try to see how it feels when their whole body lies on you.

Second partner exercise: Both partners close their eyes. One takes the hand of the other and places it on their own body. Both feel into it and notice how it feels. The hand is also allowed to explore respectfully; if it doesn't feel comfortable anywhere for the receiver, they have full permission to move the hand away. Then change roles.

After having read this, how do you feel now? How are you looking at your personal history? At your child's development? My aim in this chapter has been to offer you some theoretical knowledge combined with practical examples so that you might not only understand cognitively the complexity of the developmental process, but have a somatic experience of it too.

Chapter 10

Glossary

Notochord: gastrulation happens in the third week of development. By the third week, two layers, entoderm and ectoderm, have been developed. Through the thickening of the ectoderm, a new layer, the mesoderm, arises in between entoderm and ectoderm. The process starts with the formation of a primitive streak and the building of a primitive knot. This is the starting point for the notochord to emerge. The notochord forms a midline cord of mesoderm, which allows the mesoderm to develop.

Video link
Contact Improvisation for tall and small people

Finding Our Ground: Working with Adopted Children

Paul Beaumont

11

I want to share my experience of bringing the Integrative Bodywork and Movement Therapy (IBMT) approach to my work with children who have been adopted.

Children and young people can have a particular relationship with their body and movement. So much comes through their behavior, actions, and responses to the world. The IBMT approach offers ways to understand what might be going on and provide insight into areas worthy of exploration for development and healing.

Working with the body is profound. It involves both our conscious and unconscious processes. This is particularly so when working with children and young people, whose cognitive and reflective understanding may not be as developed or capable of being as clearly articulated. Through movement approaches we can work with a young person's quality of energy for life that is present in their bodies. We can pay attention to what is communicated non-verbally and what is signaled through their body intelligence.

In the first part of this chapter I offer a range of fictionalized vignettes drawn from my experience of this work over the last 5 years. I describe the space and resources used, and illustrate the arc of the therapeutic process, from the significance of arrivals to finding themes relevant to each individual. I make links from the developmental, sensory, psychological, relational, and anatomical themes that form the theoretical base of the IBMT approach.

In the second part I go on to lay out key principles that anchor and orientate my work. I explore the importance of nervous system regulation, working in the present moment, finding stability, and the repeated practice of returning to the body. I note the importance of improvisation and play, and an awareness of working with both the conscious and the unconscious in the therapy space.

In the final section I describe my experience of the reality of this work within the context of the perspectives of parents and social workers, and how important the self-care of the practitioner is to the effectiveness and sustainability of the work. I close by acknowledging the bigger journey of those I work with, which goes beyond my work and will continue with them through life.

In this chapter I focus on my work with children and young people who have varied in ages from pre-school through to primary and secondary school age in the UK. They have been adopted by a parent or parents and are struggling with sensory, emotional, or relational themes. Many of the children that I have worked with have suffered severe neglect, domestic violence, or generational abuse, and have had parents who have used drugs and alcohol. They may have had the experience of being removed at birth or had a period from several months to a few years of various foster care arrangements. It is important to note, then, that I am working with a particular population of adopted children.

I practice as an *International Somatic Movement Education and Therapy Association* (ISMETA) Registered Somatic Movement Therapist. I am also a qualified counselor and so draw on a range of skills to support the therapeutic relationship, such as unconditional positive regard, congruence, and empathy, as well as an awareness of transference, counter-transference, and process work. My

Chapter 11

practice is also influenced by play and improvisatory methods.

On the Ground

The space and resources

I usually work in a studio or community hall-type space. I aim for as high-quality and clear a space as practically possible, which is private, so we can feel safe, not overlooked or disturbed, and able to make noise. It needs to be warm and clean enough, with a floor that invites low-level movement. I have to be adaptable, working with what is available and checking that the space provides what the child needs in terms of safety. I have shifted work from a studio to a secure soft-play room in a special school, and to an outdoor field as I have adjusted to a child's different needs.

In the space I will have a range of props at the side: various inflatable body balls; lots of large and small pieces of fabric (Lycra, netting, blankets, big sheets, narrow strips, heavily weighted, and light and see-through), beanbags, hoops, soft toys, paper, and art materials. Working outside, I might have a tarpaulin to work on and use natural found objects from the environment.

The use of props can support a big part of the work with children and young people. They offer something outside of themselves to interact with and respond to. Preferences can be expressed, and the focus can be on the *thing* and *activity* rather than the internal experience of the client. This can create a feeling of safety and holding for the client and the work.

The Arc of Our Therapeutic Work

I have gained an understanding of the phases of the work and the need to give time to each, without rushing on – from arrival, through exploring themes and finding an ending.

Arrival, consent, and beginning relationships

As we prepare to take the leap into the unknown of the therapeutic relationship, the work begins.

Isaac is 14 and has been struggling to stay in school for a while, finding relationships with peers and teachers difficult. He has recently been excluded. The social worker has given me some brief information about his history and what the current struggles are. I sent a form to gather some wider information from his mum, and then met her in the studio so that she could see the space and hear more about how I work, and so that I could answer any questions.

Isaac arrives for the first session – a taster, so he can see the space, meet me, and get a flavor of what sessions might be like. He appears nervous, hanging back behind his mum. The three of us sit together and have a brief chat, as I introduce myself, and outline how we might work and what the sessions are for. I talk about the clear space, and how we will follow how we are on the day and how we can find some games and activities that feel right. I suggest we try a few things and that his mum can stay a while; then, if they want, she can leave, so that he has a chance to see what it is like on his own.

The three of us move into the space and I ask Isaac to see what is in the bag of resources at the side. He pulls out a piece of stretchy Lycra and we all take hold, finding its maximum stretch. An accidental letting go sees it catapulted across the room. We try this a few times, and I pull out a large piece of netting and then a long length of broad elastic. We experiment with what is possible and there is some laughter, noise, and banter. We talk about which we prefer and we start to explore the somatic language of sensations and feelings. Our work has begun.

The "arrival" happens in this and every session, so we can be in the space together, negotiating consent, and finding safety and a starting place. We also begin navigating relationships in this initial session – finding out whether it is right for the parent to stay in the room, as we balance safety and comfort with the aims of the work (which might include supporting the parental relationship). At times, the parent being in the room might be in the way or be used by the young person to keep the status quo. All needs to be given attention, as I reflect on the meaning and purpose of the relational dynamics present.

In the arrival my assessment process begins, noticing what might be present to be worked with or what might need to be explored. I am looking out for what is communicated non-verbally, noting how a person comes into the room, where they stand, their posture, eye contact, and state of emotional and physical energy and tone. Through the games I will be noticing the movement qualities present, reflecting these back in my own movement responses and testing the water for what else might be possible.

Finding the Themes

In working with anyone, I orientate myself and the work through noticing what themes are present. Each child and family is different, and I aim to hold very lightly any diagnosing or labeling of what is going on, while beginning to find the language to name what territory the client might be in.

I hope to maintain a softer focus, to notice what is present, while at the same time using frameworks integral to the IBMT approach to orientate myself to what is happening. The work might be developmental or sensory, psychological, or relational, and is usually a mix of all of these. The IBMT approach enables me to work with an awareness of the realms of body, feelings, and mind, as we find what needs to be expressed or what resources need to be developed.

Developmental and sensory themes

I have been working with 11-year-old Clara for a while. She is in mainstream education but needs one-to-one support. She has an autism spectrum diagnosis and is on medication. It took a few weeks for Clara to come into the studio, showing great resistance, shouting, and throwing things. She engages in a game for a time, but then disconnects and leaves the room.

Over time I reassure Mum, offering my perspective that the work has begun. Clara is showing us what we need to pay attention to.

As a practitioner, it can take time and the reflective space of supervision to gain a perspective on what is happening in the therapy space. This is invaluable, as it enables the practitioner to value what is happening and to find resources for what might be needed.

Week by week we try different things to respect Clara's choice not to come in, to encourage her to cross the threshold of the studio, to engage and connect. Bursts of play happen across the doorway. I notice that every game is turned into a pull game. We find ways to explore this, making up activities as we go: pulling on rope, elastic, and netting. We find the "twangs" as we pull and let go, and there are brief moments of delight and connection, pulling and being pulled along. I introduce throwing, then pushing, exploring the edges of what is possible from her starting point.

In this example of working with Clara, I make sense of what is present from a developmental perspective. With the resistance, push, and pulling activity I hold the possibility that we are working with Infant Movement Development patterns (Bainbridge Cohen 2018; Hartley 1995). I wonder too about birth themes that might be being played out, as she seeks movement and sensory experiences that tone the muscle-body.

After several months, there is a short series of sessions that stick in my mind. A push game has evolved with Clara and her mum as they sit on the floor. She pushes her mum with her head with great force and direction across the studio several times. In another session, she pushes her mum with her back. And finally, after further pushing, Clara is resting on her side, in gentle, soft contact with her mum, as they quietly rest together.

Our work supports the expression and integration of these early developmental patterns, as well as birth themes, of being viscerally met and received in relationship, beyond words.

Psychological and relational themes

Eight-year-old Jay arrives for his fifth session with his dad. He goes straight for the table covered by the large cloth and hides underneath. I come alongside, responding and joining in with his animal noises, and a game evolves as small beanbags become food and are passed in and out, accepted, rejected, offered, and shared.

Over the coming weeks, Jay embodies various young animals and plays out a whole range of key relevant themes: his connection with food and nourishment, as well as relationship dynamics (withdrawal, attack, defense). Rich early developmental material was covered, as play involved using the environment as a resource. Corners of the room, together with fabric and chairs, created dens and containing spaces. Through games and stories, I work with his dad to hold boundaries that are resisted, pushed away, rested into. The narratives developed as Jay embodied pets in a pet shop, where I am cast as the pet shop owner and his dad as the one who comes to choose a pet. Jay, as the pet puppy, repeatedly escapes, is lost then found, injured, and then carefully tended to. These narrative games are repeated and layers of exploration and meaning revealed.

It was deeply touching to work with Jay and his dad and to witness these young animal themes, which I have seen in a number of children I have worked with.

In this example, we let go into the image and narrative of the puppy that Jay brings. This holds the work and the embodied truth for Jay. Myself and his dad participate in the embodied play, trusting in following the path of what is meaningful for him and therefore its importance and worthiness of our attention.

It is interesting to note how, through the embodied play and held therapeutic space, earlier developmental themes are explored, irrespective of the child's chronological age, and how, in the adult's participation, being alongside and with the child's experience, relational themes can be explored.

As a practitioner, I am reflecting on what happens in a session as it is happening, and later, when I make notes and consider our work. From my IBMT perspective, the practice of Authentic Movement (Adler 2002) holds the framework of being able to discern movement, sensation, feeling, and image. I followed and guided the above work through the tracking and embodiment of those four areas. We had times where we dwelled for a few moments in the detail of a sensory experience or, while resting, we shared what a moment felt like or looked like.

The map of the body

Another teenager arrives for their session. Dean is 16, not in mainstream education, and struggles

a lot with emotions and relationships. We begin using the physio balls, as he kicks one away and across the room.

We join together in an evolving "kicking away" game, finding what is most satisfying – which ball, how it arrives, whether it is caught or bounces off a wall, whether it is kicked into the space or towards someone else. The game has high energy and has engaged Dean in being here.

Here, I pick up on the expression through the skeletal and muscular systems, as well as potential developmental and emotional themes. I reflect back, through my own participation and encouragement, Dean's embodiment, feeling my own bones and muscles as we play. In exploring what is most satisfying, we are able to refine and fill out his somatic, felt-sense experience. His kicking-away energy is accepted and given space.

I shift the game after a while and include the upper body, with big bounces using both hands, launching the ball into the ground and walls. There is a rhythm in movement, sound, and relationship.

Here, the props give sensory, tactile, and proprioceptive feedback to Dean. He can begin to feel himself through the action, and a sensory-motor cycle is repeated. I aim to enable a sense of being met in the process, and a resolution and balance of experience to be found. This can be immensely valuable for those whose emotions and tensions in the body can become blocked, unacknowledged, or stuck, building up to often destructive release for the person and those around them.

We shift the game again, as we face each other across the space, using arms and hands to launch and receive the balls. Heads and eye levels are brought up into a more relational domain. I slow the pace down, holding the ball for a moment of eye contact before returning. I time the throw with an outbreath.

The session, then, moves through this anatomical territory, from bones and muscles in the lower limbs, through engagement of the upper limbs to enable some openness to the hand–heart–face relational connection. We go from the anatomical to the relational.

As we come to the latter stages of the session, I introduce leaning into the balls on the wall, squashing, rolling, bringing in a tactile experience. This shifts nicely to rolling them on the floor, arriving at resting places, front of the body supported over the curve of the ball, seeing if we can feel the movement of our breathing.

Through the use of the props and the map of the body systems, the session enabled me to meet the client where they were, support a wider somatic experience, and develop resources to begin to manage emotions and come into relationship.

As the sessions progress with a client, I might have a sense of which body systems are present or absent. **Is someone in their muscle, engaged in action and drive? Or are they in more of a fluid state?** I will be asking myself if there are any developmental movement motifs present, such as the relationship between upper and lower body. The IBMT approach gives me the ability to offer a response to the holistic nature of what is present.

Endings

As we come in to land from all that our therapeutic work has included, there is much to pay attention to. The ending of work often comes from outside circumstances. Families can extend themselves hugely to bring their child to therapy. It can involve extra travel, arranging childcare for other children, and time after school or out of their working day. Families and children may need to end therapy, then, to enable other siblings to have time, or they may simply need a break. And although sessions may go on for several years, funding is limited and dependent on the shifts in governmental priorities and budgets.

As in the arrival stages of the work, I pay a lot of attention to endings and preparing to end, finding ways to embody and acknowledge this significant stage in a relationship. Work in the ending phase can be very potent for these adopted children and young people. Themes of abandonment, rejection, and loss can surface and be played out in the therapy space. I aim to give the ending phase lots of time – giving children lists of dates when we will meet and naming when we are likely to end.

Principles and Practices

I want to lay out the principles and practices that I apply in my work and which come from elements of the IBMT approach. The principles inform the practice. The practice is an expression of the principles. They are inextricably linked. Being able to articulate them guides my work.

They are my fundamental assumptions or "truths" that I hold centrally. They provide the anchor when the work is intense or challenging and help me make sense of what is happening and guide the work. They provide the spine of my work, helping me orientate and guide its direction.

Nervous system regulation

Using my soft focus "lens," when I reflect on my work with someone I often notice what may be going on in their autonomic nervous system. Is their state a more active, outwardly expressing one (sympathetic activation) or has it more of an inward focus (parasympathetic activation)? A young person might be angry and physically aggressive or closed down, subdued, or depressed. As a somatic practitioner, I aim to draw on the ability to meet their state in my embodiment, as well as holding and modeling the other aspects of nervous system expression.

My work here has been informed by Porges's Polyvagal Theory, and Deb Dana's use of this in therapy (Dana 2018). Working with a somatic movement approach, we can notice the embodied states of being immobilized or collapsed, finding ways to move into action in some way, with the intention to find the direction in the work towards being socially connected.

Working in the present moment

Throughout this work, I come back to core practices of finding present moment connection. **How can I be with what is present? What is in the room? What is being called for, needing attention?** By bringing what is present out into the room in some way, giving space around it, we provide the conditions where it can be witnessed. From here, we can reflect back or join in, or provide the counter-point, the still place or opposite tension. I aim to allow something to come "through" in the here and now, piece by piece, balanced with ground and rest. And with children especially, I aim to do this through play, following the child's focus and energy.

Early on in working with adopted children, I realized that the problem, the "behavior" that would often make the session so challenging, was what I needed to pay attention to. The child was showing me. But such behavior was also what others (parents, teachers, social workers) wanted to go away or stop. For example, a child might be all over the place – wild and noisy, not able to stop and sit still or be in relationship. They may not have control of their movement, impulses flying, and they potentially might harm themselves or others. Or they may be at the other end of the spectrum, extremely passive and withdrawn, not able to take any initiative or express a choice or engage in play.

I discovered that I needed to pay attention to the "problem" in a particular way – to give it space, enable its expression, and to encourage some bodily, creative encounter to take place, so that change could happen. I found that "the problem" holds the solution; the problem is what needs our attention.

I have supported children in the depths of despair, feeling lost, stranded, abandoned, as well as those in huge rage. My Authentic Movement training and ongoing practice also enable me to draw on the ability to be with, to give some space around whatever is happening, and to make contact there. I draw on my inner witness. This is an ability to notice something and observe it, with some degree of separation or breathing space, simply to notice without judgment, interpretation, or projection of my story on to what I am witnessing (Adler 2002). I aim to discern what I am feeling in emotion or sensation, noticing but largely putting to one side my own images and associations. I do my best to locate what is happening in witnessing the movement and gestural quality of the person I am working with.

In many ways, this is all there is, especially with children. IBMT is a here-and-now practice. Things might be automatically in the room, in how a child is behaving and what they are doing. And part of the work might be noticing what is *almost* happening or not happening (but might be balancing or resourcing), and finding ways that it can be embodied in the room safely.

It can be a delicate balance, for it is so easy as a practitioner to be drawn off into problem-solving, focusing on what "needs to change." This is especially prevalent when there are parental expectations or wider organizational pressures.

I am also tuning into where there is flow and energy in a session from moment to moment (remembering the Mindell Process Work aspects of my training; Mindell 1985), noticing when a child is energized and engaged, where there is an alive presence of body, mind, or emotion, and when there is an ability to be grounded and in relational contact. And equally, I am aware of when the energy and connection go, and a shift in focus into a different channel might be called for, so moving from feeling to visual image or from relational dynamics into kinesthetic/movement. These present-moment tracking skills support the work as it progresses.

Stability before mobility

This principle is expressed in many ways through the IBMT approach. It has its foundation in infant movement development work (Bainbridge Cohen 2018; Hartley 1995) and is reflected in the field of developmental psychology and attachment theory. As infants, we first bond and attach. We gradually feel and fill more of ourselves in preparation then to separate, to move away and express our individual selves out into the world. This principle might be present in the work with a child whose movement organization and integration of senses are not settled. It might be valuable to explore coming to the ground with whole-body movements, finding ways to yield. This can provide foundational support for a child who is in flight – up, off, and away.

Related to this principle is working from the horizontal to the vertical, again having its foundation in infant movement development. Here, coming to the ground, lying on the floor, being able to rest and receive, before pushing away, can be key skills. Also, in coming to standing, we feel the connection with the ground and movement between our supportive back and softer front.

Chapter 11

The principle of stability before mobility is present each time we meet. We will be saying hello, arriving in the room, establishing connection, and managing the different levels of intensity around this. For example, a familiar game of batting a balloon around provides the structure, "rules," and containment, establishing our stability, before the exploratory or expressive part of a session.

Returning to the body

This principle relates to myself as the practitioner, and is a key practice in what I am wanting to support in my client.

For me, the body provides the anchor and the orientating guide that I trust implicitly. My practice in working with others is to keep in contact with my feeling body. I am noticing the ebbs and flows of sensation, allowing this space, but also working to keep my own sense of ground, my vertical and regulated balance. I also aim to have a repertoire of different body/movement states that are accessible to me to join with or reflect back to a client.

I am tuning in all the time, in the softer tissues of my body. **What am I feeling? Where is any tension or space present?** In experiential anatomy study we explore the tissues that run through the body: connective tissue, skin, bone; the key organ systems of heart, lungs, and digestive system, for example. We move from each system, letting go of the Western maps we study from traditional anatomy and physiology books, to learn something of what the body holds. This gives me an exquisite respect for the body and helps me have sensitivity to the different body systems that might be prominent for my client.

As a practitioner, I also return to the body as a resource when someone might be expressing a lot of emotion or strongly acting out in some way. Here, I will draw on feeling the contact through my bones into the floor, the verticality of my spine, to keep me in contact with myself and not let myself be swamped. At the same time, I am also softening in my belly, to feel and empathize with what a young person is bringing, and to be able to reflect this back.

I will also regularly bring the client back to the simplicity of their body. I might check if they want to be in a different position in the space, if they need another blanket or just need to have a run around the space. I am inviting them to notice what they sense and to respond in some way: to feel, then move. This is often what has got stuck in some way. Early life experiences have prevented feelings being moved out of the system, which would enable them to be integrated and other feeling states embodied.

Working with the conscious and unconscious

Working with children, I am responding to the different degrees of outward expression or inward holding that are present. In somatic work, we give the chance for some of the unconscious yet bodily held stories and meanings to surface. This has been explored by Larry Heller (2012), Bessel van der Kolk (2014), and Babette Rothschild (2000).

Children often cannot help but reveal something of their story and experience in how they are in the studio space. **Do they linger at the side or dive straight in? Do they want to find ways to be small or does every game turn into a pushing, pulling game?** Working with them, I am required to let go of knowing, for if I try too hard to work it out, to know, to try to change or sort, I can lose connection and the work can become dry and lifeless. It is this very creative being-flow that I am wanting to give the space to, offering the safety, play, and experimentation to enable what is there to come through. And it is this place that can hold so much variation from person to person. It can be messy, noisy, and dangerous. It can be quiet and subdued. It can be a place of active resistance or more subtle avoidance. My job is to meet a child where they are and keep them and myself safe. Through following the flow and adjusting/nudging the play, games, and environment, I balance expression of what is present with enough grounding and containment to enable safety.

I have found that improvisation and play hold both the conscious and the unconscious. My exploration of dance and movement improvisation earlier in my life gave me the experience of following the body and being in the moment. The relational dance form of Contact Improvisation embodies a dropping down into the basics of a relational moving body. Here, we work with gravity and momentum, as the dance spontaneously unfolds.

My work with the movement play organization JABADAO introduced me to the significance of play, beginning with a clear space, and following the child's lead and a child's body intelligence (Greenland 2000). The work of Dan Hughes (Hughes 2009) and his PACE Model, of Playful, Accepting, Curious, and Empathy, can also guide my approach. My work with Helen Poynor and Halprin's RSVP cycle (Worth and Poynor 2004) reminds me of the simple act of noticing and spontaneously using resources present, whether that be chairs and tables at the side, a puddle on the floor from a leak in the roof, or specific props I have gathered together.

My work with this client group has also been supported and influenced by my learning from my supervision by a Dance Movement Psychotherapist, drawing on perspectives from Jungian and Psychodynamic approaches. This broadened my perspectives, taking in the significance of the bigger picture, how all can be relevant or have something to offer the therapeutic process – the blue-bottle fly not settling or the sounds of the trains outside the studio. These associative aspects can also align with my understanding, from my Authentic Movement practice, of the value of what can be held in an image or memory, so opening up to a wider field, the magical and the ordinary, as the therapeutic path unfolds.

The above influences all touch on an equal respect for both the known and the unknown. As an IBMT practitioner, sessions hold the space between these two, so that we can move between them, finding the learning and personal evolution that come in this transitional space.

What is it Like on the Ground?

It can be easy when reading chapters such as this to think that the author has it sorted, that they have a way of working that is successful each time. I have selected here illustrative stories from my work that show the rich resource that IBMT has to offer this field. The approach is not for everyone, and in its nature does not provide solutions or cures, but rather offers the embodied and relational nutrients that can support someone's development.

The work takes time and is cyclical, as we return again and again to the practice of being present with people and returning to the body. We can practice noticing the moments of grace when the elements involved are aligned in a way that enables a person to grow.

I have had to be hugely adaptable to find ways to respond to and engage children and young people. I use the IBMT "maps" (movement and psychological development, anatomy and physiology, Authentic Movement tracking, and so on) to understand where a child might be developmentally or to understand what they might be seeking. As their conscious minds are less developed, I need to draw on creative means to guide their somatic work to include what might be needed.

I can have times of feeling lost, not knowing what to do. It can appear that children are fleeing from the very thing they most need. Or they absolutely need to test it out, again and again, as they find stability. It is here that I have to pause, reflect, and go into the studio to move, write, and draw for myself. It is here that I have to return to my key principles and practices.

There can be challenges and pressures from outside the therapeutic relationship, as there will be other stakeholders involved. Parents/carers may want the "problems" to go away and for the child to "fit in." Social workers and funders may want to see evidence of change as they judge whether services offered are value for money. I can often pick up the anxiety of those around a child; I have to note this but also hold it at bay to respect the container of the therapeutic space.

Unless I am careful, I can so easily be drawn into the pressures of trying to cure, or sort, or make go away the behavior that is causing difficulty. It may well be causing suffering for both the child and the parent, but therapy gives the opportunity for a safe enough place to be created, where slowly the suffering behavior can be held, contained, and acknowledged, emotions released, stories told and – gradually, gradually – new ways of being and relating can come through.

Here, I need again to trust and hold the space for the body. IBMT work comes within the whole range of person-centered approaches that are focused on relationship rather than technique, and that believe change occurs when the conditions are right.

I have also found there are many allies in the work, as I have learned to articulate to others what I am doing and why. For example, talking with therapist colleagues within the adoption field has highlighted the Sensory Integration work employed by Occupational Therapists (Kranowitz 2005). We have realized the overlap in underpinning theory, in how we understand the nervous and sensory systems of young people who have had a traumatic early life. We speak the same language and share many beliefs about the significance of how the moving body is operating and what might be needed for healing, balance, and integration. It has been empowering to find this shared language and understanding with mainstream professionals; I would recommend that any somatic practitioner makes links with colleagues from other disciplines.

Self-care

Working with children is only part of my therapy work. In my early days of working with children whose nervous system was often highly anxious, alert, and unregulated, I found I had to do a huge amount of embodied resourcing to calm, ground, and balance my own nervous system. And I found, when my caseload included adults, that this facilitated a further grounding, release, and relaxation in my system. Widening the horizon of my therapy work brought in more balance and perspective. I would recommend any practitioners notice the impact of their work on their own embodied selves, and have regular time to move so that what is received through our own tissues as practitioners can be motored out, given expression, and released. This enables us to recalibrate and discern any transference issues that may arise, so that our own material can be attended to through our own support and therapy; in this way, we can respond more consciously to our clients.

The Bigger Journey

I have to respect the children's knowing of when the time and conditions are right to do their work.

It may not be with me at this time. These children are on a big journey as they make sense of their history and early life story. They will have started this process before I meet them and will continue afterwards. In the course of our work, we begin a **meeting** together, **exploring** what is possible, finding **expression**, **understanding**, or **acceptance** and then saying **farewell**. Their arc of development will continue beyond our work together, just as mine will. This was an important realization for me as a practitioner, as I made the shift from believing early on that I was somehow going to "make it all better," to realizing the bigger journey and arc of development on which they were, and indeed we all are. I am just a small part of that process. Just as I need to connect, I need to let go, find acceptance and trust, and allow someone to be.

I hope and trust that children will find their way as they go on to meet others and do what they need to do to continue to resolve underlying feelings and embodied experiences, to find peace and connection. Somatic Movement Therapy offers a wealth of resources to support the integration of adopted children's history, together with the liberation of their potential, as they find the ground under their feet and in their bodies.

Part 4

Therapeutic Applications 1: Holding and Containing

Circle: The Nature of Containment

Daria Shamina

12

Ever since my IBMT training, my work has been devoted to the exploration and application of the "Mandala" method and Authentic Movement in IBMT practice. I became completely fascinated by the methods associated with the shape of the circle and with the magic of the circle in general. While working with clients, more and more I found the circle to be a healing form. I expanded my research on the circle and its healing nature in somatic practice and therapeutic work. In this chapter I will share the results of my research and practice around the nature of containment and methods associated with the circle.

The Symbol of the Circle

The circle is the oldest symbol. Different cultures consider various values to be inherent to it, but many of them converge on the meaning of protection. In the Slavic tradition, circle is one of the most significant mythical and epic characters, reflecting the idea of time cycles ("Circle of Life," "year-round") and the primary forms of the structuring of space – division into "their own" and "foreign," where the circle acts as a border creating a closed, protected space.

There is evidence that people used to plough around an area where they wanted to settle and establish a village; this was an act of separating "their" space from "foreign" space. Ukrainian legends also mention that the first houses had a round shape.

In mystical practices, the circle has the function of protecting against evil spirits. During ceremonies and spells, a magician draws a circle around herself, which defends her.

The natural qualities of the circle have a special healing effect for our psyche. I am fascinated to meet the circle symbol in different psychotherapeutic and somatic methods and practices. My exploration leads me to the thought that the circle is a universal symbol and natural form that helps our psyche to create a very safe and reliable structure for experiencing various processes, reflecting, expressing, digesting, and containing.

Once I led an unusual workshop, where we experienced through dance and movement different geometric shapes – circle, square, and triangle. At first, we danced and connected to the figures through movement, and after that we went straight into drawing. There was no task for the drawing part, except following the inner impulse.

During the dance of the circle, I observed many soft, fluid movements. At the end of the dance, all participants lay on the floor, motionless and very peaceful. Some were in a fetal position. After we danced and painted the "circle," there was an unexpected pause in the process of the workshop because the participants did not want to leave this state of peace and tranquility; they did not want to move on to explore the other geometrical figures. There was some magic in this silence.

It seems that these qualities and the image of a protective circle go back to our intrauterine life, when the mother's belly creates absolute safety and reliability for us, an inner paradise, where it is easy to grow, develop, and change. Or perhaps we go back even earlier, to the cellular state, when our being was represented by only one cell, when we were just at the beginning of our journey, when we were in a state of being, rest, and tranquility.

Chapter 12

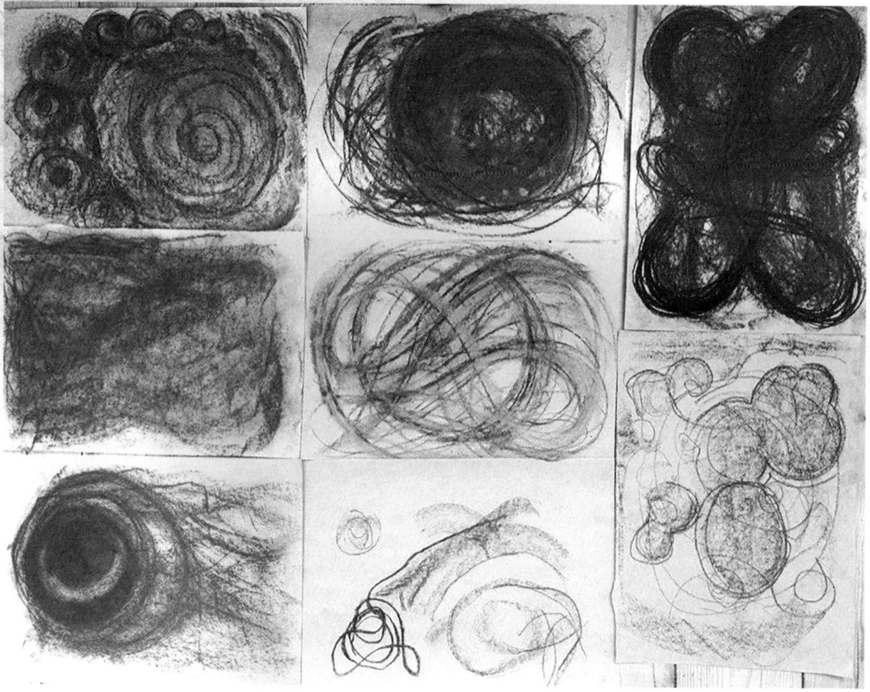

Drawings after the dance of the circle

These examples also help me notice that the circle often represents basic, beginning stages, or stages of maturation. Pregnancy represents the first Basic Perinatal Matrix (BPM I) in a spiral that leads to the birthing process (Grof 1985). This is a time of peace and blissfulness for the baby. This stage is more strongly associated with the circle, while the birthing itself (which is represented in Grof's theory as BPM II and III) is more closely linked with direct movement and transition into another state and space. The Cellular Breathing pattern is also the first in the sequence of the developmental movement processes and represents the basic states of body and mind, to which we can always return.

Containing and Holding

The concepts of holding and containing belong to the psychoanalytic tradition. Both terms refer to early childhood and concern the issue of how the mother meets the child's unbearable feelings.

"Holding environment" is a term introduced by Donald Winnicott. It describes the optimal environment for "good enough" parenting. The holding environment is the psychic space between the mother and her infant. It is the space between the inner and outer worlds. It is both physical and psychological. A key function of this early holding environment is the protection of the baby from inner and outer stress, which can cause damage to the baby and her development. And, on the other hand, this is a space where the baby can learn to experience frustrations, little by little, with the help of her mother (Winnicott 1971).

Psychoanalyst Wilfred Bion was the first to use the term "container" in the context of the infant–mother relationship. Bion writes that infants become overwhelmed by their own experience, as they do not yet have sufficient internal control. That is why the baby projects uncontrollable, most often negative, emotions on to the mother. She takes them in, contains them, and returns them to the child in a more acceptable form. For example, when a child is hungry, she breaks down in hysterical crying. The lack of food at that moment is experienced as a fear of death because the baby is completely helpless and cannot solve the situation on her own. Then the mother comes, calming and feeding her, taking away the fear of death, transforming it (Bion 1962).

These concepts are similar in the way that they describe the safe relational environment between the mother and the infant that helps the infant to mature naturally and correctly. But as I see it, holding is a long-term concept; holding is created every day by the mother. Holding is related to the environment around the baby, and containing is exactly what mother does in the moment to help her child deal with intolerable feelings. Still, it also has a long-term effect – good containing helps the infant develop a capacity for self-regulation.

The Role of Holding and Containing in Therapy with Clients

The therapist fulfils a similar function for the client to what a "good enough" mother does for her baby – she creates a holding environment and helps the client understand and contain her emotions and sensations. It is important to remember that Winnicott's holding is a developmental stage; by providing this environment for clients, we help them learn how to regulate themselves on their own. We encourage their nervous system to learn how to deal with and digest overwhelming information. We let their bodymind discover what it means to be safe and calm. We nourish them with our therapeutic presence. We encourage their Self to stay true and authentic by witnessing and accepting everything they sense or feel.

Here are some of the major functions of holding and containing that I have found in practice.

Reflecting

One client of mine has an interesting issue. On the one hand, she knows her inner world very well. She can easily name her feelings and sensations in our sessions. On the other hand, she always doubts her feelings. There is always one part of her psyche that questions everything she feels. This comes from her early treatment by her parents, who always questioned her feelings as well as her body sensations. The thing that works best in our therapy is reflecting and witnessing. When she names what she senses and feels, I repeat it as an echo and add, "I believe you." Sometimes I name what I feel when I meet her feelings, and it matters crucially to her that I do not try to change her feelings; I just name what they are in the moment. This helps her, little by little, to strengthen the part of herself where she knows clearly what she feels, and to weaken the part that questions it.

Digesting

When overwhelming emotions come to a client, the main task for the nervous system is to process them. I meet many adult clients whose bodymind does not know how to deal with emotions because they did not experience proper containment in their early childhood. They are often terrified when we move closer to the area of feelings. This function is important when we work with the client with trauma. There are usually very intense feelings, which could not be digested at the moment when the trauma happened and are held inside the traumatic experience. The therapist helps the client to experience these feelings, to stay in contact with them without being too overwhelmed; the therapist helps the client to digest something she is not able to digest alone.

Resting and being

Being contained also means simply being calmed and comforted by someone. Sometimes, it means letting go of our adult parts for a while, allowing the therapist to play the role of an adult so that the client can go into rest, into the being state, into some basic early states of mind.

Storage

Often in my practice, I meet a situation where some parts of a client's psyche are contained inside. Sometimes we say that these parts go into the shadow. What I find in my practice is that, when we explore these parts with movement and touch, it often turns out they are surrounded by a special defense, by guardians who protect the part and do not let it out. It is as if the psyche saves this part for better times. I imagine this as a kind of containment that our psyche does for us. It looks like a seed in a shell, which lies in the earth waiting for the right time to start *growing*.

Development and maturation

This function refers more to the concept of a holding environment than containing. Creating a safe long-term space for a client is necessary for her development and individuation. The therapeutic space is like a cocoon or a uterus for a client, where he can grow, mature, and transform.

Safe space for expression and exploration

When the proper container is created in the therapeutic process, unconscious material can be revealed. I remember when I was a student on the IBMT program and we were studying the organs of the upper body (heart and lungs). I was anxious to take my attention to the area of the organs. It seemed to me that there was a lot of unconscious emotional material in this area for me. My teacher invited me to stay at the edge at first, to keep my attention on the ribs that contained the organs. From that place, I could enter the organ area little by little and stay safe. Initially, we need to build a container to keep us safe and then we can explore something new or express ourselves in a new way. The "unknown" is held in our unconscious, and it takes courage and confidence to explore this unknown within ourselves.

Incubation

This concept comes from Graham Wallas's theory of creative thinking. According to Wallas, there are four stages of creativity:

1. preparation
2. incubation
3. illumination
4. verification (Graham 2017: 202)

I will not describe all four stages but will focus on incubation. This is a stage where creative thought is produced by the unconscious processing of available information. We do not have to make any special effort to solve a problem at this stage; it is solved by our unconscious knowledge, images, fantasy, emotions, and ideas. Incubation always leads to illumination, where we can find a brand-new answer or solution for our problem. The way I see it, we should put our problem or idea inside a special container or in a special state of our mind, where it will be brewed. This is right not only for mental ideas or problems we have to solve; it is the same for feelings or emotions. Our feelings in some ways are just like babies – they have to grow and mature inside us to be born and expressed.

Circle: The Nature of Containment

In the next part of this chapter I would like to describe different practical methods and techniques associated with the circle, which helps us work with containment and holding in therapy.

Mandala Method

Mandala refers to very ancient drawings that appeared thousands of years ago. Ancient Mandala was a model of the universe, a spatial map, and a schematic illustration of the places where the gods live. In psychology and art therapy, mandalas were introduced by Carl Jung. In his autobiography, Jung told the story of how, in 1916, he painted his first mandala; 2 years later, he was sketching a new mandala every day in his notebook. He found that mandalas reflected his inner life in the moment and began to use the pictures to capture his "psychic transformation." He noticed that, in difficult times, our unconscious often motivates us to draw something like a mandala or to see such figures in a dream. In addition, he believed that the mandala helps us to better understand what we are concerned with at an emotional level. The power of the mandala lies in its protective abilities: the circle, like the "dream catcher" of the Native Americans, **protects the spirit from scattering**. Later, Jung came to the conclusion that the method of the mandala is the way to open our unique individuality (Jung 1963).

In art therapy, the mandala is a drawing in a circle (or just a circular image), which can be a product of spontaneous creative activity or be established for specified patterns and instructions (Kopytin 2005).

The series of four drawings shown here were made by a participant in a workshop that I led. It was a 4-day workshop where we were practicing Authentic Movement, and afterwards I asked

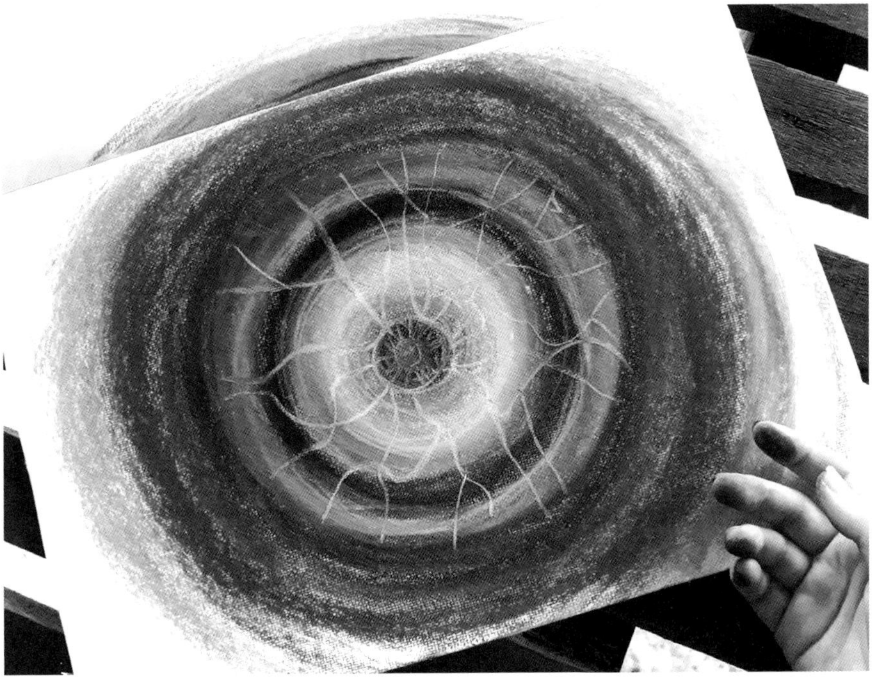

Mandala drawing by Russian art therapist Nadezhda Tuikina

participants to draw a mandala. In this series it is remarkably visible how changes in the psyche appear from drawing to drawing. The dynamics of the series reveal the constancy and variability of different elements through the forms and colors (for colors, see the video link at the end of the chapter). I invite you to look at these mandalas with your whole body – just to catch the sensation of their life and dynamic. The drawings are displayed chronologically, according to when they were created.

The first drawing is "cold" because of the color tones and the snowflake shapes. It is amazing to see how the curls transfer from the first drawing to the second.

It is easy to notice how a new story seems to appear in the second drawing. The double-color spiral appears inside the circle – cold blue and warm green colors.

In the third picture, we can see the colors combining the first, second, and fourth mandalas. A new motif appears with semi-circular lines, which "hugs" the center of the circle. The interior space of the page is completely painted over with saturated colors.

In the fourth drawing, all forms in the mandala turn into a circle. The warm yellow background uniformly fills the space outside the mandala. The purple color from the first drawing again becomes dominant, but the new colors from the second and the third drawings are added to it.

The circle is so safe and containing for our psyche that it always invites a client to capture the essence of her state very precisely in a drawing. Mandalas can be used as an instrument for a transition, or as integration in processes with a client or a group, or as a separate instrument for individual work.

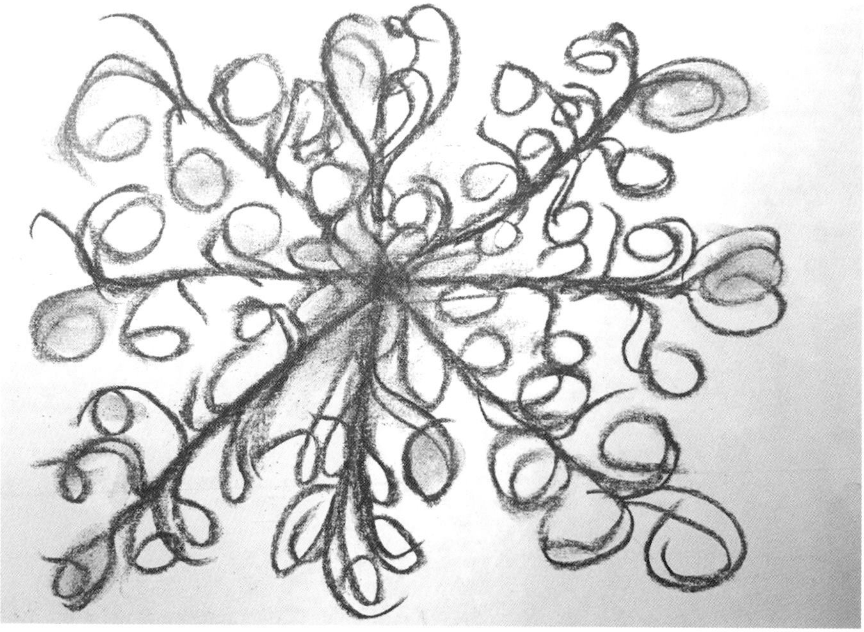

Mandala drawing at the workshop – day 1. Drawing by Daria Shamina from original artwork by Evgenia Samsonova [Orehova]

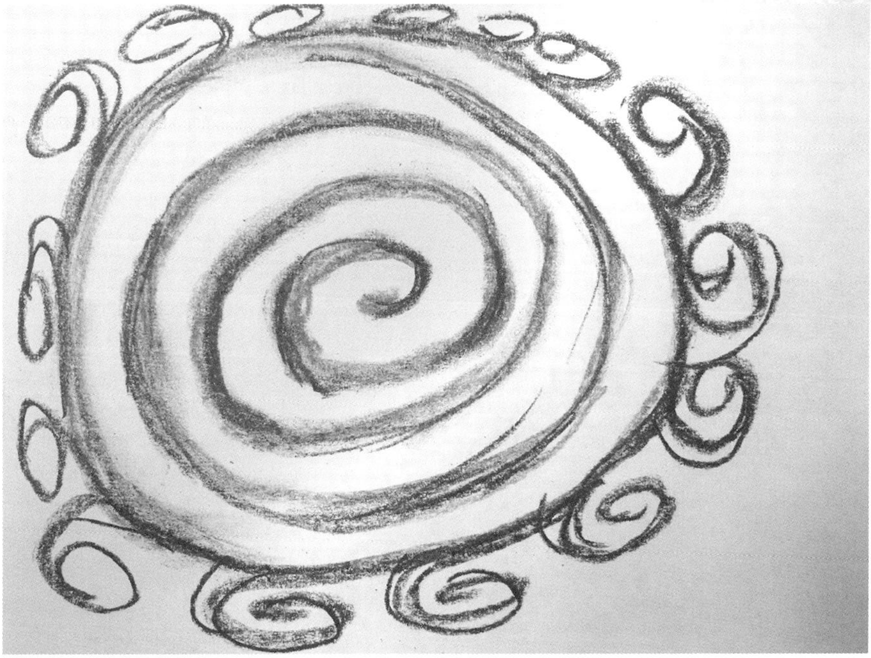

Mandala drawing at the workshop – day 2. Drawing by Daria Shamina from original artwork by Evgenia Samsonova [Orehova]

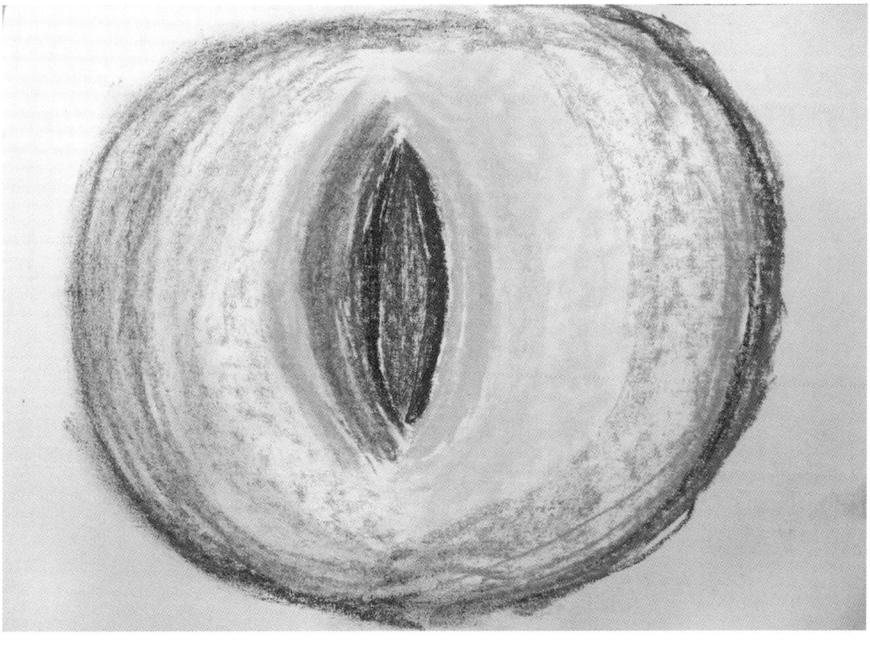

Mandala drawing at the workshop – day 3. Drawing by Daria Shamina from original artwork by Evgenia Samsonova [Orehova]

Chapter 12

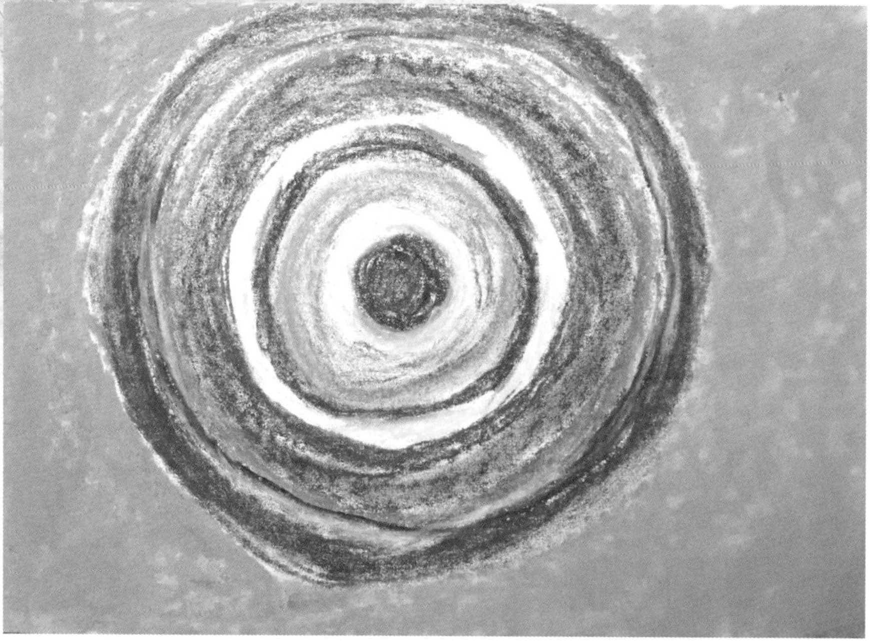

Mandala drawing at the workshop – day 4. Drawing by Daria Shamina from original artwork by Evgenia Samsonova [Orehova]

Authentic Movement

Authentic Movement is a practice in which there is a mover and a witness. The mover closes her eyes and moves, following the impulses arising from inside. The witness supports the mover with her attention, creating a safe space to meet the mover's process. When the movement ends, the process of transition starts, which helps mover and witness transfer to verbal sharing. During the transition time, the mover and the witness can draw, write, or sculpt in clay. Then comes the time to speak – the mover talks about her experience and the witness talks about hers.

This is the ground form of practice, but Authentic Movement is used by practitioners and therapists for various purposes and in different formats.

Authentic Movement can be practiced in a group and can also be applied in individual sessions. In a group, there is a real circle of witnesses, which creates a strong sense of a reliable container. In the individual format, there is a feeling of an invisible circle, which is created by the therapist's or witness's attention.

The witness creates and holds a safe space, the witness circle, into which the mover enters and begins to move, usually with eyes closed, following her own internal impulses. Both mover and witness attend to their own experiences as the mover's process unfolds.
(Hartley 2004: 62)

I have a client who experiences a lot of shame in our sessions, even in very common situations. We found out that she often looks at herself through the eyes of her mother, who was toxic for her. We started to practice Authentic Movement. It helped her to express herself in my presence and see herself through the eyes of my non-judgmental witnessing. Her shame has started to go away, little by little.

Circle: The Nature of Containment

Cellular Holding

In psychotherapy, we often turn to holding as a process that begins with the contact of mother and child after birth. Yet the uterus where the fetus evolves is a container in itself. Moreover, the embryonic period, when our bodymind was represented as a cluster of undifferentiated cells, opens up another layer of self-containment that expresses itself in the properties of the cell itself. It significantly expands our understanding of holding, as described by Winnicott, and of the container, as described by Bion.

In the notion of holding, Winnicott includes the idea of both physical holding – the mother holds her baby in her arms – and psychological holding – how well the mother can recognize the needs of her baby and respond to them. But the same thing happens in the womb, although the mother holds her baby in her belly at that point, and not in her arms. And I am sure that the baby recognizes and responds to the mother's womb as a safe and supporting environment or a dangerous, unsafe, and even hostile place. This type of holding lays the foundation for the holding between mother and child after birth.

I had a client who could not stay in contact with me for long during a session; at some point she "disappeared" – in other words, dissociated. She noticed it herself and always named it when she was dissociated, but she could not change the process. We kept looking for a form of contact where she could stay with me. We tried different things – changed the distance between us, attempted different kinds of touch, searched for the right words and messages about my presence: for example, "I'm here and I support you" or "I'm here and am not going anywhere." Once, we spent a session not looking at each other, with our backs turned. All of that helped for a short time only or did not help at all. But at some point, I remembered reading that a baby feels the presence of the mother on a cellular level (Hartley 2004: 105). I suggested we try that. She was familiar with the cellular bodymind, and I offered her an image that I was not "me" but rather a cluster of cells, cells that were present with her. I felt that I was surrounding her with my cellular presence, where she could stay, rest, and be nourished by that. We remained like this till the end of the session. At the end, she said she felt safe as never before. She even drifted to sleep for some time, as she was feeling deeply relaxed. We did this a couple more times in our sessions, so she could be nourished by this fundamental sense of safety and presence in contact.

If we look into the cell itself, into its essence, there we will find the magic form of a circle. Our body knows this shape very well because it is our first body shape as we are in this life. At the moment of conception, we are one cell that later on keeps on dividing and growing. Before that moment, there were two different cells from the mother and the father, and at this moment – one new whole. This first cell and all the ones that follow have the same basic structure: nucleus in the center, gel-like cytoplasm, and surrounding semi-porous membrane. The structure of the cell itself creates a container inside of it. This self-contained whole exists in all our adult cells, as well as in the very first cell, from which the embryo grows. By applying cellular consciousness through work with touch and movement, we turn to these early pre-conscious forms of awareness where there is wisdom, rest, and a state of a simple being. Turning our attention to the membrane can activate all kinds of issues connected with boundaries, a sense of wholeness, a container, and communication with the environment.

In my own therapy, where I was the client, there was an important period connected with the maturation of boundaries and inner support structures through cellular presence. I had several sessions with my therapist where I was lying or sitting in the darkness of a room, with my attention going into cellular awareness. My therapist's attention stayed on the outer layer of the membrane of a cell. Sometimes she touched me; sometimes she was simply present with her attention. I did not move. I noticed my barely heard breathing. But I sensed constant little movements inside of me – inside my cells, as it were. I had an image of movement from inside a cocoon; on the outside, the cocoon, where the caterpillar turns into a butterfly, looks still and unmoving, but there is a lot of movement inside, where a total transformation takes place. So mostly we just sat there quietly, sometimes talking a little when it was needed. After this series of sessions, there was a great change in my sense of boundaries: they became less vulnerable, and I stopped feeling alert all the time and ready to defend myself to prevent bad things getting inside. It seems that this sense of wholeness and inviolability, and at the same time flexibility of my boundaries, integrated into the body. I started feeling less social anxiety, as if my inner sense of wholeness embodied and matured in this cellular presence and being.

Methods of Containing in Individual Work with a Client

I will now write about some methods for containing that I use in individual work with clients. They are all based on the shape of the circle or an enclosed space. The methods are also connected with the issue of boundaries, within which important processes can take place.

Time and space

The first simple method relates to space and time. The space and time of the session are connected to boundaries and create a very important container for both client and therapist.

Time is about agreement around session timing. On one hand, it demands from a therapist extra attention and skill to finish the session on time (usually after an hour); on the other hand, it creates clarity and teaches the client to trust that the most important things will happen during this time.

The space of a room is already a container; it separates therapist and a client from the outside world. I had an interesting experience when I was leading psychological development groups for teenagers in a summer camp. When the weather was good, we used to have our classes outside. It was easy to notice the difference in working in an open space: the attention of the group easily became unfocused and work became superficial. The boundaries of a studio helped participants to stay more focused on themselves and the group process.

When I work with a group or a client, I enjoy preparing space for a session. In the practice of Authentic Movement, there is a ritual where movers and witnesses look into the empty space before the beginning of the process, greeting the emptiness that movers are about to enter and from which everything emerges. For me, preparation of the space is the same act of witnessing the space where things will soon happen to us.

Circle of relationships

This circle relates to the traditional understanding of containing in the psychoanalytical tradition: a client projects her unbearable feelings on to a therapist (in the same way that an infant does). But I like to think about it as the client placing her feelings into the space of relationship between client and therapist. Good, trusting relationships can be experienced as a safe and supportive space that can hold a lot of things – like a circle. And when a client knows that the therapist and the relationship are stable enough, she can let herself address feelings or unconscious states, sensations, projections, and processes that are difficult for her to handle on her own, and place them into the space of their interaction.

In this process, an important method is reflection and witnessing.

To reflect means to allow a client to place her feelings and process in the circle of the client–therapist relationship and to mirror them, name them, acknowledge them, and give them back in an adapted and contained form. Reflection is also important when a client has difficulty recognizing and naming her feelings, emotions, and physical sensations. If that is the case, a client needs to learn an "alphabet" of feelings and sensations through the therapist. I like the way Carl Rogers writes about reflecting on feelings in therapy: "The feelings and personal meanings seem sharper when seen through the eyes of another when they are reflected" (Rogers 1986: 376). Rogers also mentions the importance of suggesting and asking about the feelings of a client but not giving an interpretation while reflecting on the feelings. He proposes that we ask a client: "Is this the way it is in you?" (Rogers 1986: 376).

Witnessing is similar to reflection, yet different. The term comes from the discipline of Authentic Movement. In this practice, the witness does not interpret or suggest what is happening to a mover. She notices her own experience as a response to a mover's process. The witness can say: "When you go on the floor, I feel relieved." And that is the difference from the reflection method. In the witness role, we do not try to work through or interpret a client's experience.

Yet it often happens in a process of witnessing that, because of the mirror neurons, we tune in to the body of the client so we can sense and feel the same way as they do. Babette Rothschild writes that the therapist can directly experience the client's feelings, emotions, and experiences when she passively observes her or actively copies: for example, taking up the same body position. The more attentive the therapist is to her own body, the more she can activate the work of mirror neurons. But in this case, it is still important to check in with a client about her experience to avoid mistakes. For example, if you have an anxious feeling in your chest during the session, it is better not to guess but to ask the client about the sensations in her own chest. Feelings and sensations experienced through somatic resonance help to formulate questions for the client (Rothschild 2005).

Imaginary spaces

Another way of containing that I use a lot with my clients is creating an imaginary capacity, where it is possible to place everything mentally that does not fit inside the client. Usually, clients choose the image that suits them best. In my work, I have met images like boxes, bags, bathtubs, bowls, closets, suitcases, and wardrobes. It is also possible to place the container at a safe distance from the room where you are working. The offer to the client not to hold the overwhelming feeling inside can be a great relief for her.

I once had a client with depression, who felt very overwhelmed at finding a sense of life force and love energy inside herself, her nervous system reacting by giving out an alert. It was important for her to keep the connection with this new feeling but it was hard to bear. She felt torn apart and energy was going upwards (dissociating). We looked together for a space to place this energy, so that she would not be overwhelmed and could keep on feeling it. She mentally placed the energy in the next room and closed the door. She immediately felt better and we kept on slowly experiencing it through the body.

Chapter 12

Natural containers in our body

There is a great capacity in the body to contain our feelings. This is one of my aims as a therapist – to help my clients learn to contain their feelings and sensations in their body. And as a somatic therapist, I know that there are many spaces and structures in our body that can help us contain an overwhelming experience. I will name some of them.

The first is the **skin**. Skin envelops the whole body, holding everything together. In some ways, the skin is like a cell membrane: it helps us feel the wholeness and the entirety of the body. Just like a cell membrane, the skin is a place of communication between the inner and outer worlds. On one side, the skin protects everything that is inside; on the other side, it is the place where we meet the outer world and other people, where we can feel touch, temperature, pressure, light, and so on. As a primary boundary, the skin helps the infant distinguish herself from others through touch and to start identifying herself as a separate individual. Bodywork with the skin through touch can help the client to feel containment physically in the body on the one hand, and your presence on the other.

The **ribcage and pelvis** are the spacious places of the body. I prefer to trace their bones as, in my perception, they are more grounding and containing. With your touch, you can help your clients to feel the volume of the ribcage or pelvis so that they can place their feelings in these spaces. Bringing your client's attention to their breathing, and the movement it causes, can also help them to feel the volume of the ribcage and pelvis. You can invite your client to explore and check if these places are secure and capacious enough to contain their feelings.

I have already written enough about cellular holding, but I want to add that sometimes it can be helpful to go into the **cells** themselves with your awareness. This can be valuable when a client needs to rest, to stay in a state of being, or to incubate something.

Groups and Sharing Circles

Bion, while extending his theory of containment, came to the idea that social groups are a type of "maternal container" (Bion 1959). Therapeutic groups are usually organized in space in the form of a circle. Within the sharing circle, when participants speak of their experience, they put their feelings and meanings in the center so that the group can contain them. While I was studying IBMT, I experienced strong feelings around the group container; I felt the power of the group presence was so significant that it could hold any process and feeling arising inside of me or inside of the whole group.

> *As movers in a group learn to witness each other and themselves, the power of the witness circles grows: it becomes strong enough to contain the energy of transpersonal and collective processes as well as material from the personal unconscious.*
>
> (Hartley 2004: 67)

I felt our collective body was very much like a circle figure – something between an image and a sensation. If I could, I would call it image-sensation (which is what I feel about all mandalas, actually).

At the final presentation of my training, I asked the group to draw a collective mandala. This mandala is not like any that I have ever seen. I suppose it contains some of the collective conscious and unconscious. It represents each of the members of the group, and some of our connections and relations; it contains our knowledge and common experience. I feel a lot of movement, flow, and power when I am looking at it. Now I keep it at home as a reminder of the safety and beauty I experienced in our group.

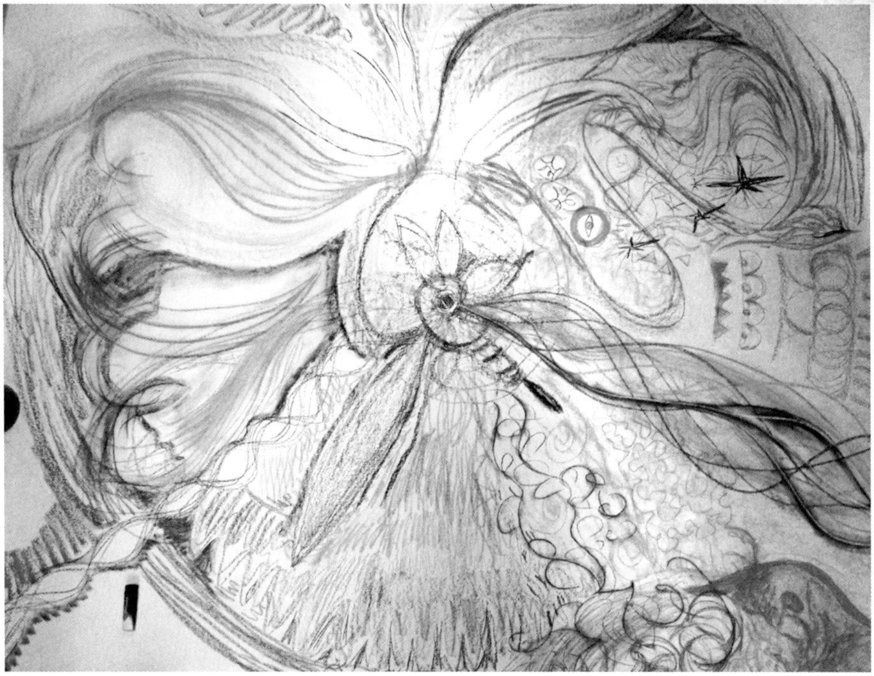

Group mandala drawing

Conclusion

To conclude, I would like to share a poem which is dedicated to the role of witnessing in Authentic Movement practice. Sometimes I have a strong experience, in the role of the witness, of the movers, of the group, of the processes arising. I feel that to be the one who contains, to be the "circle," is a privilege, one that offers an opportunity to see much beauty.

(In English)

I see you, the river, I see

Your waters falling into the stream,

Playful glare, a gentle wave, how fearlessly you lift the sand from the bottom.

I am your riverside. I'm always here, calm and still.

I see you, the seed.

I feel there is the power of a huge tree in you,

it's folded into a spiral, into a small dot in space and time.

I am your shell, I hug you tightly and confidently.

Until you want to sprout, I will wait with you in the darkness of the earth.

I see you, the body.

Blood, muscles, organs, your dance,
your breath, every cell, every form and
matter of yours.

I am here, all with you, naked, all masks are ripped off.

I am your skin, I am the impartial spectator of your Divine Mystery.

I am the womb, I am the grave, I am the circle, I am the living cell membrane.

I see you freezing and moving,

Chapter 12

Your unconditional happiness, boredom, hope, shame, wounds. I hear all your songs.

I am the witness of life. And in your presence, I am with my own experience.

(In Russian)

Я вижу тебя, река, Я вижу.

Твои воды, срывающиеся в поток,

Игривые блики, нежную волну, на дне золотой песок.

Я твой берег. Я всегда тут, спокоен недвижим.

Я вижу тебя, зерно - твою силу огромного дерева,

Свернутое, в спираль, в маленькую точку пространства и времени.

Я твоя скорлупа, обнимаю тебя крепко и уверенно,

Пока не захочешь прорасти,

я с тобой буду ждать в темноте земли.

Я вижу тебя, тело. Кости, кровь, мышцы, органы

Твой танец, твоё дыхание, каждую клетку, каждую форму и материю,

Я с тобой целиком как есть, обнажена, все маски сорваны

Я твоя кожа, Я беспристрастный зритель твоей божественной мистерии

Я утроба, я матка, я круг, я клетки мембрана.

Я вижу, как ты замираешь и движешься. Я слышу твоих песен тропы.

Твоё безусловное счастье, скуку, надежду, стыд, раны.

Я свидетель жизни. И в твоём присутствии я проживаю свой опыт.

Video link
You can find all the illustrations from this chapter in color by opening this link

Somatic Counter-transference in the Work of a Somatic Therapist

13

Anna Khasina

(Translated from Russian by Elizabeth Tsfasman)

I was led to psychology by the desire to fill my life with different emotions, to be able to feel these emotions, express them in contact with other people, and feel accepted in this. I was looking for a sense of integrity, grounding, dignity, centering, and calm. I wanted to be useful to people who came to me for help.

I have been consistently studying, practicing, integrating, and researching into many areas of psychology and psychotherapy since 1993. I am now 52, drawing on the experience of 30 years in marriage, raising and losing a daughter, raising a grandson, and accumulating more than 25 years of individual therapy, professional practice, and supervision. I have also been practicing Authentic Movement, therapeutic yoga, and dance for many years.

All of this experience informs my way of working as a somatic therapist, allowing me to move to the psychology of personality through the body, and from the body to the history of the person.

In the process of learning somatic psychology, I studied embryology, the movement and emotional development of the child, and the development, structure, and functioning of the body systems. This learning was acquired not only through literature, maps, and diagrams, but through my own experience of movement, touch, and imagination, and through the particular quality of the therapist's presence, who sees, hears, and feels as the witness in Authentic Movement practice does. Many years of training, therapy, supervision, and practice in this approach brought to my work a deep attention to the bodily processes occurring between myself and the client.

Touch has a special place in this practice: through touch and imagination, the somatic therapist can connect and interact with different systems of the body. But for this, it is also important for the therapist to be connected with herself, with her internal body systems, and through this connection to make contact with the client.

I perceive this method of therapy as a space for connection and exploration through **transference**, **counter-transference**, **somatic counter-transference**, and **resonance**.

When I am in the role of a somatic therapist, I notice my sensations, my tendencies to move in a specific way in contact with a specific client, and images that give rise to certain sensations and feelings in my body. I realize at this point that I may be identifying with some figure in the client's life or reacting in my own specific way to the client's material. Thus, I try to bring aspects of psychotherapy and psychoanalysis into somatic work.

Here, I see great benefit in being able to rely on my somatic counter-transference. Above all, it helps me to feel, learn, and empathize deeply with the personal history of a client, and to explore the relationships in his life. This happens through:

- paying attention to my own feelings, emotions, motor impulses, images, and associations in the process of long-term engagement with the client
- mirroring, observing, and witnessing the micro- and macro-movements of the client in the process of his verbal and non-verbal storytelling about himself

Chapter 13

- discerning my own body sensations and motor impulses in response to the client's movements
- differentiating sensations: detecting stresses and blocks, as well as areas of my body that feel resourced
- disclosure of movement that comes from the sensation; moving with the client – unfolding movements through amplification or deceleration
- tracking changes during sessions
- body interaction, touch.

Then we search to see how this self-exploration might help identify significant people from the client's life, and how this discovery can inform the process of the work.

Through all of the above, the somatic therapist has many opportunities to support the client, and to reveal his capabilities and resources through difficult moments in his life. This approach can be used in individual work, in group, marital, and child–parent therapy, and in training.

The client, with the right use of somatic resonance by the therapist, receives support, acceptance, understanding, and a feeling of "I am not alone," which is the basis for trust, for building a working alliance. He learns to recognize, accept, express, and regulate his feelings and bodily reactions. This gives a sense of self-respect and dignity, a support for building connection in his life.

Illustrating Theory with Practice

In this chapter I will briefly introduce some definitions. In the process of forming the theoretical part, I was particularly inspired by an article of Patricia Pallaro's, "Somatic Countertransference: The Therapist in the Relationship." For each definition I will give examples from my own practice, each of which will demonstrate the idea of somatic counter-transference through working with empathy, kinesthetic empathy, and resonance. Permission to publish the examples has been received from each client. All names have been changed.

The term **somatic counter-transference** contains a psychoanalytic concept: **counter-transference**, linked with the verb, to **transfer**.

Counter-transference

The term **counter-transference** was first introduced by Freud in 1910 as a by-product of his analysis of transference. He defines counter-transference as unconscious responses of a therapist to a patient that need to be identified and eliminated so that they do not interfere with treatment. It would take decades before the ideas of "mastery," "submission," and "taking control" were replaced by the idea of "using" counter-transference, and the ideal of cold objectivity and detached neutrality on the part of the analyst was replaced by more flexible and realistic ideas about the analytical position. Subsequently, this concept was supplemented with a description of the phenomena of projective identification and counter-identification.

R. Horacio Etchegoyen (1991) defines counter-transference as all the analyst's responses to the patient that occur within or outside of the analytical setting, but in the context of analytical relationships.

In a clinical situation, a projective identification is placed between the client and the therapist, and the therapist begins to experience either the client's experiences or the experiences of a significant person in the client's life. In this case, counter-transference allows you to access a client's experience that is unconscious, rejected, and inaccessible to verbalization.

The question is how the analyst allows himself to have an experience of the client's experience, digests it, formulates it, and reports it as interpretations. Selectively revealing your own counter-transference feelings can be valuable for therapy (cf. Pick 1985: 164–5).

Somatic counter-transference

In 1984, Penny Lewis Bernstein coined the term **somatic counter-transference** to define precisely the counter-transference reactions that occur at a bodily level. She noted the need for awareness and realization in the somatic unconscious of the patient, to help the patient in the process of integrating split-off parts of themselves, to disclose the resistances and defenses of the patient (Pallaro 2008: 9).

The process of counter-transference is now understood as something manifested in the therapist's ability to recognize and use the sensory (visual, auditory, tactile, kinesthetic) and affective qualities of the image that the patient generates in the therapist (Schore 1994).

Example from practice: 1

First session. I see a beautiful pregnant woman with a big smile and shining eyes, who wants to prepare for the birth of a child. She says it is hard to imagine being a mother yet. Now she enjoys actively communicating with people, dancing, a life full of activities. Life after birth seems scary. Elena says that she is very interested in psychology, attending training and groups. At one of the training sessions, according to her, "Behind the mask of happiness, I discovered a lot of insights."

(My internal process of analysis of the **counter-transference**, occurring as introspection and internal dialogue, appears in the text below in bold.)

I am immediately attracted by the phrase "the mask of happiness." I compare it with Elena's wide smile and feel tightness in my chest; it is difficult to breathe, I feel a tension in my stomach. I feel hurt. My first reaction – the interpretation of "devaluation of the feeling of happiness" – I decipher as a reaction of defense against attack; I feel fear. At this point, I finish building a picture of a possible conflict, where there is one who defends and one who attacks.

I wonder what is the essence of this attack, with whom is it terrible to experience happiness? Perhaps a bad interpretation from the coach on one of her "psychology clubs" that she likes to attend causes a reaction of wariness in our contact, which means that this can already manifest in the transfer to me as, for example, a possible condemning parent figure? I note these questions with lightning speed; they have yet to be answered in the course of our work in the future.

As a somatic therapist, I am attentive to how I organize myself somatically in the compression that I noticed at the beginning. I realize how I am contracting in the intercostal muscles, thereby squeezing the organs of the chest, squeezing the stomach with the movement of the chest slightly down and inwards; I am aware of the impulse to make a small backward movement with my head. I make this gesture with a micro-movement, almost in my imagination, and I am aware of the feeling of surprise, shock, and indignation. Perhaps these are the feelings that Elena stopped?

I also note memories from when I first went to a therapist. My child was 1½ years old at the time. I fell into the solution of my endless problems coming from the child being seriously ill. I'm experiencing misfortune, the bitterness of losing

the happiness that accompanies my contact with the child. I wonder how I can use this memory in a useful way for Elena.

I gently inform Elena that I want to support her in happiness, in the resource, before going anywhere. I suggest that she try to notice what she experiences in her body, in her breath. Elena replies that her breathing is shallow. I gently suggest that perhaps she is afraid, afraid to be happy. Elena says with a deep exhalation that she is afraid of losing happiness, that it is very important for her. I say that I want to support her in happiness.

Perhaps at this point I fall into the role of a mother. We have yet to reveal the essence of Elena's basic relationships with her parents together.

The bodily tension goes away with the exhalation. Elena sits in her chair more widely and freely, relaxes her muscles. The smile softens. Her cheeks turn pink. Elena is grateful for my humanity and depth. Together, we experience the depth of revelation, trust, and heart-to-heart contact.

Internally, I register and evaluate the somatic reaction: I feel relaxation in the muscles of my body, I stretch my spine up, I release my stomach from the pressure from above the chest, my nervous system comes into balance; I feel calmness, relaxation, warmth in my body and in contact. A good basis for building further long-term work. A good foundation for experiencing a healthy pregnancy.

Example 2

The therapeutic technique of **self-disclosure** supports the process of experiencing the client:

Catherine is 35 years old and has been in therapy with me for months. She is in a relationship with one man, but constantly remembers and thinks about the relationship she had before. There was love, betrayal, disappointment, loss of trust, separation. At the same time, there are regular meetings with her ex and hope remains. However, at this stage, it is not possible for her to be satisfied in any relationship or, generally, in any events in life. She either feels anger and resentment or seems only half-involved in life. She feels a lot of dissatisfaction with herself and her current partner. She cannot decide to marry him and have a child. She often thinks at such moments of the meaninglessness of life, of a dead end, of death. When she talks about it, she looks down to the right.

I empathize, feel myself going inside my body to the bridge of my nose. I think about the possibility of grieving. Suddenly I remember that in family therapy, when a member of the placement looks down, you need to check if there is a dead family member down there.

I ask: is there a loss that you have not overcome? I see the surprise on her face and then hear the confession: "dog." The most beloved creature in her life. Almost like the closest friend and child. She cries and tells me that she cannot forgive herself for putting her to sleep when she was sick. I am there for her, empathize, and support her feelings.

As I think about it, I also put my cat to sleep not so long ago. I feel despair, guilt, grief of loss. I feel a desire to cry, a heavy heart, something very unbearable. It is difficult to make your own decision, even if it is caused by objective reasons. Through my own experience, I feel sympathy, empathy for the feelings of Catherine. I decide to share my own experience in order to support her, to bring her out of the experience of loneliness and shame.

I tell Catherine about my own difficult choice and decision.

Catherine looks at me in surprise, smiles, and is grateful for my openness. There is a sense of connection, warmth, and open-heartedness between us. It becomes easier to breathe. Catherine says that the former partner is somewhat similar to this dog. And in general, she herself feels somewhat similar to this dog. Now there is an opportunity to find the new qualities of a dog in herself, come to an internal resource, and also more profoundly experience the grief of loss. The road is open to experiencing complex feelings. I make the assumption that, after a loss, it is scary to become attached again and make a life decision, and, perhaps, there are even deeper losses that affect today's life. Catherine agrees.

Empathy

By **empathy** we usually mean the ability of a person to put themself in the place of another. To experience empathy, it is vital to be able to live in the moment, to be able to switch from observing to participating (Pallaro 2008: 5). Victoria Stevens (2005: 9) thinks that communication between the patient and the analyst engages the right-hemisphere state of receptivity. It allows them to tune in empathically to the affective and bodily states of patients. This subsequently creates the opportunity for resonance or a moment of synchronicity between the analyst and the patient on an unconscious, pre-conscious, or conscious level

The recent discovery of "mirror neurons" shows that the ability to respond to and understand another person's emotional states is actually a function rooted in the body (Bauer 2009). The ability to mirror depends on the experience of parent–child relationships. It can be developed, through therapy, but might decrease during stress (Bauer 2009).

The empathic quality of the therapist is considered crucial in successful therapeutic relationships and interventions of any kind, no matter what theoretical approaches are used (Basch-Kahre 1984; Kaplan 1990; Kohut 1971; Winnicott 1958).

Example 3

I am approached by a mother with a request to resolve the conflict between her and her 6-year-old daughter. The mother is worried that she does not interact correctly with her daughter and that this might traumatize her. She feels powerless to cope with her own feelings and confusion. She feels offended by her husband, who, in her opinion, distances himself from these conflicts. At first, meetings are held only with the mother and child. Then the husband joins our sessions, with great resistance. As a result of the work, it is found that each of them experiences loneliness, misunderstanding, despair, anger, and resentment at the time of the conflict. My task is to help build a harmonious relationship in the family so that the family can feel the joy of being together, the pleasure of communicating with each other. Here, I will give an example of two sessions using somatic counter-transference in working with the family.

In the first of these sessions, we worked with the parents' relationship, applying **empathy and somatic counter-transference**:

> **Before the next regular session, I notice unbearable feelings of burnout, fear, powerlessness, the desire to cry. As if I am being pulled to the ground, weakness in my hands and feet. I want to sleep. Constriction in the stomach, heart.**

At the start of the session, the husband and wife look in different directions. Silence. The wife puts the paper handkerchiefs on the table. *[I recall my feelings before the session.]* I ask: "Are you getting ready to cry?" She immediately starts crying, complaining of powerlessness, feeling tired. *[Before the wife starts crying, I feel a lump in my throat. When she talks and cries, I feel relieved.]* I inform her of my reactions. She breathes out, continues to cry. She says she is not crying at home. She needs support.

> **At the same time, I feel heaviness in my chest, the feeling that the heart is drawn to the ground. I support myself by stretching my spine up. And I touch the ground with my feet, alternately rolling each foot from the heel to the toes and back again. I see that the husband also makes a movement with his feet. I realize that I am unconsciously mirroring him. Understanding that I support and empathize with the spouse through this movement brings me peace. After all, thanks to this movement, this situation is bearable for both me and him. It is interesting that I simultaneously resonate with both spouses, thereby supporting and uniting them in resolving the conflict.**

Externally, the situation is also changing. You can see how the contact changes on a non-verbal level. The husband turns to his wife at this moment, looks at her warmly; he leans slightly towards her, makes a wider gesture with his hands, as if embracing at a distance. The wife gradually calms down, slowly turns to him. There is a feeling of energy, warmth, care, tenderness in the field between them. I assess the results of the session as creating a good basis for mutual support between the parents.

In the next session, the work with the child–parent relationship continues, supported through the use of **somatic counter-transference**.

The session is attended by the same couple with their 6-year-old daughter. The girl first complains angrily about her mother, saying that her mother screams at her, then stamps on the floor, loudly banging her feet, attracting our attention. This causes irritation, anger in the parents and me. Then she comes to me, stands next to me, and starts crying. I put her on my lap. She begins to sob and says, looking at her parents, that she would cry forever because "no one pays attention to me." She really touches me with her words; the irritation goes away. I feel movement in my chest, my heart. I support her crying and worry, and this calms her down. I create a model for the mother to communicate with her daughter when the girl is upset. The mother at this point reports that she feels confused. At home, she would have interrupted her daughter's crying because she herself was forbidden to cry as a child. She says she could not have calmed her daughter down like that. "I believe you can," I say, and I feel confident about it.

[At this point, I remember the previous session with the parents, when the husband listened to his wife and expressed his willingness to support her in her experience.] I remind them of this. My reminder quickly changes the atmosphere in the room. I see the eyes turned to each other. In resonance, I feel the inclusion in contact, readiness, ability to communicate.

The next session begins in an atmosphere of joy, shared excitement, more contact, describing what mom and daughter sang on the way to me. Dad at the same time was nearby and smiled. The experience was of community, warmth, sharing experiences with each other.

Kinesthetic empathy

The term **kinesthetic empathy** means that the therapist physically embodies (reproduces, imitates, copies) states of feelings and motor qualities of the client, achieves self-awareness in this movement, and through this, understands the internal affective states of the client. At this first stage, the therapist may have images that are triggered by unconscious bodily responses. Imke Fiedler calls them "kinesthetic images" (1989). Fiedler describes the second "inclusion phase" by means of emerging associations (in motor, figurative, and verbal modality) associated with perceived bodily experience. In this second phase, as Fiedler understands it, a counter-transference reaction occurs because, through empathy, the therapist opens up more to unconscious processes and deeper internal sources.

Pallaro (2008: 9) said that there are specialists utilizing movement only during the sessions, and there are others using it [dance improvisation] afterwards, to understand their reaction in the session better and thus understand the client better. I would like to think that I belong to the latter.

Example 4

Kinesthetic image involves supporting a new quality through repetition of the movement and awareness of its meaning in the communication between husband and wife.

I see a husband-and-wife couple. The husband is a religious man. The wife accuses her husband of not meeting her expectations. They have no shared interests. She has hoped to grow closer to him, to his interests, to religion, to God, but there is no possibility; communication does not work out.

I empathize with the wife's experiences: frustration, despair, pain from lack of contact. I feel oppressed, depressed, desperate in the role of a wife. But I am in no hurry to voice my understanding to the wife, so as not to take her side. I am sure that the husband also needs support.

I ask the husband to show how he perceives God through movement. He begins to say that he experiences it as a dome around himself and makes movements with his arms stretched out over his head and to the sides. I interpret this movement as a sign of personal space.

When I repeat this movement after the husband, I feel the volume of space around me. These movements bring more mobility to my body, more liveliness. I slightly extend the movement to my whole body and feel a greater inclusion, a connection from the center, from the stomach to the heart, the head; a sense of connection of all body systems: bones, muscles, fluids, nervous system, organs ... Through this movement I have the opportunity to feel and understand the husband's need for greater expression, vitality, safety.

The wife says: "Now I understand why I can't come closer to you. You are protecting yourself from me by God." Then comes the work about their relationship, what the husband is protecting himself from. Themes of fear, defenselessness, vulnerability, confusion, and self-doubt come up. There is an opportunity to support the wife in voicing her feelings when there is not enough contact. There is a space for both, in which there is more trust, openness, understanding, calmness, and life.

Example 5

The following example illustrates working with **somatic counter-transference** through reproduction of the client's movement, in the child–parent relationship, after the session.

A mother and son with cerebral palsy come to the session. The child is 6 years old. He cannot sit, crawls only by rolling over to the side; movements of his hands and feet are limited. Because of spasticity, the legs are crossed and stretched out. However, the child looks me in the eye, smiles widely, and is in emotional contact. Mom shares her anxiety and annoyance: "When will he grow up and become serious like his peers!? Everyone is already so serious." She says that when he behaves like this, she loses hope for the child's further development.

At this moment, I feel confused, shocked, unable to change anything, desperate. At the somatic level, I feel a compression in the center of my chest; it is difficult to breathe. I feel the area of my heart and lungs. My words – that when a child smiles, it creates a positive background and a response of sympathy for him – have already been said more than once. I am feeling powerless, thinking that the mother and the son feel the same way.

My suggestion to the mother, to try experiencing the world like her son does, seems impossible at the moment. A few days later, I go to a group supervision session. The supervisor invites us to feel ourselves as a client, making the usual movements for the client. I decide to play the role of a happy child with cerebral palsy. I lie back on the floor. I strain my whole body (I move the muscles of my arms and legs to the bones, which creates a feeling of spasticity and numbness; I squeeze the muscles of my ribs to the organs inside, minimizing the movement of the diaphragm) and try to move with this tension. The result is very limited. I imagine that I always move like this, 24 hours a day, for several years. I feel horror, despair, lack of hope. I try to smile broadly, joyfully, expressively, like the boy does. In this moment I feel the joy of life, joy of movement, joy of the slightest change of position (I feel the extension in my upper torso, inside the head–neck–chest–diaphragm. An image of orange color, a feeling of warmth that fills and expands from top to bottom and is very soothing). Then I meet the serious, self-focused faces of my classmates in the roles of their clients. They look at me, turn away. I feel abandoned and alone. I focus on the smile and the joy. Strength comes from the heart, I feel openness, empathy for others, the ability to wait for the situation to change and see me. I open to a huge resource of joy and inspiration in my heart and the heart of this little person.

During the next session, I tell the child's mother about this discovery. She smiles, expresses gratitude for my involvement and understanding. She calms down for some time.

Resonance

Originally, the concept of resonance was a technical term and was normally used in physics. In scientific language, resonance is defined as the coincidence of the vibrational frequency of two or more objects, as a result of which they begin to "sound" synchronously.

The idea of resonance is also applied to human communication. When the sound of two subjects coincides, there is a resonance between them. This coincidence is expressed in an emotional uplift on both sides. If there is no match, then there is a dissonance with the loss of energy.

In psychology, there are many different concepts related to resonance. Joachim Bauer argues that "mirror neurons" are essentially the core of resonance (2009).

Drawing upon the work of David Boadella, Hartley writes:

"David Boadella (1980: 1) uses the terms interference and resonance to describe … different levels in the therapeutic relationship. For him, a resonance pattern is the natural state of bonding between the child and parent, or between two adults, when a healthy relationship allows energy to flow freely from the core of each person. Transference and countertransference are reflections of early interference patterns that arise when resonance is disturbed; the disturbance can be on the part of the client or the therapist, respectively. Transference and countertransference are seen as disturbances in bonding."

(Hartley 2004: 204)

Counter-transference in Somatic Therapy

Boadella uses Reich's three-level personality system, where the deepest essential layer expresses the true Self (core, authentic self) and creates the conditions for the establishment of resonance. The superficial "mask" layer, as a rule, expresses positive transference and countertransference, while the middle layer, the "shadow", expresses negative transference and countertransference. Boadella believes that therapy should "lead the client beyond the transference, both positive and negative" (Hartley 2004: 205), in order that the core can be touched and resonance recreated.

Example 6

Work can be done through the bodily reproduction of a **kinesthetic image** of the client. Body interaction and touch give an understanding of the process in the client's life: the search for resources and life solutions through the therapist's **kinesthetic empathy** and **resonance**.

John is 30 years old, raised by his mother since childhood; he does not know where his father is and what happened between his mother and father. He has been going to therapy for several years. John lives with a woman but cannot decide on marriage and the birth of a child. He perceives a woman's intention to get married as pressure.

At one session I ask him to tell me how and where the pressure is felt. He says, in the back area. I propose to become this pressure. He agrees.

I approach him from the back and begin to press my hands on the top of his back, first lightly, then with all my body weight, under the guidance of the client. At some moment I notice that I can barely keep my feet connected to the ground.

John bends under my weight and informs me that this situation is similar to his life.

I say that I feel great discomfort, uncertainty, fear of loss, tension, a sense of suspension, shame …

John says that what I am voicing is reminiscent of the experiences of the women in his life.

From the context of our work, I understand that these feelings and states are also John's feelings. But at the moment of this bodily exploration, he is in a different role, and I remain with this knowledge within me. Recognizing heavy feelings as your own is a separate part of the work.

I suggest that he find a way to change the situation physically (with his body).

He says, "I want to straighten up," and starts to do this.

I am glad. Then I stand steadily on my feet. I listen with my hands to the movement in John's back and accompany with my fingers a small movement in the area of his spine, back, torso – to the right–left, forward–backward.

John talks about the experience of freedom, joy, pleasure.

I feel a similar experience, as well as a sense of pride, self-respect, dignity. I feel strength in my feet, relaxation in the muscles of my shoulders, chest. I feel a great ability to expand my lungs and inhale–exhale fully, connectedness, calmness, balance at the level of the nervous, endocrine, and immune systems. I voice feelings that were not named by John (self-respect, dignity). John finds them a kind of discovery in himself: what he has yet to master and what he is interested in.

I assume that it will also be much easier for his girlfriend if he finds a way to "straighten out" their relationship: not to run away, but to stay and find another way of being in contact. John is ready to think about it.

Summary

In this chapter we briefly reviewed the following related terms: counter-transference, somatic counter-transference, empathy, kinesthetic empathy, resonance. They give us an understanding of the client's unconscious feelings and motives of behavior, and are used as a way of deepening awareness in the search for solutions to life's difficulties.

In the above examples, as a therapist I mirror the client, most often **consciously**, identify myself through imagination or movement with the client, empathically interact with him, resonate with his emotional and bodily experiences, verbalize or help the client to verbalize his consciousnesses and discoveries. I maintain communication, including through body contact and touch.

However, some of the examples above present elements of a counter-transference that are difficult to comprehend, corresponding to the concept of projective identification; they reflect the client's unconscious intrapsychic conflict that has been brought into the client–therapist relationship. The therapist **unconsciously** identifies with either the client's role or the role of a significant other in the client's life. In order not to act out this conflict but to deal with my own experiences in relationship with the client in a useful way, I, as a therapist, monitor my bodily and emotional reactions, analyze the way they are used in a session, and investigate it in supervision. This is done in order to process the emotional and somatic information received qualitatively in the counter-transference before bringing it into the client's therapeutic space. The task of the therapist here is to create a safe, accepting atmosphere, different from the usual environment in the client's life; to help the client find resources; and to accept their own rejected feelings, pain, and vulnerability.

Thus, in my understanding, a professionally honed capacity for empathy and resonance helps us to feel the somatic counter-transference, both positive and negative, and find a way through it into a state of warmth and contact. Here, it is possible to experience a deep understanding of the inner world of another, empathy and sympathy opening the way to further strengthening of trust, intimacy, and connection. This is what really heals pain, loneliness, and detachment from the world and others.

The ability of the therapist to notice and reveal, at the right time, their physical and emotional reactions allows the client to reach a deeper level of feelings, come into contact with rejected experiences, share and express them in relationships, expand the possibilities of contact, and improve their attitude towards life.

Nourishing Ourselves: A Somatic Approach Towards Deep Connection and Healing

14

Maren Hillert

Throughout my years as a teacher, through my work with clients as well as my own research, I came to see that a lot of us who live in highly developed industrial countries suffer from a neglect of high-quality self-nourishment (I use this term, widespread in the somatic field, in the sense of self-care and self-love). This alarming development affects people regardless of their professions, including managers as well as people working in social care and teaching, for example. As a result, the autonomic nervous system (ANS) is often out of balance, which can cause various physical and mental diseases. This can lead to suffering that is often reflected in financial loss. When people are not secure in their inner power and in their right place, following their own rhythm, the work they do and the life they lead is less effective, unfulfilling, and full of sadness. Burnout, depression, fear and anxiety, back pain, tinnitus, and maybe even stomach aches, heart attacks, and strokes might be some of the results of this imbalance.

As the parasympathetic state is a healing one, I focus a lot of my work as an Integrative Bodywork and Movement Therapist and Educator on balancing the ANS of my clients or students, seeking the balance between rest and activity, play and focused work. There are a lot of possibilities for working towards balance on the somatic path: for example, encouraging pure movement, inviting play in our lives; awakening all of our senses, sensing our bodies and moving outdoors, in nature; and connecting to the fluids of the body. Strengthening the early foundations of our human development, our relation to earth and gravity, early movement patterns, and, through this, the sense of self and inner coherence can cultivate feelings of safety and trust. All of these create a safe ground on which we as human beings can release, and then draw on to support our inner resources. Related to the start of our life as social beings, I have guided different research projects with groups of students and interested explorers. Some of them have been around the context of birth, perinatal, and postnatal issues. Others addressed the nourishing of the inner child and the development of a responsible, loving, and respectful inner parent. In this chapter, I want to share some moments of my work, focusing mainly on balancing the ANS.

I will show in the following text why placing the focus on the parasympathetic part of our ANS could be life-changing – and a good base for being able to take action in a calm and centered way. In my experience, this is also the basis for being able to create a loving relationship towards ourselves.

Preface

March 2020: Sitting at my desk, not knowing where exactly to begin, during a special time in which a virus moves the whole world and leads to unexpected measures and unknown possibilities. I will start by simply inviting you, the reader, to join me for a moment of entering into bodily awareness, after reading the next paragraph.

Let us start with an empty

SPACE

Now, I invite you on an experiential journey inside of your bodymind:

Chapter 14

Be aware of your sitting bones touching the surface you are sitting on; allow the weight of your upper body to drop down through your sit bones into the ground.

Breathe.

Release tension in your neck and shoulders, and let your arms hang heavy for a moment.

Take another breath in; rest a moment.

Allow the air inside of you to release out of your body again, while your spine lengthens towards the ceiling, and your head gently swings on top of your spine like a flower opening to the sun. Just sit there and observe the movements your breath creates inside your body for a few cycles of breathing.

Be aware of any thoughts or expectations about reading this chapter now – any bodily tensions or released areas. Just be aware, without trying to change.

Gently bring your awareness back to your body sensations – the ripples of movement through breathing in and out – without changing your way of breathing.

After a few minutes of sitting and breathing, take a bigger breath in, and when you are ready, open your eyes again.

Stretch out your arms or turn your head, allowing your upper body to follow into a spiral; repeat to the other side, if you wish.

After experiencing this short journey inside your body, I invite you to write down a word to express your sensations. Take a moment to reflect on your own experience:

How often are you aware of your breath, of your body, in everyday life?

How do you feel inside your body now? Ready to go on reading?

Below I share my own experience, sitting here and writing now:

After doing this exercise myself, I feel much more present, calm, and ready to jump into the unknown: writing a chapter for a book about collected material and experiences of Integrative Bodywork and Movement Therapy (IBMT). I have the sensation that a lot of the weight of my upper trunk drops down into my hip bones and sitting bones, and some of the tension in my neck area loosens at the same time. My breath calms down and my thoughts become clearer. I have a feeling of groundedness, from where it is much easier to start and to focus my prior wild, jumping thoughts.

In my training with Linda Hartley, more than 20 years ago, we started nearly every day sitting in a circle and being guided into clear body awareness. I appreciate the many aspects of this ritual: the connection to the ground which carries us, the connection to our body, the connection to surrounding space and inside space through the simple exchange of air, the possibility of coming to rest inside of the body, even if thoughts are still running. We can always come back to the breath and witness the fine movements of our ribcage or belly. Through breathing and sensing the ground beneath us, we can also gain a sense of safety and calm through our whole system. With more and more training, our thoughts and emotions will calm down as well. This is one way to enter the parasympathetic state, one branch of the ANS, and through consciously resting here we can support the recreation of a healthy inner coherence.

Developing an inner witness during a phase of sitting in stillness, being aware of our bodily sensations and tracking our thoughts and emotions, is generally refreshing for every human being. But especially if one is suffering from frequent experiences of dissociation, which can be felt as the inability to sense certain parts of the body or as a sensation of not really touching the ground, breathing, sensing one's body, and seeing the environment clearly are the basic tools to heal frozen and fragmented parts of ourselves caused by earlier traumatic experiences. Entering into the parasympathetic state can be very supportive of recovery and is often the first and most effective step towards healing most kinds of physical or mental imbalance. In the following section, I will briefly explain the mechanism and influence of our ANS on our bodymind entity.

Encouraging a Parasympathetic State

Most of the work I do in somatic classes aims to establish a more parasympathetic state. This means a more inner-focused, process-oriented, sensing, and feeling state, as opposed to a state of outwardly oriented action. The parasympathetic state can be considered a state of rest or relaxation, a state of refreshing the bodymind system – creating an open, wide view. Often perceived as a state of digestion, the parasympathetic state brings our tissues, as well as our minds, into a receptive place. For a lot of people, being in such a state creates feelings of calmness, joy, and trust, of safety and home, sometimes even of satisfaction, wellbeing, and happiness.

A Short Overview of the Autonomic Nervous System

Fortunately, the ANS works involuntarily, as the name describes. We do not need to think about how much more blood is required during muscular activity or focused mental work. Our ANS automatically supplies the right amount of blood to the part of our body which needs it at that very moment. In the case of increased mental or physical activity, the ANS activates a response in the sympathetic branch. When we are at rest, after eating or sleeping, the ANS will activate the other branch, the parasympathetic nervous system. Both branches of the ANS are in charge at all times, but one is usually the active player in the foreground. Our ANS at all times controls our breathing, heartbeat frequency, blood circulation, digestion, metabolism, and excretion activity, as well as our body temperature and energy balance. It stimulates the striated heart muscles and most gland activity, as well as the smooth muscles inside of all organs. The ANS is subdivided into the sympathetic, parasympathetic, and enteric nervous system. The sympathetic and parasympathetic branches act antagonistically, as described earlier. The enteric nervous system, as a third part of the ANS, was discovered later than the other two branches. Known as "belly brain" to some people, the enteric nervous system has an effect on the whole of the gastrointestinal tract as an independent part, but its function is influenced by sympathetic as well as parasympathetic activity. Our digestive tract functions and sorts out a lot of important information, for our body as well as for our mind. If we train ourselves, we might listen and benefit from this information. Our belly often shows clear signs of a need for rest, even if our mentally directed will has plans for focused activity. For our long-term health we would benefit greatly if we listened more often to the wisdom of our belly.

The following overview is inspired and adapted from the book *Sensing, Feeling, and Action* by Bonnie Bainbridge-Cohen (2008: 177), combined with experiences from my own practice.

Chapter 14

Sympathetic characteristics

- Nerves originate in the thoracic and lumbar spine area (thoracolumbar chain of ganglia).
- Breathing and heartbeat frequency rise, bronchial tubes widen, more oxygen is provided, and peristaltic movements of the intestines slow down.
- Blood flows directly towards the skeletal muscles and into the periphery of the body; blood pressure rises.
- The whole body is in a "state of alertness and activity, awake and stimulated" (Bainbridge Cohen 2008: 177).
- Energy is ready to be used: the eyes are fully activated and focused outwardly; there is orientation towards fulfilling goals.
- Expanding and stretching of the whole body, and push and reach patterns (as in the early Developmental Movement Patterns), can support a sympathetic state; active fingertips and toes and open eyes lend their support.
- Embodying the arterial blood flow and its staccato rhythm can bring us into a sympathetic quality of movement.
- In my experience, sympathetic activity can give us a feeling of easy flow, strength, focus, clarity, and readiness.

Parasympathetic characteristics

- Nerves originate in the brainstem and sacrum. 75% of all parasympathetic nerves come from the brainstem; so does the nerve vagus.
- Blood flows mainly to the digestive tract and organs; the blood pressure lowers.
- "State of rest and recuperation, eating and sleeping, storage of energy."
- "Inner focus, self-orientation," process-oriented (Bainbridge Cohen 2008: 177).
- Condensing and folding in the body, and yielding into the ground invite a parasympathetic state.
- Embodying the flow of venous blood, cerebrospinal fluid, or cellular fluid can bring us into more of a parasympathetic frame of mind.
- In my experience, the parasympathetic state creates a feeling of satiety, fullness, being nourished, and deep release.

Alternating focused and unfocused work or states – Doing and Being – as well as movement and stillness, counter-balances our ANS in a very healthy way. We all know how difficult this is in a goal-oriented society, but it is possible to create such a structure in which activity and rest mutually influence each other. We are able to learn to be more aware of when our ANS is out of balance, and how we can rebalance this system, to heal ourselves. At the end of this chapter, I will propose an experiment to explore your own rhythm of rest and activity.

When we are in a calm, parasympathetic state, which feeds nerves and organs, it is much easier for our nervous system, fluids, and other tissues in our body to reorganize, to reach for balance, as every cell and every tissue naturally do throughout all of their lifespan. For example, if the tissues of our body are hurt, certain bodily fluids and other helpers like white blood cells (depending on the injury) regenerate and heal us. Healing is more effective when we are able to give time for the bodies' inherent "tissue repair." In craniosacral lectures, I have learned that, even with a severe injury, the rhythm of the ground substance – a fluid in our body – remains healthy. In craniosacral terms, we speak of the "long tide."

This long tide has the ability to regenerate our damaged cells so that the human being can fully regenerate again (Seitz 2015).

Charles Ridley speaks of "primary respiration" (Ridley 2006: 79, 83-7). I wonder if the "drone", which Bonnie Bainbridge Cohen perceives as "some essence that is us" as part of the ANS, could be compared to the "long tide" mentioned in Craniosacral Therapy and also to the "primary respiration" in Bioenergetics. Bainbridge Cohen describes "the drone as cellular-based and relating to the enteric and parasympathetic nervous systems in terms of the ground. As such, it is the background or baseline nerve tone throughout the body, deeper than physiological tone" (Bainbridge Cohen 2008: 178).

Much healing would take place if we, as human beings, would allow – or better, actively balance – our daily structure into clear phases of activity and rest. Phases of activity or focused attention – *Doing* – require short phases of unfocused relaxation or rest – *Being*. This rhythm of alternating from activity to rest can be created most easily by giving ourselves a break. For people who feel that they are beginners in terms of sensing their own needs clearly, I recommend the following (approximate) timings: take a break of 5 minutes *Being* after 45 minutes *Doing* (high-concentration forebrain work or another activity); or 25 minutes *Being* after 90 minutes *Doing*. This can be a first step on the way to supporting healthy balance of the ANS.

Different Qualities of Rest and Recuperation

Above, I mentioned that there are different qualities of rest. If we are looking for rest and recuperation, we often think first of sleep, or maybe some of us take a break to have a coffee, candy, or cigarette, take a short look at our smartphone (which often ends up being much longer), play a game on the screen, or watch a film. If you do not feel refreshed and inspired by doing this, I invite you to make a list of your favorite activities where you do experience a deep and relaxing state, including a feeling of recuperation and maybe a desire for activity afterwards. The quality and the rhythm of our breaks from concentrated work or activity influence a well-balanced ANS enormously, and with it our wellbeing.

Below are some possibilities which bring me easily into a parasympathetic state and contribute to rebalancing the ANS. See if you feel inspired by any of these, or feel free to replace what is missing for you personally:

1. **Sleeping** regularly.
2. **Sensing** the body, **breathing**.
3. Having **short breaks** between focused work.
4. **Touch**: cuddling with loved ones or receiving a massage.
5. Integrating **silence**/meditation/contemplation as a daily ritual.
6. **Playing with visualization or memories**: imagine sitting next to a flock of sheep and listening to the sound of their chewing, or sitting by a fireside and listening to the crackling sounds, gazing into the flames.
7. **Contemplative activities**: gardening or being in nature, observing a snowflake dancing to earth, or looking at the ornaments of a mandala, or into the depth of a flower or a piece of art for a while. Take a barefoot walk in the woods or a bike ride along the riverside, swim in a silent lake, or walk in a huge park.
8. Allowing my **creative side** to blossom: painting just for fun, writing, knitting a small and colorful unnecessary thing, cooking with my favorite spices, playing guitar, repeating newly learned picking patterns on

the guitar, or just simply singing or humming my favorite song.

And again: which are your favorite ways to relax and recuperate? I invite you to write down at least three of them here and now:

____

____

____

You may observe what happens if you integrate some "personal refreshers" or inspiring contemplative states into your daily life. As you certainly already have experienced for yourself, a lot of different activities besides sleep can create a restful and refreshing state.

Excursion: Key Methods and Tools for Somatic Movement Educators and Therapists

In the following section, I will share some methods and tools which I use in my somatic-based work with clients and students. I find that they calm down the whole bodymind system, which, in my experience, usually invites a parasympathetic state. I include a first but very important step: the preparation before starting work with a group or with an individual.

Creating a safe and trustful environment

- Creating a safe (and, to me, holy) space before starting to work. This includes a clear and tidy space, plus simple rituals, repeated each session: clearing the inner space by centering myself through meditation before the session begins and preparing the outer space (with flowers, candlelight, cushions, or whatever creates an inviting, safe environment).
- Being there as a therapist in full authenticity.
- Offering myself as a person with open heart and full trust into the goodness, multiple abilities, and choices of my students or clients. Being open to listen and resonate with what I hear. The state of "beginner's mind" often supports me: being open and curious about all that will arise or want to be expressed by my clients.
- Holding space and giving time – a lot of time; being fully present and patient for whatever wants to show up. A lot of the work as a somatic-oriented body therapist is to offer an open, patient, and trustful space, and to witness the development of the client, encouraging her at all times to access her own inner wisdom.
- Entering the work with empathy and compassion, non-judgmentally. Staying open to the unknown, as well as to the diverse possibilities for each person in every encounter.
- Looking for and feeling the potential and talents in others, which are sometimes hidden, while trusting and staying connected to my intuition.
- When working with touch: listening and fully sensing the other's bodymind beforehand. I stay connected to my own bodymind and give space to the person to sense and feel herself. Listening with my full skin and all cells, fully embodied. Checking in from time to time with my client to see how she is feeling. I may ask myself – or her – if there is any need to change the quality of my touch or the place I am touching.
- In cases of strong trauma, touch might not be the method of choice and is sometimes contraindicated. (Touch in therapy with

traumatized clients will be explored in Chapter 15.) I will always stay in contact with a client: sometimes in verbal dialogue, and sometimes by using other tools such as body dialogue, guided body journeys, writing, painting, and other methods.

Strenghtening the inner base, creating a feeling of safety and stability

- Creating a strong and welcoming container through offering a clear outer framework, including rituals and repetitions (such as opening circle, meditation, movement, sharing, exploration, clear beginning and end); this is an important step that I always take, whether working with individuals or groups.
- Teaching precise body awareness through different exercises (including guided journeys); movement and stillness on the ground; exploring the skin through rolling or self-touch; becoming familiar with and exploring the most earth-like structure inside the body – the bones.
- Developing a trusting and delicious relationship to the ground (including exercises to become aware of gravity and anti-gravity, such as body journeys; rolling or being rolled; leaning towards walls, balls, bodies).
- Working with and strengthening our early ground, seen from an evolutionary perspective as well as from our ontogenesis: embodying a cell, an ameba, a sea star, and so on, and exploring the movement patterns we create in each of these animal-like states.
- Re-embodying early developmental movement patterns, which ideally all of us practiced *in utero* as well as after birth as little babies till we could walk and talk, so that we are able to create new pathways and connections between body and brain via nerve cell connections (as described in previous chapters). These new pathways allow fresh possibilities for movement and behavior, allowing us to respond differently. This works well if the early movement patterns are repeated daily by the adult client for a few weeks. (For more information about this method of repatterning and some exercises, I recommend the first few chapters of *Wisdom of the Body Moving*; Hartley 1995.)
- Alternating the use of words, music, anatomical images, tissues, scarves, walls, balls, or other suitable material to support the aquisition of the learned material.

Tools to Invite Students or Clients into a Parasympathetic State of Relaxation and Recovery

As mentioned earlier, I spend most of my time as a therapist inviting my clients into a parasympathetic state, as the majority feel imbalanced in their lives. Many of them experience burnout, deep depressions, or post-traumatic stress symptoms, and with this a loss of joy for life. Symptoms are expressed in different ways: some clients are not able to sleep properly or are not aware of hunger, thirst, or the need to go to the toilet. Others feel numb for shorter or longer periods in their lives and/or are not aware of their needs. Many lose their sense of pleasure or even interest in life completely, and with this the ability to create visions for their future. In those phases, nourishment is urgently needed.

I described earlier how rest can be one way to nourish and rebalance our nervous system, but often sleep is not available in such a phase of imbalance. Quite the opposite, there is too much poor-quality sleep, which does not lead to a feeling of recharging one's batteries.

Chapter 14

Many clients respond positively to play or touch, as well as to the creation of a special time and space for releasing all felt and sensed pressure from their daily lives. This can be a starting point for change, towards deep inner connection and also different behavioral possibilities in daily life. This is why I use all of my skills as a creative dance educator and a somatic movement therapist: I propose different approaches, depending on each client.

Pure movement

I use movement, pure bodily activation, for a few minutes, which activates the muscular system and the circulation: simple running, ball games, and fast shaking movements of body parts, to name a few. When humans move without thinking and without aiming for any goal, their brains and nerves usually relax and take time out from thinking and worrying very quickly, effectively, and easily.

Stillness

After activation through pure movement, the client is often open to standing, sitting, or lying down in stillness. In that state, I guide my client through breathing and inner body awareness, and – after some time – towards witnessing their emotions. Afterwards, I invite them to feel the outer environment, nearby and further away (maybe hearing sounds from outdoors).

I might lead some clients into slow movement, often guiding them into early movement patterns. To others I would offer touch to calm down their system and to bring their awareness towards cellular breathing, experienced in their own bodies. I support this through a guided journey or through direct touch.

Spontaneous painting or writing as creative tools

After having worked with movement, touch, or stillness, I sometimes offer colorful pens and big, empty sheets of paper to give time for "digestion" and integration of the experience.

We use spontaneous painting in IBMT to support the integration of embodied experience,

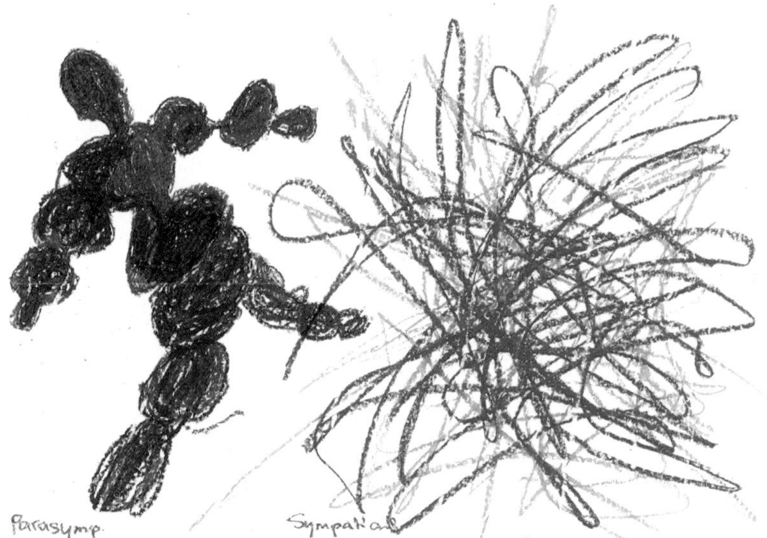

Example of a spontaneous painting made after moving with sympathetic and parasympathetic nerves, 2000. Colors in the original: left side blue and dark green, right side red–orange. Painting by Maren Hillert

without the goal of creating anything beautiful or meaningful. The act of painting rather serves as a bridge, a kind of transformational space from bodily, unconscious experiencing into more and more conscious reflection. Painting used in this immediate way can help foster the ability to share verbally with a partner later about one's bodily experience.

Senses

Another tool I often use is working with the senses, starting with the mother of the senses, which is touch or being touched (Juhan 1992: 109f.; Bainbridge Cohen 2008: 106–7). I guide clients towards an awareness of their own skin by touching different surfaces, learning to discern being touched by tissues, clothes, or the floor, curtains, or walls of the space. I might add self-touch and sometimes being touched by me as a therapist. The journey into perceiving the outer and inner surfaces of our body, through becoming aware of our skin, can provide a sense of self, of coherence. This can strengthen the sense of one's boundaries in relation to the outer world – the environment, as well as people.

I adapt the way I work with touch, according to the needs of each client: sometimes it is more playful, and sometimes I include objects to explore. I may work with or without music, with more or less movement, with self-touch or touch provided by me.

Other senses that I use to bring clients into the parasympathetic state are hearing, smelling, seeing, and sometimes taste also. I offer music to listen to or different sounds to hear. I invite them to smell different scents or imagine different smells from the memory of environments or objects they have loved, or not liked very much, throughout their lives.

Working with the senses facilitates a direct connection to the present moment. It also helps individuals to discover their likes or dislikes, through gestures of reaching towards or away from a sensory stimulus, such as a smell or a sound. These reactions, if invited and fully allowed, can recover a sense of clarity and boundaries in relation to what we want to have near to us and what we want to avoid. This ability to discern in a bodily rooted way supports us to sense our deep inner needs.

Being connected to our needs sets the base for expressing them as a second step. Self-expression and modulated communication could fill a whole new chapter. In this chapter, however, we are looking at preparing the ground for expression: feeling safe in our bodies and being aware of our own true needs in order to fulfill them in the next step.

Fluids

The embodiment of certain fluids is also a strong way to enter into the parasympathetic state. Usually, I choose between some of the slower-moving fluids (venous blood, lymphatic fluid, cerebrospinal fluid) or those you can find spread throughout the whole body, such as intercellular fluid, connective tissue, or even the very calming fluid inside a cell. Embodying the latter creates in most people a feeling of being – simply being. In some moments of life, this simple fact, **being** felt deeply rooted inside of our body, can feel revolutionary, refreshing, reaffirming. It is a little bit like a fully embodied "yes" to living. Bainbridge Cohen says about cellular awareness: "nothing to do, nowhere to go – home" (Bainbridge Cohen 2008: 70). And often this is the sensation, combined with the emotion evoked by embodying cells or being touched by the awareness of cellular breathing.

Working with the fluids can calm people down. Simply communicating the image that our central nervous system is bathed in an ocean-like fluid, the cerebrospinal fluid, might have the power to release a human being's whole system. Sometimes, I also lead my clients or students into embodying the fat

Chapter 14

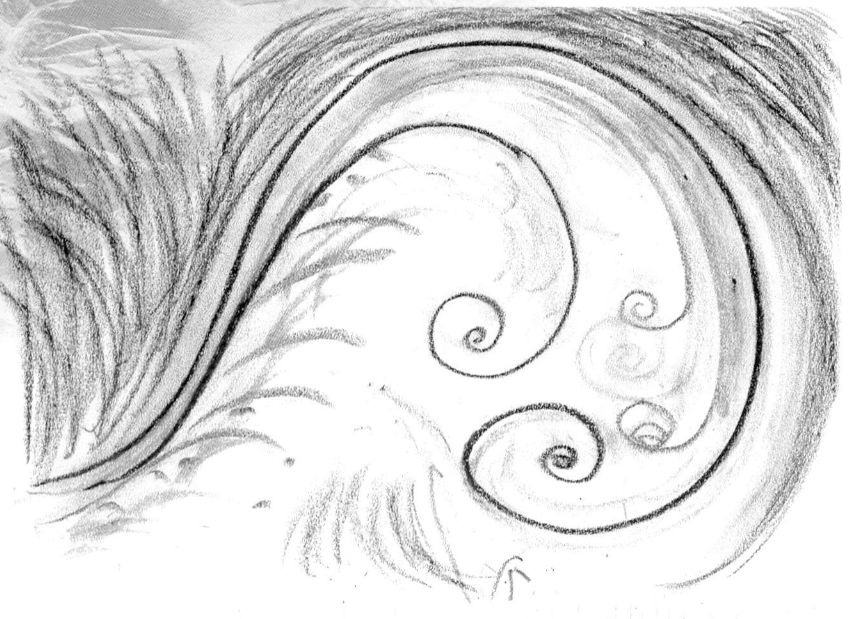

Spontaneous painting after a session with a client, using cellular breathing and intercellular fluid in movement and touch. Painting by Maren Hillert

beneath their skin – such a delicious golden coat, enveloping our whole body. This often creates a strong feeling of release, joy, and a feeling of being wrapped up, cosy and safe. A good relationship to their body fat also has the power to calm down nervous people and create a feeling of comfort.

Contacting, connecting to, and embodying the fluids inherent in our bodies: from intercellular to cellular fluid, from continuous lymph flow to pulsating blood flow, from different rhythms to stillness, from gel-like connective tissue or fat to the light flow of cerebrospinal fluid – this can be a gateway to more connectedness and a great support for contact and communication with others in an easier and more comfortable way. It gives some people a deep feeling of relief and, with this, more comfort in being able to lean back and relax.

Nature

An immediate possibility to nourish the parasympathetic state is walking, moving, or simply being in the natural environment. This can help build a healthy connection between one's inner and outer environment. I sometimes offer somatic walks in parks or courses in a still, fresh natural environment. My experience is that somatic-based work is greatly supported when courses take place out of town, in the countryside. I also love to work in and with nature, with different textures and materials found outdoors. I enjoy leading groups exploring the fluids near to rivers, lakes, or even the sea. In my experience, students embody the fluids inside their bodies more easily and connect immediately to the fluids outdoors. With this experience, they easily feel how near their own body is to the natural material of which the earth is made. As humans, we all breathe the same elements in and out; we connect to the trees as well as to sand, stones, or water, as most of the molecules we find in nature are inherent in our own bodies. This deeply felt awareness often creates a deep gratitude for life – our own, as well as that of all creatures in this world – humans and animals, as well as plants and minerals. It offers a base from which to honor and treat ourselves and our surroundings with respect and love.

Sound

Sound can provide further access to hidden places in the body, and I sometimes use it in my sessions. The vibration of sounds inside of the body is often experienced by clients as soothing or reassuring. I love to hum into certain tissues and invite people to use their voice to create vibrations in different areas of the body or to achieve inner touch through sounds. Creating soundscapes through the human voice has a calming and sometimes even healing effect on people.

Importance of Body Awareness

People who listen with an awareness of information coming from their body are at an advantage on the journey of balancing their nervous system and creating a healthy lifestyle. Cultivating a compassionate awareness and connection to our bodies is, however, within everyone's reach, as it is something we can train for.

When we are connected to our instincts and bodily needs, they usually direct us to what we would like to do (or rather not do right now). Following our inner felt rhythm can establish a healthy body–mind continuum and joy, satisfaction, and peace.

A Practical Experiment to Balance Your Autonomic Nervous System

An experiment in how to create a fulfilling work/life balance

Be aware of the rise and fall of your concentration. Follow immediately the needs that your body clearly announces: signs of tiredness, boredom, numbness, pain, and so on.

Immediately take a break from your screen if you are aware that your concentration is fading. Switch to some less focused work for a moment, maybe folding your freshly washed clothes, washing the dishes, looking out of the window, singing a song, whistling, playing guitar – whatever feels easy, nourishing, and non-focused to you.

Train yourself to be aware of the longing or satisfaction of your bodymind for resting, playing, reading, listening to good music, walking (barefoot), sleeping, silence, recovering, gardening, making music, painting, writing poems, crafting, or pottering.

Allow one or more of these things to happen as soon as you sense the desire.

Can you imagine how this would feel?

How much energy is lost just because you do not follow your own rhythm or deny your inner needs? How much life energy, joy, and creativity would be released if you followed your bodily sensations and came from there into action?

I invite you to try, for one whole day, to follow your very own needs. Why not start this project tomorrow or the next free weekend you have? If you do this experiment, you might start by marking a day in your calendar. One proposal for this first day is to switch off your smartphone, telephone, and internet, at least for the first few hours. See what comes up inside of you without being online. You can consciously choose online times for one such experiment, and choose to be completely offline in a second experiment. Observe the difference.

What nourishes you more at each moment?

Be attentive and ask yourself:

- When are my needs nourished completely? For example, after having listened to your favorite music, lying in your bed for half a day. When does the moment come that you feel: I am nourished, I am happy, I am energized?

Chapter 14

- When does a new need show up?
- Do you perceive a turning point sometimes: a point when you maybe feel bored and a wish arises to leave your bed? Perhaps you perceive a desire for movement, work, or contact, a need for a concentrated talk with somebody, or a wish to create a sculpture, write a text or a song, build a new cupboard, or whatever comes up?

Most of us rarely experience a joyful balance between rest and activity. Can you imagine what might happen if you lived like this?

I am a messenger of this vision: more and more people around the whole globe with a well-balanced autonomic nervous system. I love to serve this goal; it is a way towards a higher life energy for all humans, full of vitality and joy, creativity, peace, and satisfaction.

Part 5

Therapeutic Applications 2: Working with Trauma

Somatic Bodywork and Movement Approaches to Trauma

15

Jane Okondo

Emotional intelligence is only part of the story. The big other part is about the body's sensibility, what we can learn from our bodies, what kind of messages it holds. The body holds a tremendous amount of wisdom, not just for healing from trauma, but tremendous wisdom, because when we connect to our visceral self, to our primary instinctual centres, we connect with source.

LaPierre 2020: 22

I first tasted working directly with somatic practice and trauma at a workshop after the Breath of Life conference in London in 2009. The participant receiving the session came to a moment where bound-up energy that had been held in the muscles of her right arm since she was a teenager, healthy aggression, began releasing as diffusion of heat and shaking. I felt what I can only describe as my body becoming more liquid, a wave moving through my body. I was sitting in a room full of biodynamic craniosacral therapists, so I was not surprised to feel the release of a fluid wave. Still, I was very impressed by the insight that, as one person releases and integrates trauma, this has a ripple effect, allowing a deeper settling in others too.

Since then, I have integrated somatic movement and touch into my work with trauma as an Integrative Bodywork and Movement Therapist and a Somatic Experiencing® Practitioner, and will describe in this chapter an interplay that weaves between these and other practices. Drawing from my private practice, I will offer examples of working with individuals that illustrate how I work with somatic movement, bodywork, and trauma.

A Core Practice: Working with Counter-vortex and Trauma Vortex

One of the main principles of Somatic Experiencing, developed by Peter Levine, is working with the counter-vortex in relationship to the trauma vortex.

With trauma, a rush of arousal energy beyond our control occurs, creating what is called a trauma vortex, which is outside our everyday life experience. At the same time, the potential for a counter-vortex is formed.

In an interview with Dr Aline LaPierre (2020), Levine talked about seeing a symbol of two vortices moving in opposite directions in a profound dream. He spoke about connecting to ancient wisdom and bringing it into a Western scientific way of looking at things. I enjoyed hearing him name how Somatic Experiencing is based on connecting to our lifestream energy, as this resonates with my

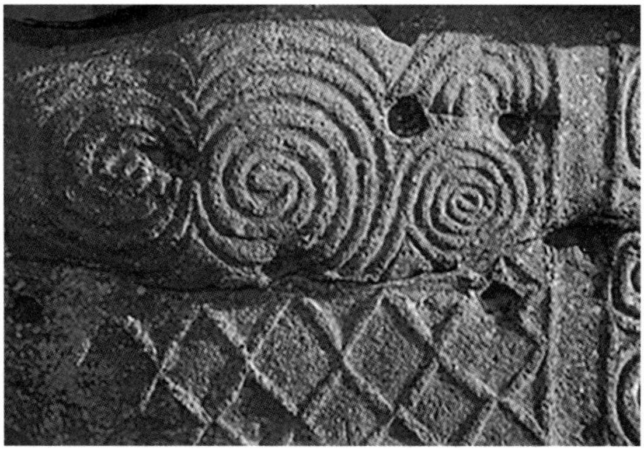

Neolithic stone spiral. Image ID: 108000095. Pytyczech | Dreamstime.com

Chapter 15

experience of the work we offer in Integrative Bodywork and Movement Therapy (IBMT).

In renegotiating with the trauma and counter-vortex, developing an ability to hold dual awareness becomes essential. Being able to maintain a sense of the underlying stability of the counter-vortex, while simultaneously experiencing the disturbance and activation of the trauma vortex, allows the possibility of working somatically. The more one can build a counter-vortex, the more the potential capacity to manage activation without becoming overwhelmed occurs. It is in the meeting of these two vortices that the energy bound in the body systems can begin to release back into the flow and motility of the body systems.

When I was training in IBMT, I had some extraordinary experiences that expressed this connection. During a weekend on pre- and perinatal development we were revisiting pre-spinal and spinal movement patterns, coming from the more fluid to the gravitational environment to meet the underlying motility of this deep instinctual knowing that lives in each of us. As we moved, we awakened the potential of inhabiting these gestures that live deep in our biological intelligence. This experience, which I connected to through the movement, emerged into my awareness as something experienced through interoceptive attention, where it is possible to receive our own meaning.

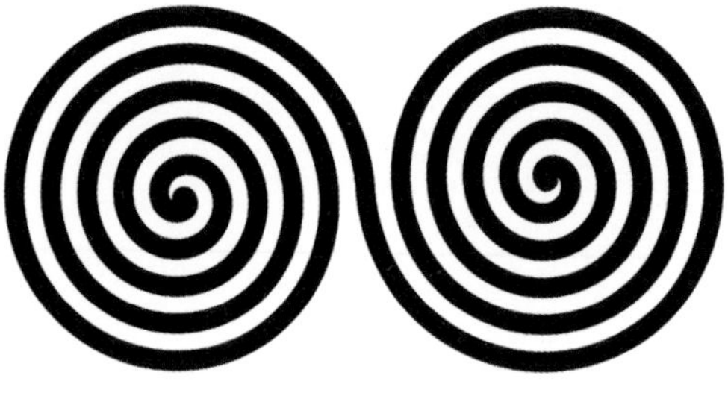

Flow of trauma and counter-vortex. Image ID: 108494918. Zina Seletskaya | Dreamstime.com

On this weekend, as I traversed these movement patterns with the support of a partner, a strong impulse to gaze at them arose. My eyes unflinchingly wanted to lock on to their gaze. This impulse continued after the weekend, my eyes taking in others without blinking, especially those close to me.

What emerged was an insight that, at my birth, there was a concern as to whether I would survive. I could feel my eyes releasing the shock at witnessing fear in those who I gazed at in the moments after I was born. It was as though my eyes were utterly thirsty for taking in and absorbing a deeper connection. I could feel this instinctual urge to bond, to receive a transmission. It was such an extraordinary experience and let me taste how profound somatic movement work is in touching into our deep body wisdom. On reflection, I understand that I was working with the counter-vortex in connecting to the more profound resource that could be accessed in embodying pre-vertebrate patterns. I was able to renegotiate the energy that was bound in my eyes.

The Relevance of Somatic Orientation in Trauma

The somatic practice and theory of IBMT increase our ability to expand our resiliency, and our ability to be present through becoming aware of and learning to follow our internal embodied process. We include studying movement *in utero*, through birth, and through the first few years of an infant's life, moving from a gravitational fluid environment into a land-based one, and learning how we coordinate our movements and find ways of rising up from the ground into crawling and eventually standing. These organizational movement patterns allow us to orientate to the environment, and shape how we take in information through our senses. We begin to create a map of our world through these bodily senses.

Somatic Bodywork and Movement in Trauma

The first learning takes place in the womb, primarily through physical sensation, and at this stage body and psyche are not yet differentiated. Here the wisdom of the body begins to develop, first through the simple and direct knowing of the cell, then through the complex sensitivity of the nervous system.

Even in the watery environment of the womb, the cells are learning about their place on earth through the sensation of the pull of earth's gravity acting upon them.

(Hartley 1995:16)

In utero, the skin is stimulated by the amniotic fluid, and this is part of the development of our autonomic nervous system. The skin and nervous system both derive from the ectoderm layer in the embryo, and in somatic bodywork we consider that when we are touching the skin, we are also in contact with the central nervous system.

Our vestibular system is one of the earliest structures to develop *in utero*, and as it does, so does our ability to recognize our environment. The foundation of spatial orientation and understanding of our self in relationship to environment arises as our senses are continuously working and assessing where we are. After birth, our nervous system organizes itself from stimuli sent to the brain by the sensory receptors in the skin, joints, muscles, and viscera via the spinal cord where the stimuli are processed. Motor neurons in the brain then send impulses back through the spinal cord to the peripheral muscles.

Our ability to orient to our environment is essential to us as we move through our lives; it is helpful to remember that, as we explore the nervous system, we are sensing through the same body system whose role it is to discern the inner landscape of our body and its relationship to the outer environment. With trauma, this ability to sense into our soma is often disrupted and the resulting disorientation creates dysregulation in our nervous system.

If we consider what this means when we explore the relationship between somatic movement and trauma, Peter Levine's description becomes highly relevant. He describes trauma not as the event itself but as the experience that is left in the body.

When we have an experience that is more than we can process physically, emotionally, and mentally, we have to find a way to adapt or to process the experience. When the experience is beyond our capacity to process, the activation has no way of moving through us and gets bound within our muscles, viscera, and joints – within our entire physicality.

The Embodiment of Body Systems as a Foundation for Coherency

If we look at this from a bodywork or somatic movement perspective, what we begin to perceive is a dysregulation that travels through the central and autonomic nervous systems and leads to a lack of coherency between the different body systems. One body system, such as the respiratory system, can no longer coordinate with another – the vascular system, for example. Or maybe the diaphragm below the lungs stays contracted, and so the breathing and heartbeat lose their ability to be adaptable. If muscles remain braced, the coherency is interrupted and the body is not able to self-regulate.

Where the body systems are coherent, we can respond to different life experiences with variation and ease. Indicators of coherency include the relationship of breath to muscle tension, the connection of breath to heart rate, the link of breath to blood volume change, thermo-regulation, and heart rate variability.

In IBMT, we include the work of Bonnie Bainbridge Cohen and her life-long enquiry into how the mind is expressed through the body in movement. We explore each of the different body systems in detail. Bainbridge Cohen often describes connecting to the "mind" of each of the body systems through a kinesthetic enquiry, where the information of the anatomy is experienced directly.

As we explore each different body system through experiential anatomy, movement, inner body dialogues, and gestures, we build a relationship with our body that comes through our visceral experience, rooted in our proprioceptive and interoceptive awareness.

Trauma can result in the loss of this felt sense. We sometimes become over-sensitized, and our sensory–motor nervous system is unable to read the signals of the current environment accurately. Ultimately, we may hold the traumatic experience in the tissues of our body and our autonomic nervous system. In an interview, Peter Levine describes trauma:

Trauma is something that not only affects the brain; it affects the mind, but I would say that it primarily affects the body. When we are frightened, our bodies tense into readiness. If we're experiencing overwhelming life-threat, our bodies collapse into helplessness. These are things that go on in the body. As long as they're going on in the body, it's actually sending information from the body to the brain saying that the threat is still occurring. So, the threat then gets, if you like, embodied. It stays with the person because they're getting that feedback from the body.

He continues,

Find ways to help people find different experiences in their bodies, ones that contradicted those of fear and bracing and overwhelming helplessness. Because when we have new experiences in the body, then those new experiences would be relaying back up to the brain.

(LaPierre 2020: 16-17)

This is resonant with the embodiment practices of IBMT, where we explore the different body systems through guided and free movement, as well as bodywork. It is in these somatic explorations that we connect, expand, and deepen our proprioceptive and interoceptive relationship.

Embodying the Nervous System

The autonomic nervous system's rhythm becomes established in week three of embryonic development.

As the notochord forms and the primitive streak emerges, a structure called the neuro-enteric canal opens up between the yolk sac and the amniotic cavity. Fluid moves back and forth along this canal, creating what Bainbridge Cohen believes to be the basis of the autonomic nervous system rhythm. This primal rhythm is imprinted into every cell.

Bainbridge Cohen offers the concept that our nervous system acts as a recorder of experience and considers that it is possible to tune into an earlier, more fluid developmental stage of the nervous system. Here, we can tune into cellular consciousness, which, in my view, is where the work of IBMT begins to offer a powerful counter-vortex to the trauma vortex.

Bainbridge Cohen writes,

When you become sensitive, you can feel when you're going against your own tidal flow. You can also change your tidal flow. You're moving within this flow. When we get in touch with this fluid rhythm, our movement is effortless, and our mind is synchronized with our body. It's a flow – it could also be through your arms, through your fingers, through your toes. When identifying this rhythm in hands-on work with others, they become effortless in their movement because they were resonating with their fluid rhythm. Resonance is the key to establishing this root rhythm, which is in every cell. This neuro enteric canal sets up this fluid rhythm.

(Bainbridge Cohen 2012: 166)

Here, Bainbridge Cohen is talking about the fluid underneath the autonomic nervous system's rhythm. This is in place before the nerves fully develop in our autonomic nervous system. After birth, we engage more with the sensory-motor and gravitational coordination, but the cellular consciousness that gives us intracellular fluid orientation remains. As we move, connection between the motor-sensory nerves of the central and autonomic nervous systems supports us in developing our gravitational orientation.

In IBMT we explore the nervous system as a whole, including the central nervous system consisting of brain and spinal nerves, the peripheral nerves, the somatic and motor nerves, and the autonomic and enteric nervous systems. In exploring these systems through somatic movement, we develop a capacity to sense and embody how the entire nervous system connects to the different body systems.

In Somatic Experiencing, practice tends to focus more on the regulation of the autonomic nervous system, exploring the balance and flow between the sympathetic and the parasympathetic branches. How this is approached will be different when working with early developmental trauma than with an acute trauma that has happened later in life: for example, in a car accident or a medical procedural trauma. However, a felt sense of the physiology is needed to support re-establishing coherency through all the different body systems.

If we look to what happens in our physiology when we consider trauma, we can see that there is undischarged survival energy bound in the nervous system and tissues of the body and this needs to be discharged before we can settle and rest; dysregulation in the body can be held within any of the body systems. Working with touch can be helpful and can encourage more awareness in the client. When using contact, I am conscious of the different aspects of the body systems, and include in my sensing both cellular consciousness and the interrelationship of all the other body systems with the ANS.

Somatic Movement and Protective Responses to Threat

Peter Levine describes different stages of a protective response: startle/arrest, evaluation, orientation, mobilization, integration, discharge. We move through these stages many times a day, which can lead to any stages of the response being interrupted. If this interruption happens with a heightened activation of threat, the body systems, as Levine described in an earlier quote, are left in a place of dysregulation. I think of these stages as movement patterns, and in my sessions bring them together with the Body-Mind Centering® early movement patterns, the initiators of locomotive movement – yield, push, reach, pull – and the gestural movement of grasp.

> *These evolutionary patterns are the organising principles. In human development, life force is primary, and trauma is secondary. By entering the pool of neurological programming at its most primal level, we can sink below the defences and resistances accumulated in our vertebrate life, and draw upon the source wisdom of our implicit evolutionary intelligence.*
>
> (LaPierre 2019: 33)

When I work with someone who is experiencing trauma, I will include an awareness of where an interruption occurred in the protective responses. I also consider which of the developmental movement patterns and locomotive initiators of yield, push, and so on could support the renegotiation and completion of this interruption.

A Client Session Working with Body Systems and Incomplete Protective Responses

This client was struggling with the ending of a relationship. He was feeling a lot of activation through the core of his body and spine, with intense energy moving upwards into his head. With this sensation came a strong feeling of not being safe. We included touch to bring in a direct experience of containment and chose to explore inviting a settling through bodywork with kidneys and adrenal glands.

The kidneys and adrenal glands are often linked to overactive nervous system responses. With the bodywork, the client can be sitting or lying on their back or front. When working to support settling through contact with the kidneys and adrenals, it is easier to go with gravity, so I often recommend sitting or lying on the back initially.

> In this session, as he lay on his back, I made contact directly under his left kidney and adrenal with my palm facing upwards and my hand resting on the ground. I asked him to sense into his body and to see how this contact was. I brought my other hand above, on the diaphragm, and tuned in through cellular touch.

I will always check with the client whether they want a lighter or firmer contact as part of the work of letting the client be proactive in their relationship to touch. Often, someone can feel the warmth of my hand, and this helps to bring awareness to this part of their body.

> I listened with openness, not bringing in any agenda. From here, we together sensed into what was happening in the adrenal and kidney. There was a constriction, and we waited to see what level of contact gave the organ and gland the support needed.

I will sometimes offer micro-movements in three elemental planes – sagittal, vertical, and horizontal. This allows the organ "mind" to sense itself in relationship to the rest of the body, inviting a release of any tension, as well as supporting the expansion and sense of motility of the organ. With numbness, you can also offer micro-movements to increase the sensation, or if the organ feels under-toned, offer a touch of containment to support bringing more presence to the tissue.

Often, it takes a while for the body to respond to touch that is offering support, especially when it has been holding bound energy somatically from a trauma. Usually, with constriction or numbness, a firmer contact is helpful. To support regulation in the nervous system, bringing touch in slowly and titrating a small amount of contact, and then checking how this is received, helps to integrate the new experience into a client's awareness.

> With this client, it was essential to let there be a connection without a demand. With this listening presence, the kidney began to soften and the constriction in the tissues released. A little discharge came through the nervous system as a feeling of fizzing. The client felt something discharging through other parts of the body, through the legs and psoas muscle. An emotional release through the breath came, and his back could soften more easily into the ground. His breath continued to expand.

> I then went to the right kidney. It was much tighter than the left one. As the kidney and adrenal gland released, there was a significant discharge of heat. I felt a strong pulsing and some agency through movement down through the right leg came to the fore. I had offered a micro-intention of motion in different directions to support an awareness of sensation. He felt an impulse for both legs to move and allowed this, completing a cycle of mobilization.

> After some rest, he came into crawling and then walking, enjoying the new sense of vitality in his legs.

With the containment of touch, his kidney and adrenal were able to yield into gravity and discharge the energy that had been bound as a constriction. My sense was that this was also held in the psoas muscle and diaphragm. As this constriction released, a discharge of heat spread through the surrounding tissue and a surge of energy moved down through his leg, supporting him in completing an interrupted mobilization of flight. He was then able to reconnect to the felt sense between his core and in his muscles, moving through the developmental stage of crawling and then coming into the vertical, experiencing how it was to walk with more expansion in his core and legs. This illustrates the interconnection between the body systems and movement, and how it supports the return of coherency.

Dr Aline LaPierre describes how vital it is to take time to listen in to the body:

The real advance in trauma treatment is the knowledge that the irrational, organic responses of the body cannot be changed except by becoming deeply involved in noticing the internal world, by becoming deeply involved in interoception. This means spending time turning inward, listening to messages from the body, and noticing how the body is engaging life. It means learning to tolerate unknown, often frightening sensations and emotions for which there are as yet no words.

(LaPierre 2019: 55)

Presence

In IBMT work, we also include the practice of Authentic Movement and Therapeutic Presence, rooted in the Discipline of Authentic Movement, as developed by Janet Adler, and integrated into the training as a foundation for bringing mindful presence and compassionate attention into our work with clients. This practice, involving a witness and a mover, creates a safe space without judgment, where a client can bring their awareness inwards to attend to their inner world. In the space of moving while being witnessed, they are invited to follow the flow of impulses which arise from the unconscious and to bring these into expression through movement. In this way, unconscious material is embodied. In my work with trauma, I am conscious that activation or threat creates a speeding up in our responses. I find that bringing therapeutic presence that comes through the practice of Authentic Movement allows regulation, inviting clients to find a rhythm where they can slow down and have space to process what is being shared by including body awareness alongside emotions and movement impulses. In somatic practice, we focus on working in the present moment, even though what is arising is often in place from past experiences.

On another occasion, I was working with a client who was exploring her experience of not being able to stay centered when somebody asks something of her. Her experience was that she could not retain her own sense of agency or embodied presence, describing it as getting "pulled out of myself and my own wishes, for fear of being selfish or demanding."

In this session, I was drawing from the IBMT approach to somatic psychology, working with gestures as a movement, and also conscious of how gravity plays a part in the ability to feel and begin to trust support. The phrase that I heard Susan Harper say in a Heart of Belonging Continuum workshop, "we can only rest as fully as we could in the lap of our mother," comes to mind.

When we looked back at the client's early years and her early relationships, we uncovered that this meaning arose through her relationship of touch with her mother. While exploring what touch meant to her and how she had embodied touch as a child, she discovered the meaning she gave to touch – being demanding or selfish. This meaning made it very difficult for her to have safe or enjoyable contact with others, and she could become disoriented. The following extract from a session

Chapter 15

shows how staying with the present felt sense enabled the flow between the trauma vortex and the counter-vortex, and also illustrates how movement gestures supported this.

I invited her to come into a more direct relationship with gravity. I was curious about accessing yielding as a way to bring in more somatic presence, alongside calling forward parasympathetic responses.

I asked, if there could have been more support present, what would this have looked like?

A body dialogue opened up between her left hand and right hand. In IBMT, we allow gestures that emerge to express what was not possible in these earlier years, either because there was not yet the ability to speak or because the experience was held as a somatic shock in their physicality.

Her elbows began curling in, and her right hand rested inside the cupped fingers of her left hand. She felt herself relax and sensed the support between her hands.

With this thought, her left hand got a feeling of being wrong. She stayed with following impulses, and the left hand realized it could touch or move away and touch again and the other hand was still there. It did not leave or get angry or collapse. Her right hand continued to be there, and this felt okay. She had a memory, from a workshop she participated in, where the trainer said, "the supporters are also being supported." This is one of the foundations of somatic movement: without support, there is no possibility of action. As we continued with the exploration, she played with dialogue between her hands, and the left hand discovered that it had become more substantial and could even at times rest into the right hand. With this embodied experience, the meaning changed and her embodied sense around yielding into or pushing or resisting began to evolve. She was working somatically and, from a Somatic Experiencing perspective, "bottom-up," where a new meaning emerged. "I am safe to be here as I am."

In letting the gestures express an internal experience, she was able to witness, through the movement and relationship of her hands, how her internal experience of touch and relationship to her mother could take on a new dynamic and meaning.

Titration and Pendulation in Somatic Movement Sessions

Another principle in SE is to work with titration and pendulation, supporting a client to manage the stimulation, and find ways to pendulate between active sympathetic and the more restorative nature of parasympathetic, or freeze of the older parasympathetic. When a client shares experiences that are activating, it can stimulate an intense sympathetic response in them that can lead to the freeze response. We want to support them in slowing down or reducing the stimulus, so that it is a titrated process where the pendulation engenders a flow between these two aspects of the nervous system. This can also be about working with resources.

Working with titration, we can gradually begin to soften any immobilization without the flood of hormones that are still bound within the tissues of the body overwhelming the client again. As they meet the trauma vortex with the presence of the counter-vortex, the bound energy begins to release back into the body systems, giving an expansion or release of energy. This can look like shaking or waves of heat moving into the surrounding tissues, and it can be an emotional release. It is this release that allows the body systems to begin to self-regulate.

As clients begin to share their experiences, you can see where the energy is held within their body systems: there may be changes in their skin color as the blood vessels dilate or constrict, or changes in their breath as they move from social engagement to sympathetic or vegetative parasympathetic activation. Trauma can compromise our ability to engage, at times replacing the ability to be in connection with protective patterns. If there is no opportunity to resolve this trauma, the early adaptive survival responses can become habitual.

In this extract from a session with a client, I illustrate how, in a somatic movement process, we work with titration and pendulation. As a practitioner, I think about the skin's response as a primary defense. Tightening and pressure of the chest are often associated with panic attacks, including tension down through the digestive tract and diaphragm, and into the solar plexus.

In this session, a client speaks to feeling pressure in the chest. The tension pulls down into the stomach and there is a tightening through the skin up into the head. This is a very familiar feeling for her and is accompanied by a sense of not feeling connected.

Asking her if she could associate this feeling with anything, she identifies an experience when this first began to emerge.

As I listen to my client sharing what she is experiencing, I ask, "When was the first moment you sensed there was something wrong? As you name that now, what do you become aware of in yourself?" We include any images that come forward, or emotions, along with the body sensations.

She gives me a clearer picture of what is happening and how it relates to two events. She could feel herself wanting to be in control, with a wish to stay connected but struggling to do so. We slowed things down and explored, allowing her to follow an impulse of movement, coming to the ground.

Very often, this can be the case, where something that is already stressful but manageable is then followed by another upsetting event. This creates a sense of overwhelm or the experience that there is more than one can cope with. As it comes too quickly, there is a sense of things happening too fast, activating the sympathetic response.

With this client, we had done a lot of work previously with the sense of yielding into the support of the floor and playing with pushing to build tone through the body muscle. As she went to the ground, she lay on her back. From previous sessions, I knew she liked weighted cushions on her feet and along her midline and asked if she would like this, to which she said yes. She felt reassured but a memory of not being in control of the situation and feeling very alone surfaced.

I use the weighted cushions, as they can increase the ability to sense and can also help clients access regulation by themselves, an exercise that they can again do at home.

Here in this moment, her body having the weights was offering a counter-vortex, the feeling of not being alone. She shared that she could feel something else there, and this movement towards regulation allowed a deeper feeling of not being clear about being here, which also linked to this memory.

I asked if she would like touch, to which she said yes, and I made contact with her left shin to bring a quality of bone into awareness. Bones are the densest system of the body and can support feeling contained. Asked how it was to have this contact, she said she felt more present. We returned to the experience of her skin's tightness around her head.

Chapter 15

I asked, "From here, I wonder what support you could see would help this part of you back then?"

Working with the imagination can help the nervous system respond and discover ways to complete the movement gestures that were interrupted in the upsetting event.

An image of an animal came forward, and the characteristics of this animal gave some pendulation from activation to settling, but still, the skin was feeling tight.

Seeing if this image, or another, could embody more of the expression of her skin, a bright, lime green snake emerged – grounded, elegant in moving through space, with a clear focus, expanding skin, and changing shape as needed.

It was clear one would not want to mess with this snake, and she began to let her body follow impulses to move.

Flexion from the head right down through the digestive tract, knees curling up. Rolling and extending, spreading and expanding, moving to the other side curling in again. Continuous folding and unfolding. Potency building tone in the muscle and releasing heat.

I stayed present, witnessing her as she allowed the movement. She came to rest and then came to sit. I offered words that reflected the movements. She shared that she was feeling a deeper connection to herself and more conscious of her body. We spoke about our inner untamed nature or wildness that can be suppressed and how the image supports the impulses to expand into movements that allow the more hidden to express.

Another area we include in IBMT is working with shadow, where an image can support connecting to an expression that is held in the body systems, either from unaccepting family patterns or from trauma. The impulses that arise can be embodied in the nervous system, and support coherency to establish through the fluid system and into the muscles. This, in turn, helps regulation. It is very similar to the SIBAM model used in Somatic Experiencing, where we track and follow the Sensations, Images, Behavior, Affect, and Meaning.

Imagery often emerges when working somatically and can support bridging between our innate biological intelligence and our mindful self-reflective capacity.

With this client, I was conscious that, in her movement, she was engaging in pre-spinal and spinal movements. She had spoken about experiences that happened in adulthood but the origins may have started much earlier in her life. Through allowing the movement, she reconnected to earlier patterns that may have not been entirely inhabited, or where trauma may have interrupted the development of safe connection through the autonomic circuitry and the ability to regulate and build up resilience.

As a practitioner, I am always thinking about physiological coherence, as this coherence is what shifts the trauma.

I am asking myself, "What is someone's body communicating at a silent level of expression?" "How are they able to settle and orient?" "Can they yield into the support of the chair?" I notice the flexibility within their body, the tension in their skin or limbs. "How does their breath respond as they settle?" "Are their eyes and facial muscles relaxed or holding tighter than necessary?"

Conclusion

In my experience, bringing the practice of somatic movement and bodywork alongside understanding the elements of trauma is very helpful for clients.

I have found that clients are able to learn how to listen to their body, and over time stay present to their interoceptive and proprioceptive experience.

Somatic Bodywork and Movement in Trauma

Whether this be through the touch work of body systems, or revisiting early movement patterns and locomotive impulses, or being witnessed as spontaneous movement arises, the interrupted and incomplete movements of the protective responses which arise at the time of the trauma can move through to completion. As the client expands their capacity to stay with sensations, they expand their ability to allow pendulation and discharge; this gives rise to proprioceptive feedback in the nervous system and brain, and a new experience of self. When this occurs over time, clients can tune into the wisdom that comes from the body and tap into or connect to "source."

Glossary

Flight: a term used when the autonomic nervous system triggers the sympathetic response that stimulates the endocrine system to release epinephrine (adrenaline), and the cardiovascular system and respiratory system to increase the speed of the heart and blood flow and respiration, in order to escape the perceived threat. At the same time, the digestive system is suppressed.

Pendulation: a term used in Somatic Experiencing that refers to the natural biological rhythm of the nervous system between contraction and expansion. A Somatic Experiencing practitioner will, at times, support the client with specific invitations to re-establish this natural flow if the nervous system's inherent capacity has been interrupted through trauma.

Titration: a term used in Somatic Experiencing, where the practice creates only the smallest amount of activation in the nervous system. This helps to prevent activation of an overwhelming disorganization. By breaking down the charge in the nervous system into a manageable process, it allows the activation to be integrated and renegotiated.

16

Post-traumatic Stress, Chronic Pain, and Authentic Movement

Barbara Teresa Erber

This chapter describes the value of Authentic Movement (AM) in individual and group therapy with people suffering from post-traumatic stress (PTS) and chronic pain. The connection between PTS and the development of chronic pain is explained from a theoretical perspective with references to my personal and professional experience in Integrative Bodywork and Movement Therapy (IBMT) and Dance Movement Psychotherapy (DMP). My main objective was to present my experience of being with trauma and pain in the practice of AM. I refer to clients' experiences but do not include case-study material. I give examples of felt experience in movement related to processing chronic pain. The chapter emphasizes the potential for integration of trauma and personal growth through being with pain.

My interest in this field stems from my own healing journey and the role AM continues to play in my personal and professional life. In 2008, I fully recovered from 4 years of severe chronic pain. At this stage, full recovery is very rare and it was a difficult process. My subsequent training in IBMT and DMP led me to in-depth work with traumatized clients, many of whom suffered from chronic pain. Based on my work in a pain management clinic, I published an article entitled "Growing From Pain: A Creative Process" (Erber 2015). The chapter you are reading now has developed out of an essay written in 2013. It allowed me to look back at my personal and professional journey with pain, after which my focus shifted to the processing of fear. Being with fear continues to be an integral part of my PhD studies (Erber forthcoming), where I look at how practitioners of AM feel safe and present in their bodies.

Pain is defined as chronic if it persists for more than 12 weeks (NHS Inform 2021). The onset may be caused by strain or injury, but pain persists and possibly spreads long after healing would have been thought to have occurred. Chronic pain is a major clinical challenge: across Europe approximately 18% of the population are currently affected by moderate to severe chronic pain. It has a considerable impact on quality of life, resulting in significant suffering and disability. While in many cases it is accepted that a cure is unlikely, the impact on quality of life, mood and function can be significantly reduced by appropriate measures (Scottish Intercollegiate Guidelines Network 2013: 7).

The majority of chronic pain patients have a traumatic history but often do not relate their physical state initially to these experiences (Levine and Phillips 2012; Roth et al. 2008; McAllister 2017a; Sledjeski et al. 2008; Wuest et al. 2010). The Scottish Intercollegiate Guidelines Network (2013: 7) agrees that chronic pain is caused by many underlying conditions and NHS Inform (2021) explains that "people are more likely to develop chronic pain during or after times of stress or unhappiness." During the course of my sessions, most of my clients recognized that insecure attachment and ongoing, long-term traumatic stressors, as well as overworking, laid the foundations for the development of their chronic pain. Many of them were referred to me by colleagues who knew this was my area of interest and expertise, and thought there was a correlation between these clients' past trauma and chronic pain. However, what was significant for their pain management was for the clients to recognize and acknowledge this correlation for themselves.

Galon (2019) calls for more publications like her own, which elucidate the construct and the

Chapter 16

components of the therapeutic process in DMP and Body Psychotherapy with trauma survivors. The key themes I have found essential for processing chronic pain combined with PTS are the quality of the therapeutic relationship, acceptance, finding meaning, transformation, and integration. My chapter explains how these treatment components are met in AM. Through being witnessed in a compassionate, non-judgmental way, with awareness for all their potential underlying conditions, many of my clients began experiencing moments without pain, or even pleasant sensations, instead of pain and numbness.

I am not suggesting that AM can solve all the severe physical and psychological issues by which the majority of people with chronic pain are so deeply affected. However, I wish to introduce the potential value of AM for this client group in response to the final report of the National Pain Audit (2012), which emphasizes the need for a variety of approaches and a range of specialist skills to address multi-morbidity. In addition, the report mentioned highlights the need for increased psychological input within pain management. My chapter will elaborate on how this need can be met in a unique way by IBMT practitioners and other bodyworkers or therapists who are able to carry out in-depth work with a combined somatic and psychotherapeutic focus based on the form of AM.

The Relationship Between Trauma and Chronic Pain

For the following story of a healing journey, I took into account the experiences of my clients as well as my own. It depicts dissociative states and the onset and journey with chronic pain as experienced in our inner, felt sense.

> It is not safe to be where I am. I feel trapped in my body, with the pressure increasing and increasing. I withdraw, disappearing into the deepest corner inside my body at the same time as going away from my body as far as I possibly can. This split into an immensely deep interior and an immensely faraway exterior place is a very clever way of hiding. The interior place allows me to conduct my body to move, just enough to give the appearance of me still being there. An empty shell. Meanwhile, the faraway exterior place seems like a haven of nothingness, complete and utter freedom in not being trapped by my physical state of being. Then, one day, that place deep inside my body can't sustain this split any longer. It has been deprived of the company of the other for too long, and it begins to ache. This pain begins to pull harder and harder on that thin line, which connects me in these two distant places. Eventually, the pain becomes omnipresent, with no way of escaping from it, even in the faraway place.
>
> The pain is horrendous and I try to resist as much as I can, but I learn that any attempt to withdraw further only results in more pain. My ability to function in the world has become increasingly limited. At this stage, I simply want to cut that string which attaches me to my body, to the pain. I want to cut off the painful body part.
>
> Then a turning happens... In the faraway place I begin to remember ... where I came from all this time ago. Rooted, anchored in the pain, it feels as though I am being called back somehow. And strangely, the pain becomes the strongest indicator as to where I need to go. With the deepest part of my being, I feel this reaction of my body as screaming for my soul, my life, my ability to experience fully, to come back to me. But I can't do this alone. I need a lot of help. I am grateful to have found solid, compassionate witnesses holding my process.
>
> Eventually, as I travel down the thread which attaches me to my body, I begin to discover different sensations, not just pain. I begin to

> expand again out of the hiding place deep inside my body. I learn, for the first time perhaps, to feel a pleasant tingling, the simplicity of a breath, effortlessness in a small part of my body, ... the beginning of freedom in movement.
>
> The physical pain eases, and where before I felt pain in my body, I now struggle with unbearable emotions ... In many ways I preferred the pain to this. All these feelings now are less tangible; they confuse me. I don't yet know them, nor do I know how to deal with them on my own. I rely on my external witness to help me contain my experience, allowing me to sink deeper into myself as I learn how to hold myself.
>
> I spend a great amount of time resting and sleeping, curled up like a baby in the womb. No thought, no worry – just emptiness, stillness. All the while, big changes in my inner life, big changes in my outer life. I begin to create an environment for myself, which is right for me.

The faraway exterior place I mention corresponds to the realm of image/imagination, which is one of the categories into which tracked experience can be divided. The other categories are movement, sensation, emotion, and feeling. Later, at the end of my "Acceptance" subsection, I write about how this category or channel of experience was very strong in me at the beginning of my AM practice, and how it subsided over the years and why.

Every person's process is different. We each take varying amounts of time in each of these stages. The process I have mapped out may span several decades and involves intense dedication to one's personal healing, as well as good, strong, and steady therapeutic relationships with one or more health professionals. Overall, I agree with Galon (2019: 220), who finds that "clinical work with survivors of trauma is conceptually individualised and complex."

At the beginning of the story I described PTS followed by the onset of chronic pain. The Institute for Chronic Pain (McAllister 2017a) offers a most comprehensive and concise explanation of how trauma may lead to the development of chronic pain. PTS leaves the nervous system in a state of persistent arousal or reactivity. Following an injury or illness, this can lead to "central sensitization," a state in which the nervous system becomes stuck in heightened reactivity. This means that pain persists or even worsens after the initial injury or illness heals.

Chronic pain, as seen from a bio-psycho-social perspective, is a joint creation of physical, psychological, and social circumstances (Main et al. 2008). Levine and Phillips (2012), McFarlane (2010), Roth et al. (2008), Sledjeski et al. (2008), and Wuest et al. (2010) agree that PTS often contributes greatly to pain becoming chronic. In general, it can be said that chronic pain and post-traumatic stress disorder co-occur at a high rate (Otis et al. 2003; Defrin et al. 2008). These two conditions have a negative impact on each other, with patients reporting higher levels of pain, affective distress, and functional disability. As depicted in the journey earlier, traumatic stress results in a disintegration of the sense of self. Bullington et al. (2003, 2005) underline that chronic pain itself can be seen as a form of disintegration.

Another important factor is insecure attachment in childhood and the foundation this lays for physical and psychological resilience later in life. Childhood adversities significantly raise the risk of developing chronic widespread pain by mid-life (Jones et al. 2009). Porges (2011) and Schore (2003) underline how insecure attachment leaves the individual more susceptible to the development of PTS. In the first instance of threat being perceived, infants cry or scream (Schore 2003). As adults we exhibit fight, flight or freeze responses as a reaction to threat. If another person is the source of threat, it is perceived through the social engagement system. In this case fight, flight or freeze/playing dead is preceded by attempts at calming this person by signaling safety through facial expression and vocal intonation (Porges 2011, 2017; Porges and Carter 2017).

Our last resort for dealing with traumatic threat is to dissociate from our sensory experience and our feelings by freezing/playing dead, through hypo-arousal of the vegetative parasympathetic, which releases behavior-inhibiting cortisol and pain-numbing endogenous opioids (Schore 2003). This explains why many of my clients reported that they were either unaware of their body before the onset of chronic pain or experiencing it as inhibiting. As a result of PTS, a sense of freedom and pleasure in movement may already have been lost prior to the onset of chronic pain. Moreover, Schore (2003: 68) describes an early developmental connection between our perception of threat and our experience of pain: "[In infants,] states of autonomic hyper-arousal are subjectively experienced as pain, and thus this strategy [dissociation] represents a psychobiological mechanism by which psychic-physical pain is instantly inhibited."

In my felt experience the pain-numbing effects of dissociation eventually melt and give way to painful sensations, perhaps as the body's attempt to heal and integrate trauma. I feel the starting point for healing from trauma is not when chronic pain begins to ease away, but when pain arises for the first time. I see the place of dissociation and nothingness as a place for taking time out – waiting for a safer space – before embarking on the process of reintegration. (This paragraph shows how I have personally found meaning in my journey with pain. By contrast, I acknowledge how the development of chronic pain, on top of dealing with PTS, may otherwise be seen as an additional curse, rather than a blessing. I have certainly felt this many times.)

As a result of trauma at any point in life, the nervous system is thrown out of homeostatic balance, with the individual spending increasing amounts of time in states of hyper- and hypo-arousal (Levine 1997, 2010; Scaer 2007; Schore 2003; Van der Kolk et al. 1996). Hypo-arousal feels to me like a state of retreating as deeply as possible into my own body, becoming as small as possible, withdrawing into the inside. Hyper-arousal feels like escaping to the outside; the senses become as wide as possible, hyper-alert, gathering as much information from the outer world as possible in a frantic attempt to find meaning and safety. Richman (2012) and Nijenhuis et al. (2006) agree that if safety cannot be found, we increasingly resort to dissociation, living a detached life, lost and unable to come to terms with reality.

Long-term trauma and PTS exhaust the human body to the extent where homeostatic balance is not only limited, but lost. The opposed states of hypo- and hyper-arousal pervade and pain may become a central experience in both (Levine 1997, 2010; Levine and Phillips 2012). Bullington et al. (2005: 263) write, "pain locks the body in a stiff, rigid armour." Movement is limited, breathing becomes shallow, and over time more and more energy is withdrawn from the body, leaving it susceptible to infection and illness. So often I have heard my clients speak about how empty their body feels, how they feel they are floating somewhere above or behind their body, unable to reach it, unable to get it to function. These descriptions clearly correspond to the way in which people suffering from PTS describe their sense of their bodies (Nijenhuis et al. 2006; Richman 2012; Scaer 2007).

Decreasing anxiety levels is paramount for reducing the amount of pain messages created by the nervous system in chronic pain. Just like the treatment of trauma, chronic pain management has a lot to do with fear management. In living with pain as a constant experience, the challenge lies in accepting this pain and/or trauma as a companion, rather than letting the fear of it stop us from being in the world, engaged in life. In the beginning of the process of coming to terms with chronic pain, this companion will most likely receive growing amounts of fearful and hurtful judgment, adding to the internal split. Many of my clients have described wanting to cut off the afflicted body part or simply have a new, pain-free body. There is an overwhelming wish to wipe out the old existence and start afresh. This energy can be used to fuel rebirth in a Jungian sense, the process of individuation or transformation (Harris 2011; Hartley 2001; Stromsted 2001; Woodman 1985). Chodorow (1991: 107), in quoting Eliade, agrees: "Life can not be repaired, it can only be recreated."

Bitzaraki et al. (2010) and Bullington (2003, 2005) identified "finding meaning out of the chaos of chronic pain" as one of the most important factors in coming to terms with chronic pain. The meaning I found in my personal story was essentially a wake-up call to embodiment, meaning in-depth, long-term psychotherapy and bodywork. Like some of my clients, I previously had not felt myself to be in right relationship with my environment. An inner change – more awareness of the painful reality – led to making vast changes in my personal environment, which in turn allowed me to heal.

Tending to Clients' Needs Through Authentic Movement

At the beginning of the last section, I told the story of a healing journey spanning years or decades. Here is an example of one session from my clinical practice describing part of this healing. It contains no identifiable details.

Kerstin suffers from fibromyalgia, which means she experiences unbearable pain almost everywhere in her body. I began seeing her after she had received every other medical and pain management support available to her in the years since her pain started. She experiences problems balancing and relies on a stick to walk. She prefers to remain seated during our sessions. We always begin with a gentle warm-up, feeling into and gently moving every part of our bodies. Then we talk about how she is feeling, after which I guide her into a short AM practice or another movement exploration – whichever corresponds best to what she brings that day. The following example describes an AM practice a couple of months into our weekly sessions together.

Kerstin sits in a chair opposite me. Her feet are on the ground, her back leaning against the back of the chair, her arms sometimes resting on her thighs, sometimes on the armrest. Without the chair, she feels a fear of falling and more pain. All seems as usual but I increasingly feel very different in her presence today. I sense the insides of my torso and head longing to move forwards inside my body. I feel alert and particularly drawn to witnessing her. Kerstin's breath barely moves her chest. Her head is tilted forwards, her shoulders and chest forming a nest for her head and chin, although they do not touch. My spine straight, I feel my breath; I feel ease in my shoulders expanding with every breath I take. We are not talking and yet I have a sense of her being quieter than usual; there is no sound to be heard and yet my ears are sharpened. I continue observing her body, barely moving. My hands rest in my lap. I feel patience, but at the same time I feel my insides reaching out to her, looking for her. My gaze keeps being drawn to the space behind her body. I see her sitting barely 2 meters [6 ft 6 in] in front of me, but I feel as though she is much further away, behind her chair. As I continue witnessing, I see this mismatch of sensory

information that I am experiencing more clearly and understand the confusion it causes in me. I continue witnessing Kerstin's tiny movements, her right index lightly lifting off the armrest for a moment, then settling again. I continue witnessing the space behind her chair. I remain steady as her witness, holding impulses to stretch to the sides and peek behind her body, behind her chair.

It is time to speak. Kerstin's head and eyes lift, halfway at first, her breath and voice slowly begin filling her body and the space between us. As she begins to speak, her head and eyes lift further, looking into my eyes and the space around us. She shares memories of horrific physical abuse she suffered all throughout her childhood. Every single day, again and again. She describes sitting here today with the intention and the wish to share this, to speak of her pain as a child for the first time in decades. She realizes her experience of pain now is connected to her pain then. We both feel compassion.

As Kerstin's head and eyes lift and her voice grows steady in speaking, I feel a slow-motion sensation of the space behind her chair moving forwards into the space where her body is sitting all this time. This movement feels like taking a big in-breath inwards and an out-breath downwards inside me. My insides settle there, tenderly welcoming her story, her pain, her voice.

In my felt experience I long for this inner movement from deep inside, far away behind or above the body, back into the body, into the present moment, into relationship. Sinking into the practice of witnessing, I often feel as though I can see more clearly where my clients are in their process, how far away or how deeply buried their dissociated, hiding parts are in that moment. The practice of AM allows me to communicate to these hiding parts of self that they are seen in their depth and that they are good enough just as they are. Having been witnessed thus, they are often able to move further into life, filling the person again with vitality.

Hands-on work is often not an option in working with people suffering from chronic pain because touch might amplify the discomfort (McAllister 2017a, 2017b). Desensitization techniques can be highly effective when the pain is a result of physical injury alone. However, I find that, in situations where the pain is associated with psychological trauma, they tend to be less useful. Touch, like pain, is a powerful reminder for the psyche of where to return to – the body – but neither is helpful without careful psychotherapeutic holding. Touch may be too directive and lead to intolerable pain and dissociation, whereas AM gives the client's body space to bring up any experience that is tolerable for them in this situation.

As we have seen the following key areas ought to be addressed in treating people suffering from PTS and chronic pain: the quality of the therapeutic relationship, acceptance, finding meaning, transformation, and integration. These themes correspond with Richman's (2012) description of three phases in the treatment of trauma:

1 safety and stabilization

2 coming to terms with traumatic experiences

3 integration and reconnection.

The example of Kerstin's session shows that trust and safety had been established in the therapeutic relationship, which allowed Kerstin to find new meaning and acceptance for her pain.

The quality of the therapeutic relationship

In clinical AM practice the therapist acts as a witness to the client's process in movement (Holifield 2007). The most important factor is the quality of presence and attunement that the therapist offers, as the form of AM needs to be adapted depending on the client's state. When we work with PTS, the degrees of dissociation need to be monitored in order to assess the client's readiness and ability to engage with this practice. Facial expression and vocal intonation play a crucial role in helping the client feel safe (Porges 2017).

Attunement is defined as interpreting, interacting, and responding appropriately to another in nonverbal and verbal dialogue. Being well attuned-to stimulates a healing process in those suffering from incomplete attachment processes and/or trauma (Devereaux 2008; Keleman 1986; Ogden et al. 2006; Porges and Carter 2017; Rothschild 2000; Richman 2012; Schore 2003; Stern 1985; Van der Kolk 1996). The practice of witnessing is a process of attunement, where the therapist or parent implicitly helps the client or inner child regulate psychobiological states. Recent findings on the working of the social engagement system show that somatic movement practices such as IBMT and AM are particularly well suited to establishing this sense of safety as part of trauma recovery (Porges 2017; Porges and Carter 2017; Weare 2020).

In my experience, witnessing people with chronic pain requires a readiness to bear stillness. In particular people with fibromyalgia, who suffer from pain everywhere in their body, often prefer to remain still rather than moving. Only subtle movements are noticeable in movement sessions, as described in Kerstin's session earlier. Mallon et al. (2004) and Bullington et al. (2003) found accepting chronic pain patients, exactly as they are, to be paramount for establishing a meaningful therapeutic relationship. Bral et al. (2002: 57) emphasize that chronic pain patients need to have somebody who is "authentically present" to relate to.

One of the core messages of pain management programs is to pace, and yet, within reason, to keep moving despite the pain in order to establish neural patterns, which are not absorbed in recreating pain messages. This fits well with the ways in which traumatic experiences are worked with in somatic trauma therapy, where clients are guided into experiencing good sensations and feelings, thus creating a safe space to further the integration of trauma (Levine 1997, 2010; Levine and Phillips 2012; Ogden et al. 2006; Rothschild 2000). These methods of working with pain and with trauma independently promote awareness of the pleasant as well as painful aspects of life and a conscious alternation between them. Consequently, most people suffering from chronic pain and PTS initially need to be guided in or into movement processes in order to stimulate this alternation. The personal limits of the client need to be respected at all times.

Cady (2016) urges health professionals to truly listen to their patients' pain stories, without judgment. In AM, safety and stabilization are provided by the non-judgmental, compassionate witnessing of the outer and, after time, the inner witness (Adler 2002; Pallaro 1999, 2007; Holifield 2007). Through being witnessed in this way, the client gradually begins to feel safe and to develop a more integrated sense of self (Holifield 2007; Pallaro 2007; Stromsted 2001; Chodorow 1991). If it is the environment or relationship to self and other which creates chronic pain, the relationship to self and other can be the key to its healing. Underlining this statement, Richman (2012) describes findings in neuropsychology, which show that the pre-frontal cortex is dead in severe long-term trauma, but that long-term therapy activates it. It is all down to good attachment and good therapy, being seen and empathized with appropriately.

Acceptance

The following paragraphs are as much about the accepting attitude of the therapist as the client's self-acceptance, on coming to terms with his/her trauma and pain. Through being witnessed in AM, the client/mover may learn to internalize this compassionate attitude towards his/her own unconscious. In addition, trust can be developed towards his/her body in spontaneous movement, while expressing incomplete protective movements, which had been frozen in moments of threat. This is an important part of integrating traumatic experience (Levine 1997, 2010; Levine and Phillips 2012; Ogden et al. 2006; Rothschild 2000). Bojner-Horwitz et al. (2010) describe a reduction of pain correlating with intense emotional expression. I find chronic pain to be a unique experience for every individual and sometimes containment and boundaries are needed for healing, or subtle rather than intense emotional expression. I agree with Chodorow (1991: 36), who states, "cathartic expression alone doesn't necessarily lead to psychological integration."

The better the containment, or holding environment, provided by the therapist/witness through their quality of presence and feedback, the more the client can trust and let go of ego control (Pallaro 1999). Once a client trusts the therapist and the safety of the form of AM, emotional expression can arise naturally, as and when the client is ready to bear it. The deeper the content arising from the unconscious, the greater the healing potential of expression and integration. Simply letting the body move from within, allowing bottom-up processing in a safe and contained manner can release tension and pain (Berg et al. 2010; Levine 1997, 2010; Holifield 2007), where exercises imposed on the body may be much more prone to increasing judgment, muscular tension, and pain.

Respecting the authority of the client in their own process is of utmost importance if the client's history of trauma includes violation of personal boundaries. Chang and Leventhal (1995) state that the willingness to move in a specific way has to come from the client. They also mention the danger of compliance or rebellion when faced with directive movement interventions and illustrate the importance of refraining from premature interpretation of the client's movements, instead allowing them to find their own meaning. These statements further support the value of AM, a non-directive movement intervention, with clients who have suffered from abuse.

In conjunction with the freedom for self-expression, which AM provides, it also offers the safety of a structure or form for holding a deep personal process. The form of AM initially needs to be learned and practiced. Berg et al. (2010) emphasize the creation of a safe environment, which facilitates exploration of the meaning of bodily sensations and also challenges patients to learn new things, thus increasing their sense of self-empowerment, self-assertiveness, and self-agency.

As explained earlier, acceptance is a central theme in pain-management programs. Self-acceptance stands in close relationship with increasing one's ability to stay present, as opposed to dissociating. This is practiced in trauma therapy through drawing the client's attention to the present moment (Levine 1997, 2010; Ogden et al. 2006). The Discipline of AM offers a unique way of integrating body and mind in the present moment (Adler 1999 in Pallaro 1999). A therapist who is well trained in witnessing will be able to help the mover track arising experience in detail.

In AM, as taught in IBMT, great care is given to deepening the experience of the present, emphasizing whichever realm of experience is least developed: that is, tracking the moving experience in the physical, sensory, emotional, or imaginary realm (Hartley 2012). This process of embodiment is compassionately held by the form of AM. Tracking movement grounds us in reality and attending to the flow of sensations focuses our attention in the present moment. Tracking emotions allows us to bring to the surface and integrate emotions, which may previously have been suppressed. Consequently, images and stories emerging from the moving experience can also be rooted in the body (Hartley 2012).

When I began practicing AM 13 years ago, I always more or less knew what my body was doing – like watching it from the outside – but I could not feel my body moving. I had strong images and intuitive feelings guiding me in movement, but I was not sensing my way in space. For those first years, my focus in AM practice was on tracking movement and sensation – my less developed realms, which consequently became my strength and grounding. However, the realm of imagery subsided over time, absorbed in the anchor of my body. Images are quite rare in my experience today.

Finding meaning

The ways in which we find meaning in trauma and pain lead to the question of how movement, sensations, emotions, feelings, and images associated with the body of the client are interpreted. The interpretation of the experience of the mover is an area which is dealt with in a great variety of ways in AM, depending on the context of the AM session: that is, within a clinical/therapeutic relationship, peer practice, teaching environment, or for artistic purposes. But mostly it depends on the training and practice of the facilitator/teacher/therapist. One might adopt a psychodynamic angle, offering interpretations based on the patient's history, or a predominantly person-centered one, based on the expression of the patient in the here and now in relationship with another. These often overlap and I would advise offering interpretations with great care. The witnessing in the form of AM, when offered as part of IBMT, additionally offers the possibility of witnessing the expression of body systems and developmental patterns.

In working with traumatized people who suffer from chronic pain, the hope is for pain and anxiety signals to become transformed into meaningful signals about the client's life situation instead of provoking fear. Personally, I find the most profound healing in the Discipline of AM as developed by Janet Adler, where the mover is encouraged to gain insight rather than interpreting. According to person-centered principles (Natiello 2001), the witness/therapist offers reflections of her/his own experience in relationship with the mover/client, staying as close as possible to where the client is in her/his process in the present moment. Some of my clients have independently sought out spiritual frameworks, which provide structure in the process of finding meaning out of the chaos of chronic pain. AM may offer a Jungian psychodynamic or spiritual angle to pain management, with the concept of the shadow manifesting in the form of pain and trauma.

Transformation and integration

Stromsted (2001) studied how AM facilitated transformative processes in mature practitioners. Although this article focuses on a different population, I still believe her findings are of relevance. She states that AM allows for the integration of shadow material, preceded by the development of a strong body ego. She identifies central stages in this developmental transformative process, which coincide with Jung's concept of individuation.

Transforming traumatic material in this way often involves re-enactments of very vulnerable, wounded, frozen places. This enables transformative change on all levels, from nerve pathways to the mover's sense of identity. Stromsted (2001) sees AM as a cocoon, a safe, well-held environment (Winnicott 1960) for rebirth processes as a result of regression to preverbal experiences. Bainbridge-Cohen (1993) and Hartley (1995, 2004) agree that the embodiment of specific stages of movement development can stimulate a repatterning of the nervous system. Dosamantes-Beaudry (2003) states that regression to earlier states of emotional development is often part of difficult life transitions, such as dealing with trauma. This regression is followed by a new organization of self (Chodorow 1991; Stromsted 2001; Holifield 2007; Pallaro 2007).

The final key element of the transformation of trauma mentioned by Levine (1997, 2010) and Malchiodi (2008) is to bring the re-enactment of traumatic content into relationship and reconnecting to the community after having been on a deep journey through the inner world. When practicing AM in a group setting, movers and witnesses may journey deeply in their inner, non-verbal world, which is followed by the possibility of speaking and sharing these experiences with the group. With clients whose trauma lies primarily within the relationships in their family or a similar group situation, the structure of witnessing and being witnessed within a group in a non-judgmental, compassionate way can be very healing. Over time, these witnessing skills may implicitly inform relationships in other areas of their lives.

Having witnessed people integrate and heal horrendous difficulties, Jung (1959) expressed the idea of it being pathological not to outgrow difficult experiences and situations, but to stay caught in them. Harris (2011) speaks of a creative spark, a seed for transformation in difficulties, but acknowledges that the path of individuation is not everyone's calling. I believe the emergence, transformation, and integration of unconsciousness into consciousness is not only the core of every therapeutic process, but the basic principle of life.

In theory, the growth process I am aiming for when working with PTS and chronic pain can be summarized as follows: stimulus processing is dynamic and can be integrated or segregated by cognition, meaning top-down control. Initially, impulses arising from the body and the unconscious, such as pain or traumatic memories, are uncontained and unsafe in their expression, experienced as uncontrollable and thus perhaps scary. Not being able to support this processing of information adequately from the bottom up, the ego has the sole alternative of more or less rigid top-down control or splitting from felt experience. As we develop more self-awareness and empathy towards ourselves and the arising impulses, this rigid control begins to be replaced by containment and higher consciousness (Sager 2008). As our ability to balance top-down and bottom-up processing in a healthy manner increases, the sense of safety grows and allows for more space to integrate body and mind. In conjunction with trusting ourselves in surrendering to impulses from the unconscious, we develop a sense of ourselves as the creator of our own life, rather than the victim of life circumstances.

In practice, I can offer an excerpt from my personal AM practice, which felt like a brief embodied reminder of the summary of my long story of healing from pain. The following move depicts a moment of disembodiment associated with a reappearance of pain as I come home to my body in the present moment once again:

> **My mind away, busy ... I am not feeling my body at all. Not filling my body at all.**
>
> **As my attention returns to my body, I find it sitting on the ground with legs folded loosely. My spine is straight. My right upper arm is touching the side of my torso, bent at the elbow, my lower arm reaching away from my body, palm facing upwards. My breathing is very shallow; I am very still. I can feel on my skin that my right arm and hand are in the shadow, the rest of my body in the sunshine. I become aware of the bound flow in my body; I know my body was just sitting there waiting for me, waiting for me to return.**

I feel sorry for having left it, for having left it alone when all the while it was waiting for me so patiently, in stillness, not complaining ... Just my right hand holding, holding ... Nothing. Empty. In the shadow. Holding itself in place for me.

I gather my right lower arm towards me, notice that it is in pain ... I notice that, ever so subtly, the remnants of pain have reappeared, as if reminding me that my deep body self still hurts when left by my presence for too long. As I touch my right hand, I notice it hurts more. Touch hurts. Gentleness amplifies the pain. Love brings out the hurt more, shines a torch on the discomfort, the sadness, the anger, the guilt. For life lost.

I touch my arm further up, where the pain is not too strong, just being with it. I feel sadness, and compassion, tears welling up ... For this deadly stillness, so void of life, so beyond hope. My hand feels stiff. Stiffness, grayness, emptiness, stillness.

I feel the rest of my body in relief, softly filled with compassion and patience. Grief comes along like a good old friend, taking up time and space. I stay with my aching arm, softly holding it with my left hand, gently proceeding to my right hand where it hurts more, where the stiffness, the numbness is more intense. My left hand moves my right hand slowly and gently. My left hand is the water flowing around the stone ... And with time it softens the stony edges, the pain subsides ... And yet remains in some form. My left hand gently holding my right, the two feeling so different in sensation and yet whole together. I am all here.

Conclusion

In portraying the connection between chronic pain and traumatic stress, I inferred the aims for working with this client group and gave practical examples. I explained the ways in which AM allows for self-expression in a contained environment and thus provides the ground for transformation and integration of the individual meaning associated with pain. I affirmed the central role of the therapeutic relationship, highlighting the quality of presence the therapist/witness needs to offer to the process of the client/mover.

I believe the future of pain management lies in giving space to bottom-up processing within a safe and well-resourced environment where clients can form positive, meaningful attachments to health professionals. In my experience the depth to which pain and trauma can be seen, physically (in order to acknowledge and heal detrimental pre-verbal patterning), emotionally (by therapists who are well grounded in containing pain and trauma empathically), and intellectually (integration through verbal witnessing), is extraordinary in AM and unique to this practice.

Embracing Trauma Through Performance

Leticia Santafé

17

Theatre has a role, a noble role, in energizing and mobilizing humanity to lift itself from its descent into the abyss. It can uplift the stage, the performance space, into something sacred.

Nadeem 2020: 3

A Personal Experience

Y así fue … más o menos [*And So It Was … More or Less*] opened in the Laboratory of the Arts in Valladolid (LAVA) in January 2017. This show was an ensemble creation that I directed and performed with three other people – Ana Laan, Alba Gómez, and Clara Parada – to give voice to the life stories of several women. The journey towards this performance piece began 2 years earlier with research into the testimonies of some Latin American women who were working as nannies in different Spanish families. They all had one thing in common: they had left their own children behind. I had been nursing the flame of this project for many years while taking care of my first child and spending lots of time with these childminders in the playgrounds where I lived in Madrid.

For this artistic project we used a *verbatim* style for the dramaturgy. This means we transcribed word for word the interviews that we had recorded when we met the women and performed them word for word. This was a big challenge and we embraced it with great respect.

I had been working as a professional performer for many years before this project, but on the opening night I experienced myself in a totally new way. We were on stage as the audience was coming in, and as I recall it, "out of the blue" my heart started to jump in my chest in a way I could not recognize as the performing energy I was used to. The dryness in my mouth, the huge acceleration in my upper chest breathing, and the lack of feeling in my hands first created in me a sense of panic. After a while, it was as if I was seeing myself from a distance. I started to think: "There is no way out from these sensations. I cannot manage them." My fellow performers did not realize what was happening to me and continued as we had rehearsed; the audience was in place and the lights went down. We were in physical contact, as if we were just one woman, and the performers' voices started to express huge sighs of relief. When we rehearsed this moment, we always talked about giving birth and coming from the darkness into the light. The sensation of connection with the bodies of the other three women performers and their own breathing and voices brought me back to the earth; at the same time, I expressed a huge sigh full of the sound of grief. I could leave behind the horror of not feeling myself, and the show could go on.

Later, I looked back at that moment and understood that I had experienced the body symptoms of trauma, and the way I had resolved them was through performance. The only certainties I had about that moment were:

1. I had training in voice, movement, and somatic movement therapy that enabled me to witness my experience.
2. I also knew that the trusting presence of my fellow performers helped me to reconnect with the impulse to move forward, towards regaining the feeling of agency in my own body.

The chance to research more around my wish to perform unleashed many questions: did I choose those stories in order to find a way to heal myself? Even in that first moment of the "birth" of the

Chapter 17

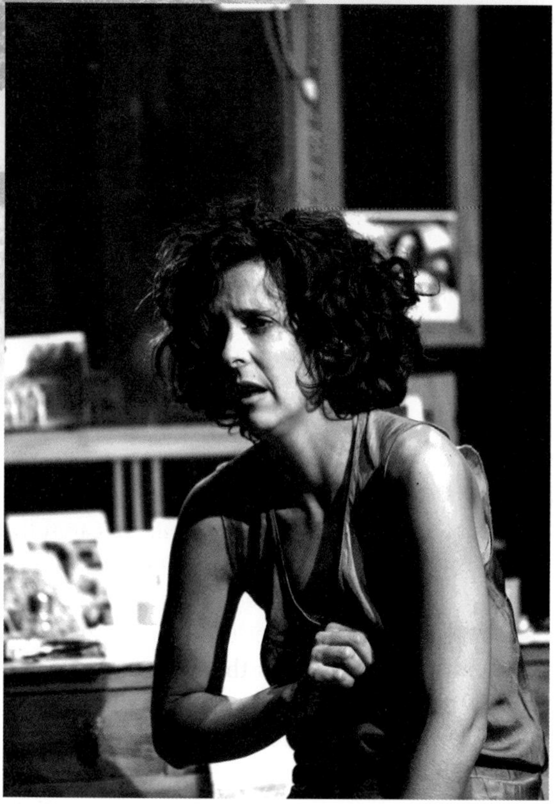

Y así fue ... más o menos. Performer: Leticia Santafé. Photographer: Eduardo Navarro

performance project that I had proposed to the group? How could my own birthing process be part of the answer? What was the role of the audience in that situation? And that of my fellow performers? Could I develop awareness with the performers/actors I worked with, and with my own self, about the role of trauma in theater and the performing arts?

The Physiology of Trauma: A Somatic Approach

Transforming the parts of us that are frozen to past places.

Schwartz 2019: 14

Trauma is a word that has become commonplace, even fashionable, in Spain in the last few years. As a professional working in the Performing Arts, Somatic Voice-Body Education, and Therapy, I have been moved by how readily the term is used by many people when describing challenges faced by human beings (without even knowing what trauma means in a physiological as well as in a psychological context). I feel it is essential, then, to clarify what we name trauma in the arena of somatic movement therapy.

When the body feels in danger, our nervous system has the capacity to deal with this survival state with a fight, flight, freeze, or even flirt response. If the feelings of danger are dealt with effectively and the body restores its sense of security and safety, we will have experienced both the challenge and the possibility of "coming back home" after it. This has the potential to make us stronger and more resilient. An alarming event that someone is unable to process, to reach a healthy conclusion in the moment (or close to the moment of experiencing it), is kept in the body, waiting to be resolved. This is what is meant by a traumatic event or trauma in the body, and it could be related to many different kinds of experience, even pre- and perinatal ones where the **social brain** is developing in relationship to the caregivers and environment (Gerhardt 2004: 35).

The consequence of unresolved traumatic experiences implies that the nervous system is unable, in those moments during or following a threat or sense of danger, to restore self-regulation, so it could become trapped in re-experiencing the feelings (mostly physical) whenever a trigger event or stimulus is experienced. The organism used the best of its resolutions available in that moment, and as a wise adviser will give cues to direct the necessary attention towards a healthy ending to that event whenever it can. This relationship with an inconclusive danger is at first physical and then a waterfall of emotions may follow. Peter Levine wisely points to the **implicit memory** (the emotional and the procedural memory) that is stored in the body in the case of trauma (Levine 2018: 58). For me, this feels as if a huge amount of energy is being kept in the body, waiting to find a way to re-enter the flow of life.

It is important for me to acknowledge that the person who lives under the influence of any kind of trauma is expending nearly her whole life energy living in the survival state through her whole body. Therefore, as a professional, I use the word trauma when the organism has lost its capacity to regulate from this survival state following a traumatic event which remains stored in the body and voice, revisiting the present moment when stirred. Through a somatic movement therapy approach, combined with other modalities from voicework or theater play, I facilitate a way to help the client carefully, first, to tolerate their physical and emotional feelings in order then to integrate the experiences. This coming back to the body will be essential to re-entering the life stream.

The Performer's Avatar: Myself and the Self of a Character in a Play

Suit the action to the word, the word to the action ... the purpose of playing, whose end, both at the first and now, was and is to hold as 'twere the mirror up to nature, to show virtue her own feature, scorn her own image, and the very age and body of the time his form and pressure.

Shakespeare, *Hamlet*, III, ii

If you watch any play or movie, from the theater of the Greeks to the Hollywood of Clint Eastwood, the variety of traumatic events, relationships, and traumatized characters is vast. The majority of the theater or screen work that an actor is going to come across in their working life will be centered either around unresolved trauma or around ways to release it. I will say that the actor's life navigates stormy waters that might not be easy.

The actor has to invite a character to live in the house of her body for a while, and will need to call on all the potential of her corporal, vocal, emotional, and mental capacities to travel the imaginary life of this guest. Entering into relationship with the play and the character is going to be full of surprises. These unexpected movements will touch the life of the actor in an unpredictable way.

Jorge Muriel is a professional actor and a dear friend. In the past decade, he has chosen some of the projects he wanted to perform as an actor and I had the gift of giving him support with workshops and individual sessions for some of them. He carefully reads and watches many theater plays and decides which roles are more interesting for him. Then he translates, produces, and performs those texts. We sometimes joke that this is the only way for him to play these characters because no casting agent will choose him for these roles. What intrigues me more in each of the projects is his initial connection with the role he is to perform and how, for most of them, he has to do his own research into the life and biography of the character. He unites with each character because he needs to reach the part of the life that wants to be heard.

Jorge: I choose the plays that move me, touch me and make me grow. For example, in one of my last roles, in Things I Know to Be True by Andrew Bovell (2019), the character I played, Mia (a transgender daughter), is full of reality and, at a personal level, I wanted to research around the freedom of being oneself, even though society and family were not very helpful. The play I am rehearsing now, Tribes by Nina Raine (2010), talks about the deafness of society and the unawareness of deaf society and culture. My character is very complex and I am feeling scared, but at the same time I want to take the risk because I know it is going to be very enriching for me as a human being and for the audience that will come to see it. So, as you can see, by working around these two characters I am confronted with myself and this makes me grow. It is as if they make me look to my own fears and help me to transcend them. In the case of Mia, because she is braver than me, embodying her I spread my own wings. With this latest character, Daniel, I am still in the process of rehearsals and his pain is touching me a lot; his insecurities, the obsession with competing, the need to be seen, his addictions ... and there my own wounds are opening now. The loneliness of this character, his hypervigilance and sense of the void, are bigger than those I have experienced in my own life and that's scary.

I gave Jorge support in individual sessions with somatic voice and body facilitation work. His own generous, resilient spirit and sensitivity allowed him to access a very rich pool of research.

Jorge: What I like about working with you, Leticia, is that I always begin from myself, my body, my emotions, the things that happen inside me, as if I can approach my visceral self and I can let go of my mental judgments. I enjoy working on very specific and important things for the role, touching themes that are stepping stones for the humanity of the character, and those themes open doors in me in a way that make me grow. So, I experience the work I do with you as liberating and very healthy. I come to know the guts of the character, and those guts echo in my own. Another thing I value a lot is that the work you offer nurtures me and brothers me with the character, and this merges me with my creativity in a more personal way. As if my own humanity communicates with the humanity of the character in a therapeutic and artistic way. And we do it in a grounding way, as if I can anchor myself into the earth, as if working in this way makes me strong because it is grounded in me and gives me the right to perform it.

During one of our sessions, Jorge experienced a proposal that I made to him as an act of aggression:

Jorge: When you told me, "try not to cry as you say this part of the text," I took it as aggression and got really angry with you and the situation. I was emotionally censored as a kid; it took me years to relate to emotional freedom and I reject any situation now that doesn't allow me to express myself with freedom. Having the time to dialogue around these feelings made me realize that I sometimes try to 'liberate myself' through accessing crying on stage or a sense of being emotionally free there. Even when I cry in my own life, anything that doesn't allow me to do this kind of liberating I experience as repressive and I assume this is part of my personal story, not the character's. Certainly, some characters in many situations wouldn't find it so easy to cry with all that freedom.

In one way or another, the performer is going to embrace the character and the story through his own body and voice experience, and often that story is going to move him out of place, even touching and activating or reviving his own trauma. Facilitating **body–mind–voice integration** (see later), or even restoring peace in the traumatized character he is dealing with, could be a kind of life insurance to enable a person to have a long and fulfilling career in the performing arts.

Graceful and Bold: The Challenge of Embracing the Actor's Personal Trauma with Awareness

María Bigeriego is a dancer, actress, and Linklater voice teacher. Our pathways met many years ago when she was my student and in the past few years we have grown quite close, professionally and personally. Knowing that, through her life, she had experienced some difficult events that became the main theme in a play that she wrote, I asked her for the chance to establish a conversation around the theme of Trauma and Performance and she very kindly opened up an honest and intimate space for this. She shared how, in several verbal therapeutic contexts when she was confronted with the exposure of traumatic events from her own life, her body felt unstable or seemed to drain all her strength; the main symptom was an inability to communicate through her voice.

> ***María:*** **I wasn't able to let the voice out, and felt very weak, wanting to sink into the ground, not feeling able to support myself on my legs.**

We discussed the process of **pendulating** instead of re-experiencing the trauma, a term that Peter Levine uses to explain the possibility of dealing with trauma symptoms in our body in order to re-establish a grounded feeling of security for the person involved (Levine and Kline 2007: 4). A couple of years ago, María wrote and directed a theater play, *La mujer de Fearon*. This play addresses the story of a woman based on María's personal experiences. She explains why she wanted to do this project:

> ***María:*** **It was a way to exorcise a period of my life though an artistic form. I needed to pay tribute to these events to be able to close the page and continue with my life.**

María also mentioned how helpful it was for her to take some workshops on Infant Movement Developmental Education that I provided in Madrid around that time.

> ***María:*** **In those workshops I allowed myself to feel contact and to decide if I wanted it or not. Noticing that I needed a lot of time to be able to say yes, and giving myself that time in those workshops, was a treasure that helped me in the theater project.**

I was especially interested in her personal experience of rehearsing and performing the play. María first wrote and directed it, then after the opening night and in the second round of performances she decided to be on stage with the performers, dancing "the shadow of the main character."

> ***María:*** **I made the transition from the huge embarrassment of being the director and watching it from the outside to feeling more weighted and grounded within a sense of lightness when I was on stage with them, also being seen by the audience. At the end of the process, I became more and more detached from those scenes in my life and a sense of humor started to appear.**

Speaking to me about how artistic forms can help resolve traumatic events in the life of the artist, she mentioned that she had talked with a psychotherapist and in group therapy about those personal events that were addressed in the play.

> ***María:*** **It was after this artistic event that I could confront the abuser, asking him for his apologies, and that helped me to finish the process.**

After this project she was able to unleash the embarrassment and found the strength to truly confront the abuser after 20 years of personal process. Certainly, the body sometimes has different timing than the mind, and giving ourselves the ability to respond instead of react with the body and the artistic work could help as well.

It moves me greatly that María's spirit persevered to find resolution and that an artistic theater space provided the context to do that, enabling her to transcend it and grow stronger and more resilient thereafter.

Chapter 17

Somatic Voice and Body Education Training to Support the Artist

IBMT and SOMArt: finding other ways to research and maybe resolve trauma

As an Artist I found that the Diploma in Integrative Bodywork and Movement Therapy (IBMT) offered me a space with enough security and support to dive into the darkness of my biography that was interlinked with my own biology. Linda Hartley's guidance and the relationship with other students and assistants reconciled me with my internal lived map that had traveled with me for years. This yielding to my own self in a loving way allowed me to open to the unexpected and to the experience of other available options. I regained a different and more fluid sense of agency in my personal life, which gave me back the gift of **rooting myself to fly** in the creative environment of the performing arts. With consciousness and a chance to respond instead of react, I could co-regulate better with the characters I worked with in the plays.

Now, in collaboration with Raquel Esteban and María Bigeriego, I have founded and coordinated my own pathway in somatic voice and movement education for the artist with a program called SOMArt. One of its aims is to provide dynamic training that allows the artist to enter into rehearsal with enough grounding in their own self to play around the character, to play with another self.

An example of this is a series of workshops for the actor called "The Unpredictable Life of the Dramatic Text." I have created this space within SOMArt to explore a character through somatic voice and body training, **Body–Mind–Voice Integration**, terminology that my colleague Pablo Troccoli and I defined when we wrote about stage fright (Troccoli and Santafé 2020: 86). One of the pathways I am developing within this training program is the marriage between Linklater voice methodology (Linklater 2007) and the developmental movement education and body systems from IBMT and Body-Mind Centering®. The awareness of somatic psychology and the principles and practice forms of Authentic Movement are a core orientation for guiding the actors' processes as well.

The training that I provide for the rehearsal and research space can be very different from that for the performance event. To give an example, during rehearsal or at the initiation of a project I take into account the possibility of an emergent self that can resonate more with pre-natal developmental neuro-cellular patterns, plus the freedom of more natural breathing based on the sigh of relief that the Linklater approach offers. All this connects the voice (sounding voice or silent voice) with a more grounded feeling of sensory vibration or the **touch of sound** (Linklater 2006: 65). On the other hand, when involved in the busyness of rehearsal, I might use an approach that gives the more instinctual and e-motional voice of the character a space by providing the organ and skeletal mind mixed with the resonating Linklater ladder (Linklater 2006: 275) to ground the desire to communicate the words of the script or the play. To offer another example, there is a beautiful work that Kristin Linklater uses in her voice training which is called *River Stories*; I use this to ingrain imagination around the life of the character in a more corporeal and vocal way. I find it is essential to this work to incorporate the witnessing skills from Authentic Movement and to provide an overview of the vibrational state of the endocrine system to hold the life stream of the character.

At the end of the process, and in relation to the performance energy that may be needed, another way of training is needed to come into relationship with the weight and pressure of the performance demands themselves. Working on more complete voice and body training, from freeing the voice in the body to strengthening and developing a range of possibilities, the performer needs to keep enough balance in her nervous system and to come in contact with the clarity and determination of the immune system. (For descriptions of the "mind" and qualities of the anatomical body systems, see Bainbridge Cohen (1993) and Hartley (1995).) Access to both systems is a way to contain and surf the energy of the performance in dialogue with whatever energy the audience brings each night.

The information that moves the actor when acting with a dramatic text is huge. When she can "ride the horse" of the character and the context of the play, with enough agency to support whatever is necessary in rehearsals and to finish the experience at the end of each performance, she will have the energy to sustain herself in the task and will be able to process and have a deeper experience of her work. For this purpose, I want to provide the actor with Body–Mind–Voice Integration training: to enable them to navigate their sensations and feelings, and practice the ability to communicate them through movement, sound, and language that is filled with emotions, instinct, and imagination.

Conclusion: A Never-ending Story

Recently, I have been rehearsing a show about Hamlet with The Clever People Company, a group of clowns based in Valladolid (www.thecleverpeoplecompany.com). Entering the crazy, vulnerable state of the clown is always a mystery. I am playing Gertrude, Hamlet's mother. (I am still in awe of being cast as a mother, while being a mother of three children myself.)

In the rehearsal process, my clown did not want to be the tormented, abdicated mother who feels embarrassed by her actions, and the female activist in me started to rebel and came into the rehearsal room. Since the clown allows the actor to turn life upside down, the director encouraged me to be in that place. Gertrude started to assert how difficult it was for a woman to be a woman in a period of time when men alone acted on their will, and to be the mother of a spoiled child who talked incessantly and did nothing, to be the queen of a country about to be invaded, and shouting all of this to her speechless and amazed son while at the same time crying because of her need to have some bathroom time ALONE. It was hilarious and HUGE for me. I went home seeing myself a little bit better, feeling both moved and tired after rehearsals. I came to reconcile this speech with my shadow and can cry with my own sadness too.

There is no doubt that this clowning version of Hamlet is going to be crazily funny and outside of the rulebook, and no doubt that this characterization of Gertrude emerged from my own experience of motherhood that is trying to find a way to be seen MORE.

As long as we actors keep on shaking up life in rehearsal or on the stage, it will keep on moving through our bodies and creative voices, and maybe move through the universal body of the audience too. The abiding question for me remains: how do we access this movement and embrace it with enough self-care to be supported and to thrive in the unknown?

Dedicated to Paul Burge, teacher and friend, may his soul rest in peace.

Video link
Video from LAVA Artistic Residency

Part 6

Somatic Movement and Dance Research

Somatic and Poetic Movement: The Connection Between IBMT and Dance Practice

18

Maria Grudskaya

I sit on the chair in my grandma's kitchen.

I allow my attention to go through the layers of skin, fascia and muscles, and sink into my bones. The coccyx attracts my attention; here it is – the small tail of the spine. I sense heat and buzzing; it is difficult to keep the tail still. I allow it to move, tiny wiggling movements, different directions, undefined, unclear, emerging movement.

I am curious to watch this movement as a dance.

What dance is unfolding from this? Where does the movement begin, how does it develop, what rhythm emerges in this tiny dance?

The tail slows down, the movement sequences to the spine and torso. I am aware of my whole body engaged in the dance.

Circle movement from tail to the torso, rhythmic, stomping each time the circle reaches the front ... jazz.

Strong energy in the legs, a bit lazy in the torso. Legs take over – stepping, swinging, circling.

I could write a whole polyrhythmic music piece of this dance.

Strong arms and fingers opening, grabbing and pulling, chest expanding and condensing, sensuality and fire.

Dance contrasts with the space of the kitchen and also there is a certain harmony – reminding me of the flamenco movies of Carlos Saura – village women dancing vigorously in the yard with laundry hanging around ...

Here it is – my dance of the day. I feel surprised and grateful.

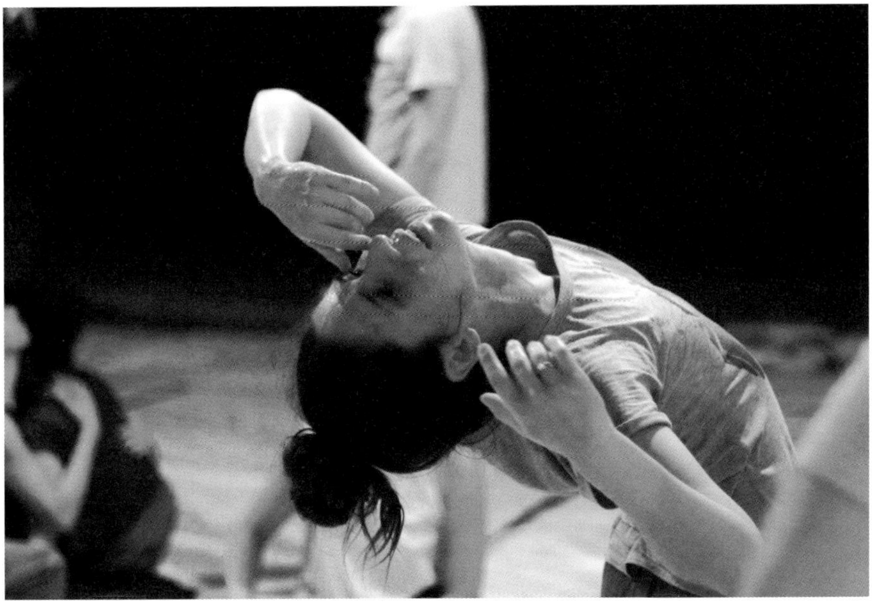

Dancer: Maria Grudskaya. Photographer: Katja Sannikova

Chapter 18

I have practiced Contact Improvisation and Dance Improvisation for over 15 years, as well as contemporary and social dances.

In Contact Improvisation I have explored elements of somatic work: for example, early reflexes and patterns of movement, proprioception and kinesthetic sense, general awareness of movement, inner experience, and connection to space and other people. At some point in my practice, I felt the desire to go deeper into exploration of my movement and presence; I joined the Integrative Bodywork and Movement Therapy (IBMT) program, where I expected to go through 3 years of practice with the support of teachers and the group. For me it turned out to be a deeper and longer journey: I graduated from my studies, became an IBMT therapist and teacher, and joined the Faculty of IBMT.

As I continue to practice both – dance and somatic movement – I observe how somatic movement supports me, informs me, makes me more skillful and conscious in dance. And as an IBMT somatic movement teacher, I am interested in how dance can support, deepen, and integrate the somatic process and how dance can be included in somatic classes.

Also, I notice the difference between therapeutic somatic "mind" and poetic "mind" in movement. I am curious how it feels to go into a somatic exploration as a dance artist and as a client or a therapist. These are the topics I would like to share in this chapter. It is not "expert knowledge," but a beginning of exploration and discussion for practitioners.

In preparation for this chapter, I talked to my colleagues, who have experience in somatic practice and dance, about their thoughts on the topic. I asked them some questions:

- How does IBMT support your dance? Does it influence your work?
- Does your artistic/dance practice deepen or support your somatic practice? In what way?
- How does IBMT support or influence you in your artistic and everyday life?

Some of their responses are included in this chapter.

I want to mention an article by Martha Eddy: "A Brief History of Somatic Practices and Dance: Historical Development of the Field of Somatic Education and its Relationship to Dance" (2009). Eddy describes the roots and lines of development of the wide and diverse field of somatic practices, mentioning pioneers and following generations of somatic teachers. She shows how somatic practice developed in close connection to dance, how both practices feed each other. It is an interesting and important view on the history and development of dance and somatic education.

The term "Poetic Movement" I learned from Stephen Batts, my teacher and choreographer based in Northern Ireland. Poetic Movement is a form of art where movement is the main source of expression; it has a certain grammar – composition in space and time – and creates poetic meaning. Poetic Movement has the same relation to pedestrian movement as poetry to everyday speech. It can be the same movements that we do in everyday life, composed to create meaning.

In Poetic Movement we can play with compositional aspects, such as:

- phrases – when the movement begins, how it develops, and when it ends
- rhythm, pulse, change of pace
- how the movement travels through space; what the relationship is to space; how it moves through vertical levels
- in relation to other people: whether we adapt, influence, or interact with each, how we play with the distance between us, what quality of touch we share.

Somatic and Poetic Movement: IBMT and Dance

Is Poetic Movement a dance? In general, dance is a wide phenomenon: it can describe a completely internal experience of movement, or a ritual, or it can mean an "exercise" or technique that can be completed without necessarily paying much attention to composition or meaning. Poetic Movement is a dance where dancers are aware of compositional and poetic aspects and consciously play with them. In this chapter, the word "Dance" will be used as a synonym for Poetic Movement.

In Poetic Movement a dancer is aware of how the movement can be seen or read by the audience; she reads her own movement as an audience would do. She needs to be aware of her sense of proprioception to track her movement in real space and real time, and at the same time be connected to the world of meanings – how the movement might be perceived and understood by the viewers. Movement may have many layers of meaning, interpretations, and connotations; a dancer and each member of the audience can understand and perceive it in their own unique way. Similarly, the audience can perceive a meaning in a poem or a musical piece that the author did not consciously put there. In a way, a poem or a dance creates itself. As a dancer, I am an audience to my own movement and I can be touched by it – amazed, surprised, mesmerized, bored, saddened, confused, and so on. This inner audience is close to the inner witness that we develop in Authentic Movement and somatic practice, and later we will talk about their similarity and difference.

Through the years of practice, I have explored how somatic movement supports me as a dancer. Somatic practice develops awareness of body and movement, the ability to tune in detail into one's state of bodymind. In IBMT and Authentic Movement, we practice the skills of tracking our physical movement, bodily sensations, feelings, and images. In dancing, this level of awareness is useful too – it allows a dancer to track the whole composition in real time. Through somatic practice we can learn to stay connected to inner experience while creating a dance, to tell a story from within, to live it. This makes the dance more authentic, resonating with the audience. The deeper the awareness, the richer the potential for the dance to unfold. Embodied presence is the field from which the dance is born. And this is what we develop in somatic practice.

Part of IBMT work is experiential anatomy: exploration of body systems and developmental patterns. Through hands-on work and movement, we develop body connectivity, find effortless movement, and widen the range of movement qualities. For a dancer, this is essential to be able to notice the smallest impulses, where the movement initiates and how it travels through the body. Somatic practice heightens the sensitivity and allows a mover to notice how she is influenced by changes in the inner and outer space. Somatic practice can feed the bodymind, nourish body systems with touch and attention. It awakens the cells, tissues, nervous system, making the bodymind more alive, available, and expressive.

Authentic Movement and somatic practice may become sources of material for dancing, revealing themes that can be expressed and explored in dance.

Presence skills that we develop as IBMT practitioners, such as grounding, centering, connection to space and other people, are useful for a dancer too. Vera Priklonskaya, dance artist and somatic therapist, says that somatic practice supports her as a person and as an artist:

Before I struggled with shyness on stage, and now I have forgotten what it means to be shy – it is me and my body process that I am aware of. I am more in contact with my feelings as a performer, my relationship to others on stage, and generally, in the dance community, this awareness gives me more resilience.

(Priklonskaya 2019)

Chapter 18

Somatic practice can support dancing, and at the same time dancing can enrich somatic exploration. In IBMT and other somatic practices, through touch and attention we awaken deeper sensing in the body. Sensing can allow us to notice little changes or tensions in the body or learn new patterns of movement. At the same time, if we focus only on sensing, it can create an imbalance in our system. At some point, the sensing needs to go into the background and give way to action and movement. In her book *Sensing, Feeling, and Action*, Bonnie Bainbridge Cohen gives this example:

the eye … was not developed to be perceived, it was developed to have an action. … when you go to look, you don't try to move your muscles and your bones, but let the eye respond to the light that's being reflected.

(Bainbridge Cohen 2012: 65)

Dancing can become a way to "change gears" and shift the focus from sensing to a solo or group activity. This helps to integrate somatic experience. Dance supports the transition from inner space to the space around. We find connection to other people, enter into communication, share our dance with other dancers and watchers. And through dance we share our experience, find support and the joy of moving and playing together.

When I enter the dance or Poetic Movement, I open myself to all layers of images, feelings, symbols, metaphors, associations, characters that may come up, connect to a rich poetic field that may widen my experience. And I become an audience to my own dance; I can observe the dance that develops, practice being a mover and a witness at the same time.

As a teacher of somatic movement, I look for ways to support the transition from somatic explorations to movement and dancing. One of these ways is to invite the transition from inner sensing to "outer" senses: what do I see, what do I hear, what do I smell, what do I taste, what do I sense with my skin? This supports the relationship to space around: we can begin with the small space around the body

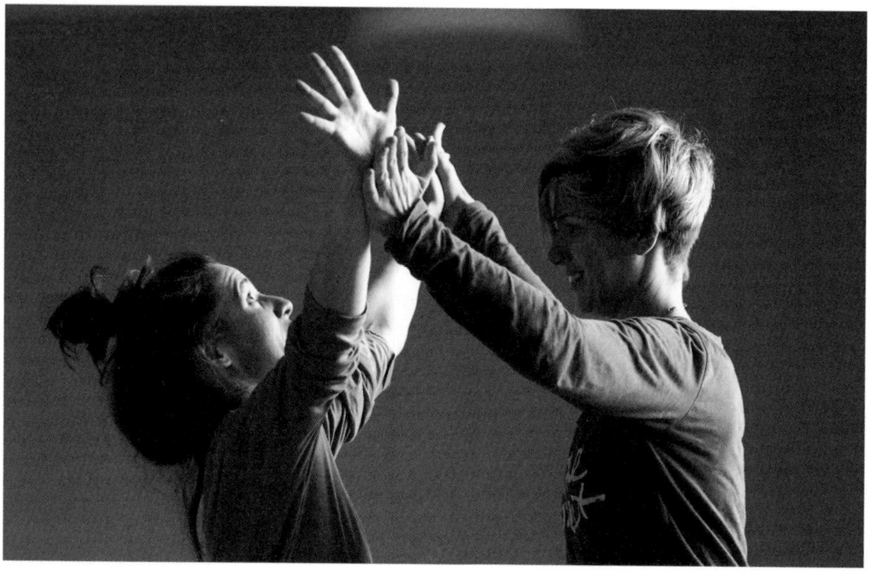

Dancers: Maria Grudskaya, Yana Sutina. Photographer: Katja Sannikova

– the kinesphere – and then the attention may open to the whole space of the studio and beyond.

Sometimes, it helps to put on music, which can create a certain atmosphere, phrasing, and rhythm. Another way is gradually to offer more compositional focuses of attention: invite students to play with speed, or notice pauses and how each new movement begins, develops, and ends, or repeat one movement – faster, slower, bigger, smaller.

Sometimes, we can find a clear ending to a somatic exploration and then create a dance based on our experience. Various scores can be offered: for example, create a movement phrase that reflects your experience and teach others.

Here is another example of transitions between different *modes* of movement. In her online course "Body and Earth," Andrea Olsen offers an exercise called "Thresholds," where we begin walking and then notice:

- What is the threshold between walking and moving?
- Between moving and dancing?
- Between dancing and raucous dancing?
- Between raucous dancing and performing?
- Between performing and meditating?
- Meditating and being? (Olsen 2015)

This exercise invites us to explore the borders between different states of mind in movement, play with these borders, and find that sometimes there are no borders.

From my practice and from sharing with students and colleagues, I notice that there are different modes of going into somatic exploration: therapeutic and artistic. By somatic exploration, here I mean any practice of conscious movement or

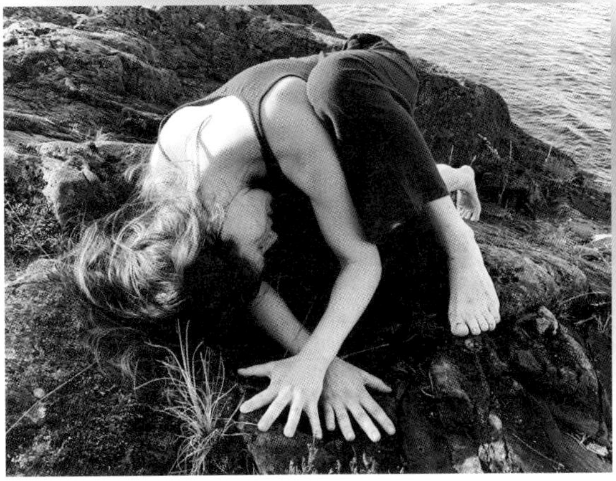

Dancer: Maria Grudskaya. Photographer: Masha Denisova

observation, when the practitioner is aware of her own experience.

In a therapeutic setting, the practitioner is in relationship with a therapist, and the purpose of the exploration can be personal healing – to find inner resources or give space to whatever needs to be expressed, seen, and supported. For example, a client can explore her bones to find grounding and structure, or to discover whatever quality they express, what message they share. A therapist creates a supportive space for the client, holds the timing, makes sure the client will find transition back to her whole adult self at the end of the session. A therapist offers compassionate witnessing to all the parts and stories of the client's bodymind. With a therapist, a client might go somewhere unknown where she would not allow herself to go on her own. It can be a healing and valuable process to be seen and supported, and gradually a client may develop her own compassionate inner witness.

From the other side, when I am in somatic exploration as an artist, I must be responsible for my own navigation, keep my own timing, find transitions in and out of the experience, and collect the harvest.

Chapter 18

If I go into somatic exploration as a performer, it means that I am potentially seen by the audience, or I explore material that I want to include later in my performance that will be seen by the audience. I enter into a relationship with the viewers, which is different from a therapeutic relationship. The audience is not there necessarily to support me; in the best case, they have interest and curiosity in what I share. I am a storyteller.

I can go to the same "places" as in therapeutic somatic exploration, but as an artist I need to be ready to play with it, to compose it, go in and out, be ready to change, sometimes switch fast to the next thing, let go easily.

It feels like a strong and profound skill – to visit different places of the bodymind and be able to navigate this journey. And sometimes artistic exploration can feel "lighter" than a therapeutic one because I keep my poetic curiosity and my center – the navigator.

As an artist I need to know my world – places that I am ready or not ready to share with the audience. Some things need to stay only in my private experience.

In an artistic exploration I sometimes find myself being braver and can go further than in a therapeutic setting. For example, the theme of death in my personal process is quite intense: it evokes strong feelings of loss and fear and can be overwhelming. At the same time, as a dancer I can explore death artistically and I do not feel instantly overwhelmed. My colleague Artiom Markov offered a performance workshop in 2018 about death where, in movement, we explored how death was perceived in different cultures; we looked at a cycle of a single cell – its death and transformation into something new. Another direction could be to look at a bigger scale – the death of a universe and what happens next, or music and artwork devoted to death, the relation to ancestors, rituals, death, and birth as a metaphor for transition, and so on. The artistic view allows us to connect to the theme of death as a phenomenon and gives a wider perspective on the topic in a cultural and historical context. We do not deal only with our personal experience, but

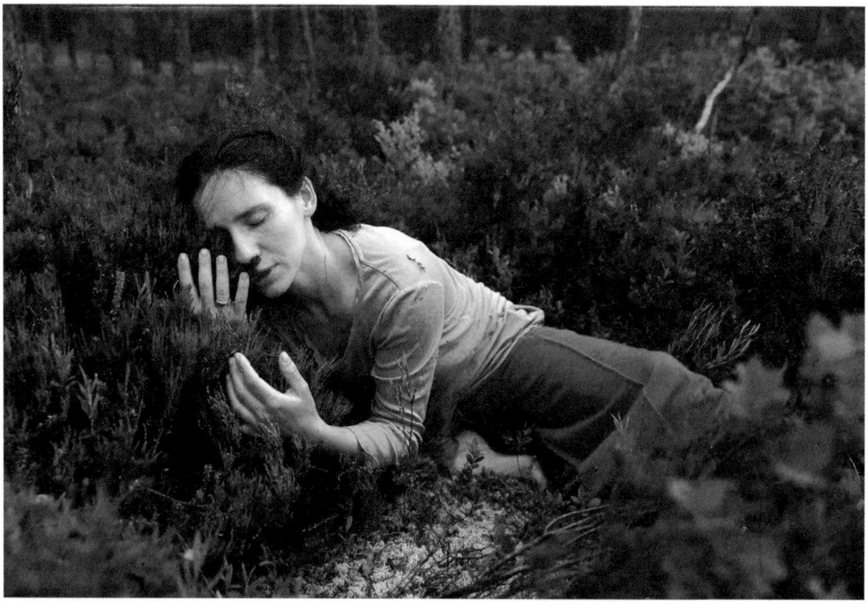

Dancer: Maria Grudskaya. Photographer: Daria Lapina

we can play with a wider field and include our personal stories as much or as little as we want.

Another example of artistic somatic exploration is the work of Debora Hay, choreographer and improviser. She offers questions that begin with "What if" and address the cellular wisdom of the body. For example:

- What if every cell in my body at once had the potential to locate and choose the oxygen it needs to keep my fire burning?
- What if my whole body at once has the potential to perceive Here, spatially, including everything I see and everything I can't see now, and now, and now?
- What if dying is movement in communion with all there is? (Hay 2000: 103)

These questions do not need to be answered or completed; they are like doorways to exploration. What if my cells know something that I do not yet know? What if my cells can perceive something that I do not yet perceive? They do not have to know and perceive, but what if? ... To me these questions are mysterious and inspiring to move with.

It is not only movement poetry that can enrich somatic experience, but a wider poetic view, expressed through different means – writing, drawing, making music, installations, and so on. Poetic process can be deeply joyful: we allow images, metaphors, and stories to arise and be shared with others. Poetic view gives freedom of expression; it reflects the complexity, chaos, and mystery of somatic experience, which is rarely linear.

As we compose our movement, we develop inner witness and inner audience. And we enter into relationships with other movers and viewers, which is a great gift – to be seen as we tell our story.

Mediating Resonant Spaces: IBMT as Support for Dance Making and Expanded Artistic Practice

19

Gaelin Little

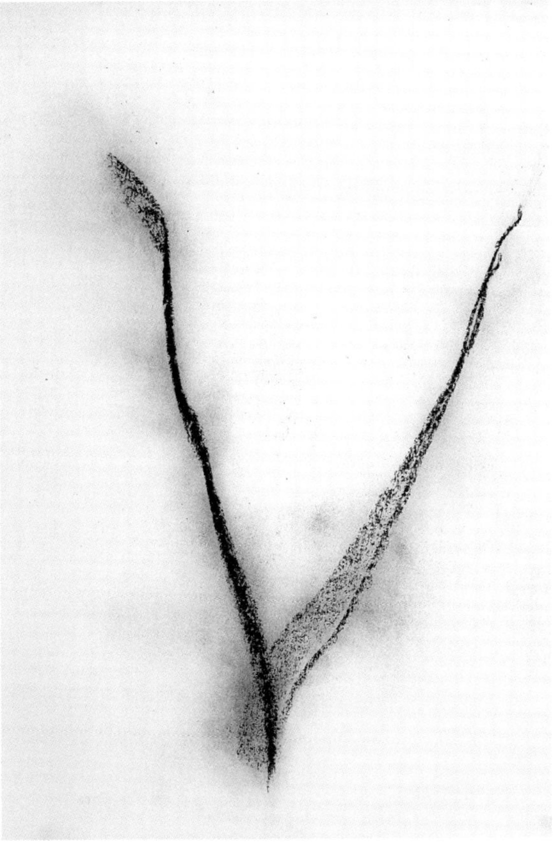

Beginnings. Artwork by Gaelin Little

Form and Formlessness Within IBMT

I originally trained and worked as a dance artist and performer. Somatic movement therapy fundamentally changed my relationship to dancing and dance-making. Through somatic practice I rediscovered an inner intuition or deeper knowing about why dancing and creating is integral to my life and wellbeing.

Integrative Bodywork and Movement Therapy (IBMT) weaves together somatic principles found within three main practices: Body-Mind Centering®, Somatic Psychology, and Authentic Movement. In the Discipline of Authentic Movement, the mover enters an empty space. Here she remains open, letting go of preconceptions; she attends to experiences arising, and responds moment to moment, allowing movements and gestures to emerge. Body-Mind Centering traces a journey of embodiment through formative movement processes in our human development: from the growing and differentiating of the intricate anatomical body systems that make up our whole organism (organs, skin, bones, connective tissue, blood, muscle, and so on) to the complex series of movement connections and pathways that evolve towards enabling us to take our first independent steps in the world. Revisiting these developmental stages in therapeutic conditions offers an experiential insight of coming into form that reveals something about our journey into relationship with the material world. Linda Hartley describes the combination of these two practices supporting each other through the interplay of form and formlessness (personal communication 2015).

Paradoxically, investing my awareness in the realm of form creates much freedom in my body; more options or ways of being in my embodied self become available, as I learn to follow ease, find healthy movement pathways, and draw support from the different embodied qualities offered by each body system. Authentic Movement develops a capacity to track the details of experience and expressions unfolding out of an empty open space, through an awareness of sensation. This often begins with acknowledging our own unconscious patterning manifesting in the body, which in turn enables us to move away or grow beyond it. Somatic Psychology offers a therapeutic understanding of these complex, somewhat intangible experiences that can be integrated into our lives to

Chapter 19

support deeper insights into our patterns of relationship and being in the world. Drawing on this specific combination of practices creates a holistic somatic process that is unique to IBMT.

The chapter that follows draws from and includes written and visual materials from unpublished practice as research dissertation with Trinity Laban Conservatoire of Music and Dance (2020).

Somatic Practice as a Support for Creativity and Art-making

Somatic practices heighten an awareness of my moving body, revealing something hidden from my "ordinary" perception. The mover could be seen as an explorer who practices the fine-tuning of her senses and turns them toward a renewed discovery of the world around her. However, I have often felt a sense of loss in the transition from dancer–explorer to dancer–dance-maker, exposing a tension between a somatically informed movement practice and approaches belonging to traditional choreographic and dramaturgical processes.

When a living process is subject to artistic critique before it is ready, what gets shut down, folded back into the shadows, affecting material from the birth of its becoming, in the pivotal and delicate moments of finding and defining the work?

It has become my understanding that somatic movement *is* a creative process in its own right and therefore the ever-unfolding nature of experience it points toward can be not only "applied" but embedded *within* the fabric of an emergent creative process.

This is relevant to all creative practices, not only dance, as I am referring to creativity in its broadest sense, as a state of being that does not assign itself to a particular medium. Each of us has a rich inner landscape that has the potential to become a unique expression in the world.

Between Understandings

I am interested in Buddhist practice and philosophy, and although this is not an official part of the IBMT training, as a Buddhist practitioner herself Hartley seamlessly wove in core principles that influenced my understanding of somatic practice. In my work I find myself sitting in the porous membrane between therapeutic, educational, artistic, and spiritual contexts. Most things are more interconnected than the categories we create for understanding, and more often insights have arrived to me in the connection between things rather than the separation.

While I acknowledge that these different practices do have different aims, it is this very dialogue between developing a healthy sense of self and the ability to transcend the ego that makes them important allies. In movement, our capacity for levity must first come from a deep relationship to the earth and an understanding of the body's relationship to gravity. Once this is practiced and integrated, we can fly.

A key way that we can find ground is through establishing a sense of safety in the body. For many individuals living with trauma of some kind, no matter how big or small, this sense of safety is not a given. Developmentally, for each movement stage to be fully achieved, the baby needs environmental support though loving nurture and encouragement. If these conditions do not meet our needs, these stages of development might feel incomplete, affecting how we move through life. In a therapeutic context we cultivate the resources to come safely into fuller *relationship* with ourselves and the worlds around us: "What we create first is ourselves and it is out of ourselves that the producing comes" (Starks Whitehouse 1999: 40).

In my experience, the desire to create artwork has been a healthy outcome of time spent in therapeutic process. As we come into greater alignment with our understanding of ourselves, creative energies that may have been dormant can be released. Creative work in turn benefits from the integrity of an embodied honesty as we include the multi-dimensional body (physical, psychological, emotional, and spiritual selves) within the making process.

A Solitary Journey

My body benefits in Solitude.

Hay 2000

A sense of loneliness and vulnerability can be an integral part of the artist's journey.

The somatic movement therapist supports the client to enter the not yet known safely, supporting a transition where the client develops a confidence to meet life's experiences and challenges creatively.

This mirrors the Authentic Movement trajectory that begins as a relational practice, whereby the presence of the witness is in service of the mover's experience. The witness's refined attention is an anchor that supports the journey of descent and ascent, where unconscious materials can come into fuller consciousness. The visceral body is the vessel for all experiential phenomena, including the parts of our being in the shadows of our everyday awareness. Eventually, the felt presence of the external witness becomes integrated, strengthening the awareness of the mover's internal witness so that she is able to make this journey on her own.

Studio notes – on solitude

Sometimes it feels such a long way out there, as I lie here feeling the weight of my body spread across this one bit of land

Body and tide.

On the edge, waiting for the water to come, to be washed.

It may take a while.

I whisper softly into the abyss, imagining out there other creatures that will come to meet me; we will share stories about what happened while we were all waiting to be taken.

The experience of longing to belong to the other, to feel connected, to come home, reveals the palpable sense of separation. In Adler's trajectory of Authentic Movement practice, we move from individual consciousness to the consciousness of the collective. The awareness of my individual body enables me to open to the other and differentiate movements and materials that arrive from an experience of connectedness or "oneness" of us and all things. Moving between individuation and connection in mutual dialogue has its own sense of natural timing, like a tide.

Remaining receptive to this rhythm is deeply healing and restful. It is so easy to panic and readily grasp for the familiar, pulling us away from the relational aspect of the present moment.

Artworks that evolve in sensitive communication with the materiality they are situated in (including the political climate and wider societal conditioning) speak to us of what it is to have a body consciousness in this world.

The body is our sensation, our felt emotion. The body is our experience of ourselves, our temple in which the light of our spirit burns. Unconscious worlds, numinous worlds can become known within the body because of the body.

(Adler 2002: 6)

Letting Go of Our Axis

On establishing our sense of self, we bring this perceived center in relation to something new in order to let it go again, a continual forming and reforming.

Chapter 19

"Turning" score – studio notes

Turning embraces new information that enters my body moment to moment, offering a change in relation to my surroundings, and/or a shift in the inner environment, a moving perspective. The smallest of turns is assuming a unique axis, however momentary or temporary, creating a fluctuating center that adapts to shifting sensation and arrests perception. I find myself somewhere – somewhere else entirely.

I have a desire to free myself from the pressure of being the creator who is in control and to see what happens if instead I fully trust in a creative process where what is made will be an outcome of the work revealing itself to me.

In this approach, form does not precede content; there is no separate articulable form or concept that exists independently from the work, but instead it is an approach where making and the made are in mutual dialogue.

This requires getting the "I" out of the way to be in service to the work unfolding. Adler describes "an absence in the density of her personality when her moving self and inner witness are one" (2002: 29). Ultimately, I am attempting to depersonalize the creative process so that the **work itself** becomes a living process of discovery and revelation.

Faith in the Ground

In the empty space of the studio, begin from where you are: "You have to be where you are in order to get to the next place" (Bainbridge Cohen cited in Olsen 2014: 225).

The old saying "look before you leap" implies a deliberate preparation for the departure, first checking the direction of travel and that the landing will be safe.

As with venturing on any new journey, safety in an artistic context could be seen as a futile occupation. Expanding perception requires a movement into new territory. This can be terrifying.

Leap Before you Look: Black Mountain College 1933-1957 was the title of a 2016 exhibition curated by Helen Molesworth, featuring the work of Cage, Cunningham, and Rauschenberg. Molesworth's inversion of the phrase, "leap before you look," points to a departure from preparation, suggesting a trusting in the process, in one's ability to navigate the landing in the present moment, adapting to time and space as it happens. Leaping first is an act of faith.

What if we entered this space between the naming of things and their being known from a place of inner confidence? What if feeling lost in a void was a place of familiarity and one where we had the tools to navigate, explore, dig deeper? Rebecca Solnit articulates a process of being lost where we can lose the expectation of knowing exactly where we are. The skill is in understanding your instruments and knowing your trajectory.

> *Lost, was mostly a state of mind […] The question then is how to get lost. Never to get lost is not to live, not to know how to get lost brings you to destruction, and somewhere in the terra incognita in between lies a life of discovery.*
>
> (Solnit 2006: 14)

My experience of Authentic Movement practice is one of returning to the unknown again and again, so many times that this place begins to feel familiar; it becomes a state I can welcome, soften into, draw out, and where I can stay longer.

> *All of it, all of this emptiness, is a reflection of our own potential of emptiness within. I invite you to enter this emptiness as a mover. Here the emptiness can fill and empty because of you. Here you can fill and empty because of it.*
>
> (Adler 2002: 9)

Perhaps the leap of faith is about a confidence in the tools I take with me to navigate the journey, developing an inner orientating compass in service of the artistic process.

Resonant Space and a Different Kind of Knowing

[N]on-knowing is not a form of ignorance but a difficult transcendence of knowledge.
Lescure cited in Bachelard 1994 (1964): xxxii

The **resonant space** highlights a space-in-between which mediates that which we know and perceive, in relation to the murky territory that arises through staying with sensing.

A practice of attending to the resonant space between sensation and perception will also acknowledge the things that might disturb it, including personal and cultural tensions.

This resonant space is often under-acknowledged and misrepresented within a cultural climate where knowledge production through the articulation of concepts and views is prevalent. Robin Nelson states that "the privileging of theory might be traced back, at the beginnings of the Western tradition of thought." He describes a schism between theory and practice that was inaugurated by Plato's division of the body and mind (Nelson 2009: 114).

Somatic experiences that include the whole bodymind value other intelligences cultivated through the interplay of received knowledge and embodied exploration.

The "overarching" influence of knowledge becomes malleable, making way for less pre-determined forms to emerge: "The imaginal reality is a place where our creative processes and methodologies live and prosper, where intellectual thinking turns from stone into putty" (Bacon 2010: 1).

Bonnie Bainbridge Cohen describes a deeper kind of "knowing" within the process of embodiment that gives weight to experiential understanding.

Embodiment is a being process, not a doing process, not a thinking process ... it is the cells' awareness of themselves. You let go of conscious mapping. It is a direct experience, there are no intermediary steps or translations. There is no guide, no witness. There is complete knowing. There is peaceful comprehension. [...] The source of this process is love.
(Bainbridge Cohen 2008: 157)

Love is affiliated with this inner knowing as it includes an enormity of experience through surrendering to something other than yourself. Hartley describes this phenomenon: with "surrender to the path comes a sense of inevitability, of the 'rightness' of a gesture" (Hartley 2015: 157). Adler refers to an "offering from the conscious body" (Adler 2002: 28).

I am no longer outwardly searching or overreaching but experiences are effortlessly moving toward me.

"Moving without searching" score – studio notes

A score with no direction, no destination,

how can my moving become directionless? But not lost.

Signless. But full of meaning.

How can I be deeply invested in the non-searching?

Are there still things to find in the non-searching?

Pre-empting as a signal for pausing, letting things be.

How do I recognize that I'm "achieving" a score that celebrates non-achievement?

Does it matter?

Non-searching as non-holding.

Chapter 19

The Loving Witness

The loving witness does not aim to impart knowledge or wisdom; she simply attends to the resonant space, and her presence welcomes all that comes into being. She is powerful because you are being seen and felt within a process that is still unfolding. To be seen here fully, without judgment, is to give that place a voice, to bring it softly into consciousness. She provides the confidence to stay longer in the unknown space and the courage to stay with difficult experiences. This is not a sentimental witness; compassion is not without discernment but she holds the space for the good, the bad, and the messy all to be present, nurturing an environment where the multi-dimensional body has the space to live and breathe.

[The witness] imparts an attitude of non-judgmental acceptance and compassion. Through practice, the witness has learnt to own her projections, interpretations and judgments, and seeks to not impose these onto the mover's experience. […] By witnessing even the smallest detail, which might feel inconsequential to the mover, with care and respect, the witness communicates to the mover that every moment has significance, is of value to her, the witness.

(Hartley 2015: 303)

We can transfer these qualities of loving attention to a witness consciousness that is in service to the creative work, suspending judgment from the making process so that we can come into a deeper relationship to subtleties and discoveries within the embodied process itself, beyond preconceptions.

I have found importance in naming the different parts of my experience, gently drawing things out into words even if they are ideas from which I eventually move on. If I remember every part of the journey as significant in the first instance, I can then look back and decide what it is important to explore further through reflection and a process of distillation. Jane Bacon describes a practice of Authentic Movement where:

The mover waits and then allows herself to give shape or form to whatever arises, not checked or mediated […] What was once unconscious has now become conscious, and can be brought to the service of creativity rather than self-censoring.

(Bacon 2010: 67)

Only remembering the parts that I think are "good," or worth remembering, is an act of self-censoring and consequently the place I arrive at may be missing creative vitality.

How to Keep Sensing and Stop Making Sense

Staying longer with sensing quiets the part of my rational mind that instinctively makes sense of things. Tarkovsky views poetry as "an awareness of the world, a particular way of relating to reality" (Tarkovsky 1991: 21). Sensorial intelligences, freed from making sense and instead seen through a poetic sensibility, can empower artwork that is not bound to becoming demonstrative.

Sensing grounds us in temporal reality. It is the gateway into our experience. "Through the senses we get insight" (Bainbridge Cohen 2008: 65). Bainbridge Cohen differentiates between the functional acts of sensing and **feeling**, which is about our relationship to that information. Through feeling, we can let go of the effort of sensing and allow the fluid body to be in freely flowing movement. Too much feeling without sensing and we can no longer maintain a conscious relationship to our movement. Dancing between the two, Bainbridge Cohen writes, "We began to experience 'feeling' as a non-doing state – as a state of being" (2008: 38). And Starks Whitehouse writes, "[T]he core of the movement experience is in the sensation of moving and being moved" (Starks Whitehouse 1999: 43).

Staying with sensing nearly always starts with slowing down until I am almost still. If I begin with lots of movement, all the "surface" sensations are ready to guide me in habitual ways. But what happens if I let go of being the one who is so ready to be guided by sensing – if, even among faster and more expansive movements, there remains an inner stillness, not busied with directions and decisions, a signless realm? Here there is a just-is-ness to sensing. In other words, if I let go of the awareness of the body's response to sensation through cause and effect, then I can also let go of making sense of it, so that the relationship between movement and sensation does not involve perceiving a connection. When awareness and movement exist in parallel to each other, separate streams existing in the same timeframe, it paradoxically reveals a more intrinsic connection of the two. There is a *sense* that these two things are related rather than a *thought*. I think this is what Buddhism points towards in the practice of "direct experience" – letting things be as they are without adding or narrowing, an immediacy that opens out the resonant space.

The Nervous System and the Resonant Space

The function of the nervous system offers an anatomical image for the communication between sensation and perception, prompting an imagining of what could be happening in the resonant space.

Information we receive through the senses arrives from the peripheral nervous system (PNS) to the central nervous system (CNS), which acts as a site of information integration, making sense of the signals that are coming to us from external and internal environments. Sensory nerves take in and transmit sensory information and motor nerves enable action in response. Interneurons send information between sensory and motor neurons.

As described in Chapter 14, the peripheral nervous system is divided into two parts, the autonomic nervous system (ANS) that operates below conscious level and the somatic nervous system (SNS) that communicates between the CNS and the PNS. Information received through the back of the spinal cord moves through the center of the spinal column, where it either travels up to the brain and then out of the front of the spine (SNS), or motors straight out of the front (ANS and reflexes). The direction of movement from back to front is much like the leap, with the spine being the central point of suspension and mediation. **Mediation** is derived from the Latin for "in the middle," informing an approach to dancing and making that is mediated from the middle or from within that space. Together, the ANS and the SNS mediate the relationship between conscious and unconscious habits and revolutions of our actions and behaviors. They are responsible for finding homeostasis for the space between inward and outward states of focus and activity, between being and doing.

Cellular tone

Through the exchange of fluids, the porous cell membrane lets in what it needs and lets go of what is no longer useful. Cellular tone underlies the tone of all the tissues of the body, regulated through the ANS. If the cell membrane is stressed, holding on too tightly and creating high tonicity (hyper-tone), it loses the ability to take things in fully. In collapsed or exhausted states, there will be low tonicity (hypo-tone); the gates are left open, overwhelming the cell. In either extreme, the membrane becomes dissociated and less active in choice-making.

Chapter 19

Breathing tonifies and balances the cell, helping it to return to homeostasis. Through expanding and condensing, breath is a beautiful metaphor for the gentle receiving of sensation, broadening and opening of perception, and then distilling down to what is needed. Here, "there is a dialogue between the needs of our body and the outer demand of the world" (Olsen 2014: 124).

Elastic Membrane

The membrane is a container, but also a space – a resonating space, a movable space. Not one thing; elements of both. A site for communication, play and interplay, providing a flexible skin that acts as mediator for the resonant space via the "elasticity of sensation" (Deleuze and Smith 2008: 29).

Included in the resonant space is **environmental** space, which sits between subject and object, giving a tangible sense of something "other," to which the dance is evolving in **relation**.

Nothing is ever one thing. Bainbridge Cohen explains, "It turns out that the first cell is two. You have two identical daughter cells encased in a membrane instead of one primary cell. It's yin and yang. It's not one its two" (Bainbridge Cohen 2008: 164). I have an image of the membrane as a tightrope between two opposites of past and future, allowing me to balance in the present but equally keeping both channels open.

The skin

> *[U]ntil the body* feels *something different it cannot* act *differently.*
>
> Juhan 2003: 162

The skin serves as the primary boundary for the **environmental space** between inside and outside. It is "the largest, most varied, and the most constantly active source of sensations in the body" (Juhan 2003: 28). Deane Juhan names touch as the "mother of the senses" (2003: 29) as "[a]ll the other special senses are actually exquisite sensitizations of particular neural cells to particular kinds of touch" (2003: 29). The skin membrane enables a **dialogic relationship** where I can be internally receptive and at the same time more sensitive to my surroundings. Through the permeability of the skin, the body "gathers information about the tactile world and the electrical field around us" (Aposhyan 1999: 123).

I become a loving witness to my own environment.

Processing information through the membrane

We cannot take in the vast and constant sensorial stimulus being received in each moment. Juhan states that "Encephalization has given us the ability to edit sensory information," so that "any particular bit of sensation may be highlighted or suppressed, as it is more or less relevant to our present activity or interest" (2003: 270).

"Exercising many kinds of discrimination" (Juhan 2003: 376), the membrane can represent our physiological boundaries, our "yes" and our "no." It actively discerns the information that filters in as our attention shifts or drifts. "We see that there is an intelligence running things. It's not a matter of energy acting on matter to creative behavior, but of the intelligence in the form of information running all the systems and behaviors" (Pert cited in Juhan 2003: 376).

This intelligence of the membrane becomes an interchangeable metaphor for the loving witness in its ability to discern with a complete loving knowing, moving towards a sense of coherency and ephemeral translation felt at an experiential level of making artistic choices. Rethorst describes a "choreographic mind" that speaks to this interior knowledge:

IBMT as Support for Dance Making

> *[Y]ou might feel out on a limb working without a thought in your head, something has to be operating, leading you to make the decisions that result in the thing you make that is from you, of you, about you. Your Choreographic mind is at work.*
>
> (Rethorst 2015: 13)

Stuckness

With most creative processes and within the act of dancing itself there are moments of feeling "stuck." These places can be rich, full of creative potential, or immobilizing and debilitating. In the artist there is a connection between a strong "inner critic" and this feeling of debilitation. Finding movement in the places one feels stuck and responding creatively will be reflected in our ability to meet, understand, and heal through traumatic experiences.

Levine (2017) describes a hierarchy of responses to sensory overload and/or trauma within the ANS. We can be flung into an extreme of either flight or fight response (SNS) or freeze and shut down (vegetative PNS). The third response, proposed by Porges as part of Polyvagal Theory (1994), is the social engagement system, a playful mixture of activation and calming (being and doing) that operates through the ventral vagal nerve. On supporting the vagal nerve, Levine writes, "You have to create a sense of relative safety – to help the person feel just safe enough to begin to go into their bodies – and support the initial exploration and acceptance of sensations" (2017).

Sensory-motor loop

In Bainbridge Cohen's articulation of the sensory-motor loop, she names the traditionally acknowledged model as: "Sensory input – Perceptual interpretation – Motor-planning – Motor response – Sensory feedback – Perceptual interpretation" (Bainbridge Cohen 2008: 114). She goes on to say that there are two more initial phases, "Preconceived expectations" and "Pre-motor focusing," that reveal a pre-existing momentum and patterning.

Bainbridge Cohen's practice of "sitting in the synapse" describes a rupture in the sensory-motor loop when information coming in through the sensory nerve is overwhelming and cannot be fully processed. Instead of motoring out, it reverses and flows back to the cells and is stored. This creates a cellular memory that can be checked against other experiences and processed gradually when the system is ready, restoring flow through somatic processing:

> *[B]y accepting, not having to act prematurely, and not adding flames to the fire, just letting things filter through, the nerves little by little de-reverse until finally there is no reversal. It's no longer being stored in the tissue. It means you now have a response instead of a reaction.*
>
> (Bainbridge Cohen 2008: 180)

This is not only about meeting our experience with awareness, but about how we meet it; by meeting difficult feelings in the body in a loving way, our nervous system can slow down and start to feel safe enough to be with whatever is happening, thus supporting the body's availability for change, to find a new pathway. Love as an inherent aspect of awareness develops a plasticity in the neural wiring of the nervous system that mediates previous experiences with the new, creating more responsive actions and the ability to move between things, energies, and states with ease.

Olsen writes: "[T]he heart is yielding to and absorbing the moment of change" (2014: 225). The act of bringing something into my conscious awareness causes me to change. Your awareness

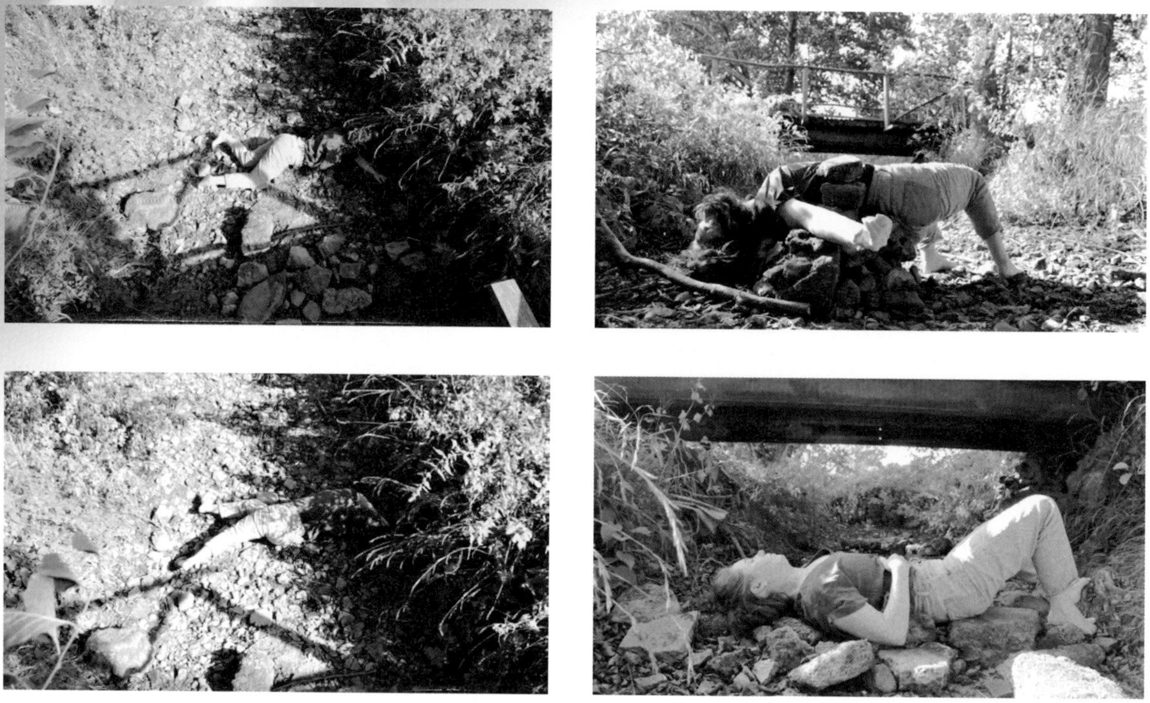

Rolling over stones of the dry river bed. Dancer: Gaelin Little. Stills from film: *TURN*, Videographer: Basil Marples

also causes me to change: moment to moment, feeling my way into a new form that has not yet been imagined.

Going through: writing from the dry river bed

The water has already left this riverbed

and so I will be the river ... going through

We all go through differently

Going through is about ... my body softening to the sharp hard edges, adapting, rolling over and around

Going through is about ... my body continuing its journey downstream, all the way until it meets the ground.

Going through is about ... leaving some things behind and taking some things with me

Going through is the space between leaving and having left.

The permeability of the membrane helps facilitate a transition or crossing over the boundary I can feel between somatic exploration and the process of art-making. What if this boundary could be traveled over, back and forth many times, without losing information from both sides, so that they might better inform each other, in a journey of descent and return?

Imagination as a Membrane

Authentic Movement differentiates three fields of experience: sensation, imagination, and emotions. Imagination can act as a portal from the external to the internal world and vice versa. The external use of imagery and visualization can be visceral

gateways into new embodied experiences, or images arriving out of the internal movement process can be a message from the depths.

Within the embodiment process, new awarenesses become integrated as a place of familiarity within the cells themselves. This cellular recognition becomes part of your embodied knowledge as a new conscious dimension to your experience of being in the world. Staying longer with sensation does not aim to diminish perception or fabrication through imaginal and emotional dimensions, but rather aims to open up and enrich their potential.

It's raining from my ovary: notes from solo dance work TURN

My right hand, it hovers above my right ovary. My thumb and first two fingers press lightly against my body as my hand carves out a scooping gesture. I imagine I am picking a tiny white translucent egg out of my ovary, an ameba, the starting cell. It rises to just underneath the surface of my skin. I trace my fingers against my skin, leading the ameba through my internal organs until I find an opening in my neck where I can take it out of my body. I peel my arm away and open my fingers, discarding the egg. My hand floats after it, following in a ghost motion down toward the ground. The action of discarding is accompanied by a feeling of emptiness and numbness that paradoxically thrills me and recharges the body with a new emotion. I become filled, leading me to perform this gesture over and over, emptying and filling.

Artistic Materials Arising out of Resonant Space

Tarkovsky describes "an organic link between the subjective impressions of the author and his objective representation of reality" (1991: 21) for the artist to achieve authenticity and inner truth. Here, there is a mirroring in the relationship between sensation and perception, truth and beauty. This is not a one-dimensional beauty but the kind that is guided by the fullness of the love – love as the witness who provides a space or a womb to grow into, where the potency inherent within certain materials that bear a sense of significance to the artist can be nurtured. This potency is akin to Amy Voris describing "a tendency to return to material which possesses a slightly 'charged' constellation of kinaesthetic, emotional and imaginal cues" (Voris 2018: 102). Voris also references dance-maker Barbara Dilley, whose material has to do "with vibrational intensity, with clarity, with something being seen beyond the ordinary, but being able to hold a kind of metaphoric drumbeat" (Dilley cited in De Spain 2014: 123).

At a cellular level, the synapse is a space between a pre-synaptic (sending) cell and a post-synaptic (receiving) cell. It is interesting that "Excitatory neurotransmitters increase electrical excitability on the post-synaptic side through modulation of the trans-membrane ion flow to facilitate transmission of an action potential" (Speller 2018). The higher vibrational activity of fluid chemical neurotransmitters just before the action speaks of a resonant place that is not empty but full of potentialities, a fully active web of communication pathways. It is the space of **almost** but not quite yet, or **just before** knowing, that makes space for multiple layers of perception, a complexity that is closer to reality.

I feel this to be the space from which artistic materials are born. Albright describes "dwelling in the 'gap' as a heightened experience of inhabiting – fully and consciously – such a space that becomes more than the sum of its parts, such that that space *makes things happen*" (Albright and Gere 2003: 260).

Chapter 19

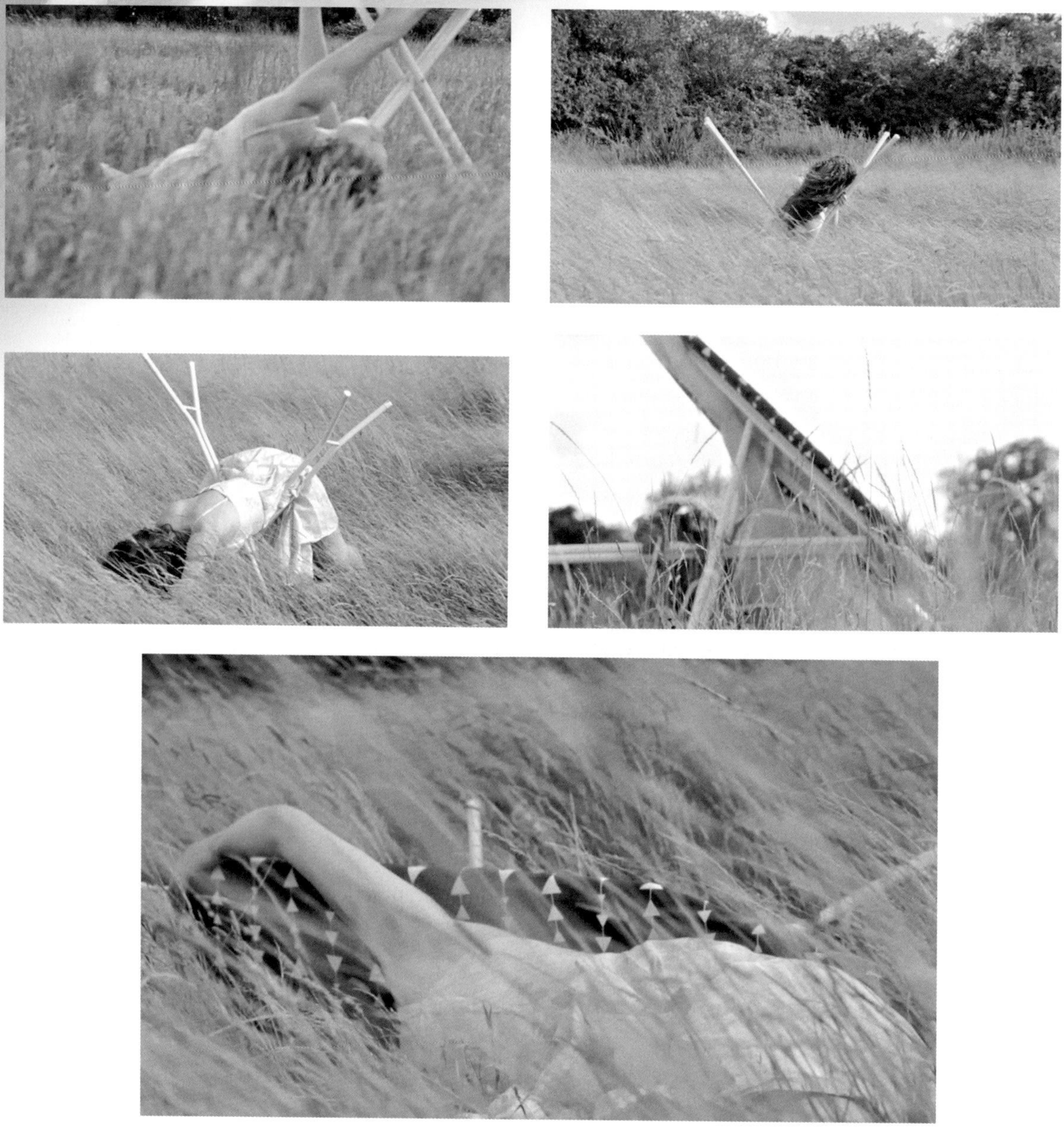

Grassy field with the ironing board. Dancer: Gaelin Little. Stills from film: *TURN*, Videographer: Basil Marples

IBMT as Support for Dance Making

When was it born?

Was it born at home? When ...

I looked for something to dance with, to be in relationship to, with a longing that drags on my limbs. I discover the contours of the ironing board, lying next to it for a while. In a removed way it mirrors a body. It was made to fit the clothes that fit us and so it sort of fits me.

Was it born in the studio? In the many hours of lying around doing much of nothing, resting in the sunny patch of the floor. A faint hope that something might be manifesting. Struggling to find any will or supportive structure, the "creative process" feels like a faraway land I might visit tomorrow.

Was it born in the imagination? As I stretched out my hand to find a metal pole I walk my fingers up it; they begin dancing in a field enveloped in sunshine and warm grasses.

Or was it born when Basil and I came to a grassy field close to his home? The wind made the grasses look like the sea, reminding me of that Tarkovsky film. We moved on.

On our way home we circled back to the field. "You wouldn't happen to have an ironing board at home, would you?" I said. "I don't but my Mum who lives next door might." Basil went to check.

Was it born then?

Or was it when he returned with a pale-yellow ironing board the same color as the grass?

In the field I danced. I danced for discovery, the ever-evolving shapes and angles disappearing in and out of the grass, as I shifted the board and it shifted me. Perhaps it was born then "in the center of the dance."

Or through the camera lens – my witness moving to meet me in the edit – within the what and how much to keep? And what bit sits next to what bits?

Or did it come into being in the seemingly arbitrary or insignificant choices – returning to the house after lunch – choosing work on that windy day.

Dailiness requires a simultaneous tuning into time and the absence of time. One had to know to not know, prefer and not prefer, empty oneself and acknowledge one's fullness, be passive and charged. It has to happen to you and from you. [...] embracing the excitement of being led by a stranger – the unmade dance.

(Rethorst 2015: 7)

The "dailyness" that Rethorst describes is for me about turning up to the container membrane so that the process can be uncontained.

Conclusion

[I]t is never at the beginning that something new, a new art, is able to reveal its essence; what it was from the outset it can reveal only after a detour in its evolution.

Deleuze 2012: 41

Somatic practices sharpen my awareness of moving, whereas Buddhist practice supports me to track the movement of my awareness; I believe both are pointing to the same thing. My artistic practice supports me to expand on the beauty of experience and cultivate an awareness of the resonant space as a place of possibility.

All of these disciplines can be articulated as practices which lovingly witness the unfolding of experience, an awareness that brings light to overlooked dimensions of experience that can be dominated or restricted by a pre-formed and self-orientated understanding of reality: "To seek an answer is to narrow the immensity of the question" (Hay 2016: 20).

The loving witness is a membranous layer for the live communication within resonant space, moving towards an intuitive multi-layered sense of knowing that lends itself to a practice of art-making with an expanded range of conscious choices that do not have to provide a rational justification. "Much of my knowing that emerged felt wordless" (Hartley 2017: 19).

From a vibrational cellular level, to skin, to the mediation of **experiences** as a conscious and creative act, the resonant space becomes a fluid and active permeable "passage," where experience can be **distilled** to precious and significant elements. In art-making the indescribability of these elements acts on us in the way that it does, perhaps stirring something deeper inside of us or provoking new thoughts and feelings.

Somatic movement practices tend toward a receptive approach as they are aimed towards the health and alignment of the organism, whereas an artistic process has a material outcome requiring it to be more active. Here, there is a relationship between activity and receptivity, ultimately searching for the space in between, a deep listening place that is inherently not divided but rather belongs to both.

This process evokes a deeper understanding of the drive to make, as a desire to know something outside of one's own understanding initiating the journey into not *yet* knowing. This active force provides a compass to the activity of the membrane.

Love was my chosen tool for orientation, in the hope that any discoveries, distillations, or perceptions will have maintained a sense of purity or truth to the visceral experience of the multi-dimensional body along with the beauty of the mystery.

20

The Best Present

Aistė Kriukelytė

The Idea for the Research

I came up with the idea of dancing to one spectator through a combination of many observations and experiences I have been through during the last 8 years, or maybe even longer. Here are some of them:

> **I teach contemporary dance to a group of schoolgirls. We started our usual class half an hour ago. One of the girls reveals that she is sad because she would like to congratulate the administrator of the school on her birthday but has no present for her. Another girl also says the same. And another one. I ask whether they think they all could dance for her as a present. They agree it is a good idea. I invite the administrator to the class. The girls are ready. I put on the music and they dance with small, colorful scarves in their hands. After the dance the administrator tells me: "You know, I have never received a dance as a present."**

I felt it was a special experience and conceived a wish that more people could experience this.

Mirror neurons are "a type of brain cell that respond equally when we perform an action and when we witness someone else perform the same action" (Winerman 2005). During my studies in Integrative Bodywork and Movement Therapy (IBMT), I was fascinated to observe our bodies communicating and sharing speechless messages without asking us whether we want that or not. It showed we all were connected much more closely than I had previously thought.

The Discipline of Authentic Movement is one way to experience the operation of mirror neurons and the resulting kinesthetic empathy directly. The basic form is when one person moves with their eyes closed, following the impulses of their body, and another witnesses, afterwards sharing their experience. I experienced how this practice can touch both the mover and the witness very deeply. I also noticed that if a person moves truly authentically – without "editing" the impulses – it is very interesting to observe such movement; even the simplest movements or positions can be so involving that you almost feel hypnotized. I became interested in using the practice when creating and performing dance art. However, as soon as we want to put Authentic Movement into any kind of form, so that it looks more like art and less like therapy, there is a risk that it will become less authentic and its power will decrease.

Having a strong passion for, and long years of practice, in contemporary dance, I am keen to explore how my new skills and knowledge gained during my IBMT studies could be used in the dance world. Exploring kinesthetic empathy is an intriguing option. In the dance world, kinesthetic empathy is usually analyzed in terms of reactions that the dancers' movements evoke in the spectators' bodies (Thiran 2015; more information also can be found here: http://www.watchingdance.org/about_us/). I would like to explore the opposite: what reactions does the spectator's body evoke in the dancer's body, and what happens if the dancer follows those internal impulses to move? How does the spectator perceive what he or she sees? Many people nowadays are not used to paying attention to the messages sent by their bodies. Can someone else hear these messages? And, if so, can another person translate them into a dance in such a way that the spectator would feel "it was something about me"? Would people want such a dance to be danced for

Chapter 20

them? What kind of invitation would seduce them to try it?

I also want to research myself by looking for ways to arrive at a state of mind in which my body attunes to the body of another and can respond to it. What helps me to stay in this state of mind and, if necessary, to come back to it? How different will my dances be to different people?

When looking for a present for someone, we focus on what kind of person they are and what they like. Thus, when exploring dance as a present for someone, it feels natural to see the person, to let my body respond in whatever way it wants and to follow wherever it leads me. Will such movements be perceived by the audience as dance? At the beginning of the research project, we asked this question of some of the observers of the movements. They all said a definite "yes," so we stopped worrying.

The Contemporary Dance World and the Somatic Movement Therapy World

A dance for one person, improvised by following the internal impulses that arise – is it therapy or a piece of dance art? The more I work in the two areas, the more I see them overlapping and intertwining. And yet, if I am to invite people to an event, I have to label it somehow. What, then, is the difference between art and therapy? If you look at definitions, the main difference is the purpose of the activity: the purpose of art is to come up with a piece of art and the purpose of therapy is to help to solve a person's physical and/or psychological problems or otherwise to improve his or her wellbeing. In practice, however, the process of creating a dance piece may be healing and, on the other hand, during a therapy session true art may start to emerge.

Still, being a therapist and being a dance artist feel very different. I want to name some of those differences here. When speaking about the features of contemporary dance art, I am aware that it can be (and is) extremely diverse. Thus, I do not aim to take into account the full range of dance performances ever made but rather keep to those features that I encounter most often.

1 **Safety**. This is one of the key concepts in many kinds of therapy. For changes to happen, one must feel safe. It is not enough to *be* safe; the client must *feel* safe. Only then can they get in touch with the pain and wounds that have been waiting, sometimes for many years, to be healed. It is the responsibility of the therapist to help clients feel safe during sessions and gradually allow themselves to be more vulnerable.

A dance performance is a place where the audience can come in whatever shape and mood – they do not have to be vulnerable (although in some cases they may feel so) in order to enjoy or otherwise benefit from it. They come to watch; the performers are there to impress them in one way or another. Dance artists are not expected to take care of the audience's psychological safety.

Generally, the audience members do not reveal anything about themselves and this protects them. As a result, dance art is something you can often go and watch with ease, while therapy, to many, sounds like something much scarier. Among other reasons, this is because it is often still seen as something you do when there is "something wrong with you." If I label my offer as "therapy," I am responsible for ensuring that the "client" feels safe and I can expect some input from him or her. If it is dance art, I presume the audience will take care of their personal issues themselves; I do not expect any input from the audience and feel some pressure to show something worthwhile.

2 **Artist's ideas versus client's problems**. Artists are there to express themselves and their ideas; therapists are there for others – the clients – to express and solve whatever troubles them. Thus, an artist can be in a creative process without having an audience (it is usual to have an audience only at or towards the end), but it is not possible for a therapist to do therapy without a client. The therapist will reveal his own thoughts or feelings to the client only when, to his belief, it is beneficial for the client to hear them. Artists are much freer to express their thoughts and feelings whenever and in whatever form they like. The therapist aims to be connected to himself and to the client and listen attentively; the artist can freely explore how different states of mind (being attuned to their body or not, paying attention to this or to that, and so on) affect what they are doing.

3 **Confidentiality**. Artists are free to talk about what they are doing in any form and to anyone they want; therapists usually commit to keeping whatever happens in their sessions confidential.

4 **Relationship to one's body**. The last difference I want to mention is a dancer's and a therapist's relationship to their bodies. Although I have seen some great dancers who practice a friendly, attentive, and caring attitude towards their bodies, the dance profession seems to be a place where it is often difficult or impossible to do that. The fact that the body is a dancer's work instrument does not necessarily result in the dancer being interested in the body's messages, let alone listening to them in order to change their habits or behavior. The approach is often exploitative: the body is like a slave, which must do what it is told. If it does not do that properly, it must repeat the action until it does do what it is told. The body is not a colleague with whom you consult, nor a friend about whom you care when dancing (you care afterwards – by having a massage, and so on). The approach depends on the dancer's personal beliefs and preferences and/or the requirements of the choreographer, but in many cases what the dance piece requires is more important than staying connected with the body and keeping it healthy.

   In a therapy session, the body's role depends on the type of therapy. In dance therapy, IBMT sessions, or body psychotherapy, the body's messages provide a very important source of information, which often cannot be obtained in other ways. The therapist will be attentive both to her own sensations and feelings and to those of her client. Much more time is devoted to listening to what is happening in the body right now than to where I want my body to be in terms of appearance, functioning, or absence of pain.

Coming back to my question of how to label what I want to do, I realize that having the freedom to pursue my personal ideas and experiment in any way I wish is key to me in this case. I want to discuss this process and share with other people freely, and I also dream of making a performance out of it one day. Thus, I put the label of "art" on it and say I am doing "artistic research." However, I am also conscious that I will use some tools and practices from the therapy world. First, being the only spectator of "the show" is already being in a vulnerable place – much more vulnerable than usual. To encourage people to go there, I may need to offer some additional safety. Second, I will be attentive to my body. Not only will it lead me to movements, but its messages can provide an important part of the research findings.

Chapter 20

I want to do this with someone else and so my dance and movement therapist colleague, Rasa Birietė, whom I first met many years ago at a contemporary dance workshop, joins me. We take turns to dance to an audience and witness each other dancing; afterwards, we share the experience.

I see Julia and Rasa standing in front of each other. Rasa is looking into Julia's eyes for a few moments and then starts to move. I see them both. Rasa is moving. Julia is watching her. After a minute, Julia's face changes. In less than another minute, I see tears on Julia's face. I can see she is deeply touched. Afterwards, all three of us talk about the experience. Julia says she hardly saw the dance. The mere fact that somebody was dancing FOR HER moved her to tears.

This experience touched all three of us deeply. Julia was our first audience and I did not expect the idea of a personal dance to be so powerful right from the start. I thought the research would involve looking for ways to make this dance more powerful, but the first try showed it could potentially be too powerful – bearing in mind that there is no therapeutic relationship that could guarantee safe processing of the experience. My inner therapist was not sure whether it was appropriate to do this. My inner dance artist was absolutely fine with it. That probably confirms the need to label it as "art" and not to give people any reason to expect any therapy.

A couple of months later, I share the above idea of the experience being too powerful with some dance artists and some of them strongly disagree. They are convinced that the purpose of art is to impress, maybe even to shock, the spectator, and use any means that help to achieve that. The artist should not care about what the spectator does with those things afterwards. On the one hand, I can see this point. On the other hand … well, we are using, maybe partly unconsciously, therapeutic tools: how to connect, how to create a safe space, and so on, which we know can be very powerful, and I feel that with the power comes the responsibility of using it safely. Dance art can have lots of different forms and goals. One of them is to impress, maybe even shock. Can there be another type of art – art which cares about the spectator?

I ask myself again why I want to care about the spectator. Does it come from my personal desire to be liked and loved? From a belief that, this way, I can make the world a nicer place? Or from my observation that I see little dance art which thinks this way and it is appealing to do something in this seemingly less explored area? Maybe the answer is a bit of all of these and maybe there are other reasons which I do not understand myself yet. And yes, maybe it also comes from my desire to connect to others. Stephen Porges says connection is the preferred way of coping with everyday stress and long-lasting trauma (Porges 2018). I have noticed that a feeling of connection makes being seen less scary.

Another reason why I want to care about the spectator is that maybe this way I can make them feel safer than usual and thus more open to the subtle experiences and subtle beauty that I myself enjoy so much. This would enable me to share what is dear to me.

Throughout this journey, I occasionally come back to these questions. What is art and what is not art? What is therapy and where does therapy end? I find some insights in external sources: conversations with art and therapy practitioners, listening to public talks on the internet, reading articles and books. At their event "Private Drama to Public Healing," psychologist Jack Saul and couples therapist Esther Perel express the idea that, in some cases, art can help people more than therapy (Saul and Perel 2019). This is true when the trauma is a collective event. "Collective traumas require collective responses," Saul says, and engaging with a piece of art can be an important part of such a collective response. When you go to individual therapy you may think it is only your problem or that you are the problem, but when artworks speak publicly about your troubles, you see that you are not alone; you feel part of a big group of people who all have suffered. This may be healing for the whole of society.

The search for connection with another person and often the inability to create that connection and/or to enjoy it seem to be common in our society. It appears to be a result, not of one big event, but of many small ones happening in our families; thus, by definition, we probably cannot say it is a collective trauma. However, it is often a result of unresolved personal traumas that many of us share, and I am asking what role dance art can have in healing them.

The Research Process

One of the key principles of Authentic Movement is to witness without judgment, without labeling things as "beautiful – not beautiful," "interesting – not interesting," or "good – bad." The aim is to look at lines, shapes, colors, body parts, and their position as if you are seeing them for the first time in your life, curiously noticing the details and not knowing how it "should be," what is better or worse, what is right and what is wrong. It is through this lens that I aim to see both the spectator that I dance for and myself dancing: without knowing what comes next and whether what is happening is good or bad – just noticing what it is. I want to meet the spectator in this moment without assumptions and judgments: to meet them with my whole body and give it the freedom to move in whatever way it wants, to let those movements evolve and change as they wish.

Throughout the research, this main idea remained the same while many other things changed. The project had two phases:

1 **Live performances** (November 2019 to January 2020). We experimented with different spaces: from a tiny 12 square meter (130 square foot) room to a spacious dance place, from galleries to dance studios to a Pilates studio. Almost every performance session happened in a different place and each time we had new spectators of different ages – from children to elderly people – and each dance was completely different from all the previous ones. At one point I realized that the only constant element in this journey was Rasa. It felt supportive.

At first, we also experimented with the form of the session: giving a dance to one spectator who was the only person (besides the dancer) in the room, or dancing to one person and having others watching both the dancer and the spectator for whom this dance was performed. We settled with the latter version since it allowed more people – including those not wanting to receive the dance themselves – to participate, and also because this format felt further from a therapy setting. Usually, we would go to one of spectators and ask, "Would you like to receive a dance?" Occasionally, we also asked, "Who would like to receive a dance?" We saw that there was a huge difference between these two approaches.

Around 30 people received their "personal dance" in this phase and around 30 more witnessed the process without receiving their own dance.

2 **Online performance sessions** (April to June 2020). Initially, just the two of us danced to each other on the screen via Zoom. We were exploring whether it felt similar to dancing in a live encounter and were looking for ways to support the connection in these changed circumstances. After a while, we felt we could

Chapter 20

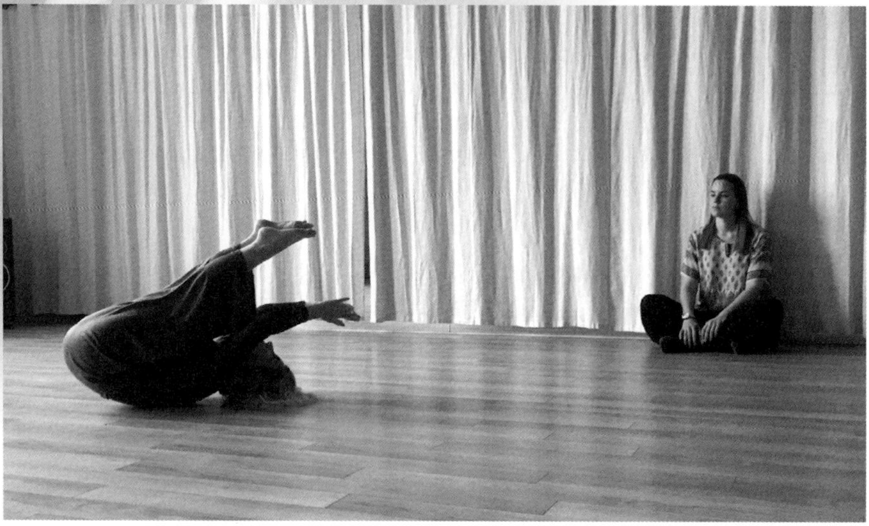

Dancer: Rasa Birietė.
Photographer:
Aistė Kriukelytė

offer such online dance to anyone and about 15 spectators received personal dances on the screen. During our experiments, we noticed a number of differences from the live meetings. We received less non-verbal information from the spectators because we usually saw just their heads and shoulders. To compensate for this, we invited them to play and share music or other sounds, which would correspond to how they felt at that moment. The form of these sessions also changed naturally to having only the spectator and the dancer on the screen without any additional observers.

The Findings

I did not aim to do a scientific piece of research, so the findings are a subjective noting of different things that emerged: both from my own and Rasa's personal observations and from participants' feedback.

Vulnerability and connection

During the first phase of the research, the most common comment from the spectators was "it seems that it was about me." Sometimes, this was pronounced as a question – as if waiting for confirmation, sometimes with surprise, sometimes joy, pleasure, or another not always easily identifiable emotion.

"It made me uneasy to see you dancing about me in front of other people. It was awkward that they might see what is inside of me."

"Would it be better if I danced just for you – without other people watching?"

"No, that would be even more scary."

A few people mentioned this in their feedback. The only way I can explain it is a fear of seeing what is inside of them.

We did not explain beforehand how the dance was created – just asked whether the person would like to receive a dance. Thus, the impression that the dance was about them could come either from mirror neurons and kinesthetic empathy, or from the fact that they knew it was for them – or a mixture of the two and maybe some other factors. Initially, the mirror neuron part was interesting for me, but in later stages it felt less important and the connection between the dancer and the spectator became key. Nevertheless, a few times people did mention that we performed some **movements specific to them**: *"Unbelievable – that's the way I used to hold my arm in my childhood,"* or *"I came here right after giving a dance class and we all did this movement just half an hour ago."* It would be hard to explain these moments as pure coincidence since, in each of these cases, my or Rasa's body did that movement only for that particular spectator and nothing even close to it came up when we were dancing for other people.

A couple of spectators said, *"Everybody would think it is about them"* or *"It could be about anybody, but since you know it is for you, you think it is about you."* Probably, that is at least partly true. However, there might be another aspect to it: if it felt too vulnerable, awkward, or painful to admit that it was about you, phrases like this served as an escape route. I welcomed this. If that was the spectator's choice, although it was probably unconscious, I believe they had good reasons for it and thus I intentionally wanted to leave an escape route open. In a therapy session, I would probably approach that differently, but with a piece of art, everyone takes from it as much as they are able and as much as they want.

It was not just the spectator who was vulnerable in these encounters. The dancers – Rasa and I – were vulnerable as well: we stood in front of the audience, having no idea what movements we would do and whether they would like them. We trusted our bodies would give some impulses. Occasionally, it happened that I did not feel any impulses. I took this as a cue to connect to my body better and listen more carefully. It also happened that I felt many impulses at the same time and did not know which one to follow. Gradually, I learned that in such cases it helps to wait a little longer, until one of the impulses grows stronger than the others. In practice, that was not always an easy thing to do: I am here to dance, everybody is watching me – unconsciously, my body takes this as an urge to start moving. The challenge was even greater when we started using music: sometimes, it would fit nicely and complement the

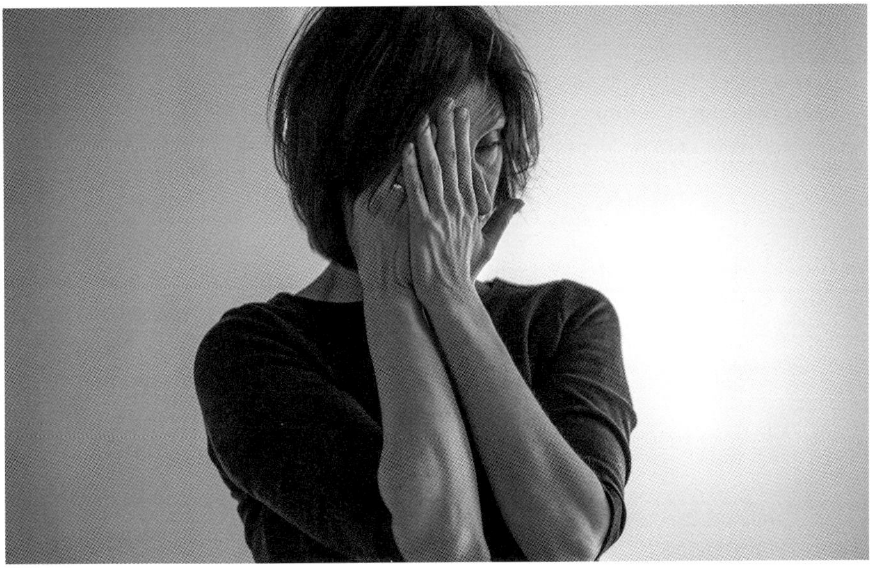

Dancer: Aistė Kriukelytė. Photographer: Dainius Putinas

impulses that I felt when watching the spectator; at other times, it would offer completely different impulses. I would have preferred to stay with the impulses I received from connection with the spectator, but then it looked as if the dance did not fit the music. Gradually, I found that, again, waiting a bit longer often helped me find an impulse that fit both the person and the music.

I feel the whole project was not so much about doing something, but more about listening – and trusting that that is enough. I needed to remind myself of this at those moments when my body was tempted to do something familiar, something that I know looks "nice" or impressive. I experienced how simple movements, done spontaneously by following an impulse, touch people much more than impressive dance tricks.

What helped me to stay in this vulnerability was a feeling of connection: with my body, with Rasa, with the spectator, with the audience in general – in that specific order, starting from my body. I suspect this feeling of connection worked both ways because some spectators commented that they felt vulnerable but safe. They said it with surprise in their voice, as if that was something new to them.

"Would you like me to dance for you?"

"No."

Some people said watching us dancing to someone was very powerful and they enjoyed watching it. Receiving the dance themselves would be too powerful. "*Then I would be singled out and would not be able to watch the dance so freely*," they said.

Being given an invitation and receiving presents

"Would you like to receive a personal dance tomorrow?"

"Yes!"

"Write down your e-mail – I'll send more information."

"Xxx. Thank you for the present."

"It's too early to thank me – I haven't danced yet."

"It's not too early because I already enjoy it."

I realized that my project starts, not when I stand in front of the spectator, but when I sit down to write an invitation to the event. I have never received so many and such warm responses to my invitations from the people that could not participate. The invitations themselves seemed to trigger warm feelings in people. It was a pleasant surprise.

Another interesting moment, mentioned many times by many spectators, was the huge difference between the feeling when you are offered the dance personally and when you yourself have to show some initiative: to raise your hand, or say or write that you would like to receive a dance. They all said that the first way feels much more like a present or something special, compared to the second.

This reminds me of Gordon Neufeld and Gabor Maté's thought that if parents want their child to be attached to them, they have to provide what the child needs or wants without the child asking for it (Neufeld and Maté 2014: 185–6). This idea resonates in my own body as well. When you are given what you asked for, it is because you asked. When you are given it without asking, it is because somebody was thinking about you, and you feel loved. Maybe this unconsciously reminds us of very early childhood when the mother guesses all the needs of the infant. This longing to be seen, understood, and cared for still lives in us as adults. Bessel van der Kolk and other therapists working with trauma say this longing is especially strong for those of us with developmental trauma: that is, people whose needs were not properly met in infancy and early childhood (van der Kolk 2005). Thus, it is a very vulnerable place, and a scary one. Neufeld and Maté speak about the fear of being vulnerable as the result of early trauma and lack of secure attachment in childhood (Neufeld and Maté 2014: Ch. 8).

One of our spectators mentioned that, at the beginning, she could not calmly sit and enjoy the dance for her because she was thinking how to give something back. It took some time for her to relax and really enjoy it. Another spectator responded by saying it was absolutely no problem for him. This made me reflect on how we accept presents and maybe even the more general idea of being loved: is it natural, does it take some effort, or maybe for someone it is not possible at all? If you have never received a sincere gift without the intention of receiving something in return, why would you believe a person you do not know will give you something worth taking? However, if you never allow yourself to take a present without giving anything back, it is not possible for someone to give you a truly sincere present.

"It was a rare present: 'my size,' 'my color,' 'didn't have one yet,' and 'I needed it but didn't know that.' I was moved to tears by the fact that somebody moves for me. Everything that was for me was very beautiful. My wedding ring has a phrase from Song of Songs on it: 'You are all beautiful, my love.' It means the part, which is not beautiful, is also beautiful. When you were dancing, I saw the beauty of my not-beautiful side."

This last sentence felt to me like the best possible feedback about a dance performance that I could ever have dreamed of.

In both stages, our dances resulted in lots of positive emotions: people were drawing, writing, and orally expressing them to us, sharing on their Facebook pages, recommending us to their friends. Despite this, not that many people were willing to receive the dance, especially in the online stage. This contradiction was one of the hardest parts to understand and cope with. At some point, I realized that it might be partly connected to the fact that the spectator is alone while receiving the dance on the screen and this adds to the observation mentioned by the spectators at the

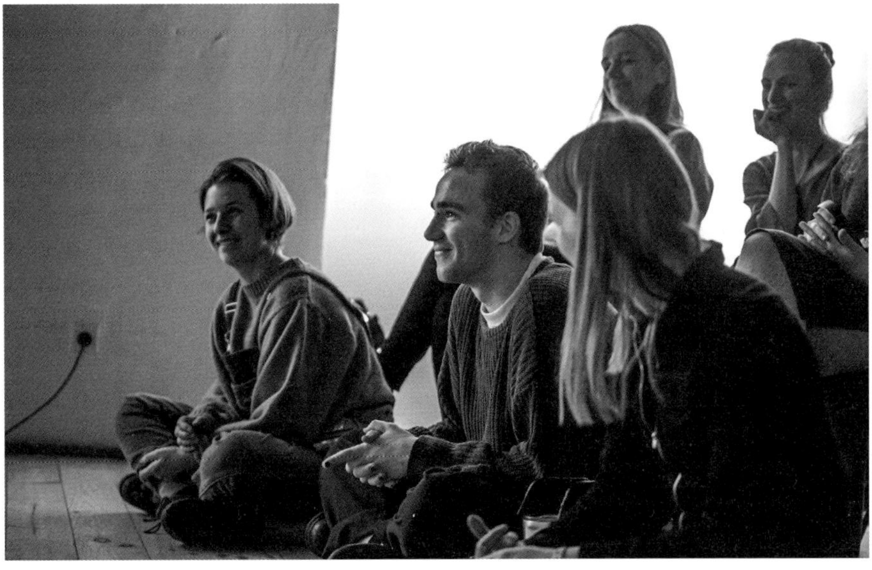

Photographer: Dainius Putinas

beginning of the project: *"It's even more scary when you're alone."* People also said that they felt the offer was something you have to prepare for or even that you need "to grow up to it." Some mentioned that a fear they might not like it was stopping them – being the only spectator felt like having some responsibility for the performance.

To me, this contradiction seems to represent the whole of the society we live in: we do not take in what truly nourishes us, even if it is easily available. It is too scary, too unusual. Instead, we try to run away from ourselves and grab anything that helps us to run away. This "anything" does not nourish, so we take more and more: more things, more food, more impressions, more activities, more contacts with people, more work … It is never enough.

The power of the feedback

We sit in a café after a performance session. Rasa is excited: "It was much better this time than the previous one." My feeling is exactly the opposite. She asks: "Why?"

It took me a while to put the experience into words. It was something about the connection with the spectators for whom I danced. I felt it did not work as well this time. While I was explaining why I felt that way, I suddenly realized that, this time, I had had much less feedback from my spectators than previously. My mind automatically reached the conclusion that the connection was not as good; and then came the next conclusion – that my performance was not as good. Once I revisited the experience in my mind, I saw that it was much better than I thought it was. I took two things from this. First, I felt how the absence of feedback works – I tend to think I did lousy work. Critical feedback is much better than nothing because at least you are seen and provoke some response. This was not a new concept, but it was impressive to notice and feel all the way how this worked in me. Second, this showed that I had to do some internal work because I wanted the spectators to be free not to give any feedback if that was how they felt. I wanted to be free of the expectation for feedback. I wanted to trust my belief that what I do is meaningful, regardless of whether I receive any feedback this specific time or not.

Spreading a love for and understanding of contemporary dance

"You told a story! There was no pantomime, no recognizable actions; however, I clearly saw the whole story! How is it possible?! I've never seen anything like this before."

The dance was not for her, but this older woman, who would probably never go to a contemporary dance performance, was greatly impressed anyway. This shows that such a personal approach works not only for the spectators who receive their personal dance, but also for the others, watching from the side. When there is no wish to show something, but just to be fully in connection with another, this speaks to others as well, and could be one way to promote contemporary dance and increase the number of its fans.

During both stages of the research, after seeing us moving, some people expressed a wish to dance to someone themselves. Sometimes this remained just a wish, but in some cases they were able actually to do it – dancing either to one of us or to someone else in the space.

Social aspect

After both the performance and the discussion are over, none of the eight spectators leaves the space. They stay speechless, as if waiting for something. "I feel a small new community has just been born, who do not want to leave," says Rasa.

They stayed as if something was keeping them in the space. Maybe this was a wish to stay with the impressions a bit longer, maybe a feeling of being seen and understood, maybe a feeling of connection to other people, maybe an opportunity to share, maybe a feeling of safety and peace, or a combination of any of these. At those times, I felt the quality of yielding in the space: yielding to where I am, yielding to what I am, yielding to my boundaries, yielding to the unknown. Yielding is a place of rest – a true deep rest that most of us lack so much. Yielding is also the place where the feeling of power comes from – without yielding, neither pushing nor reaching nor pulling is possible. Yielding is a place of connection to oneself and I believe the only way to feel a deep connection to another is to connect to oneself first.

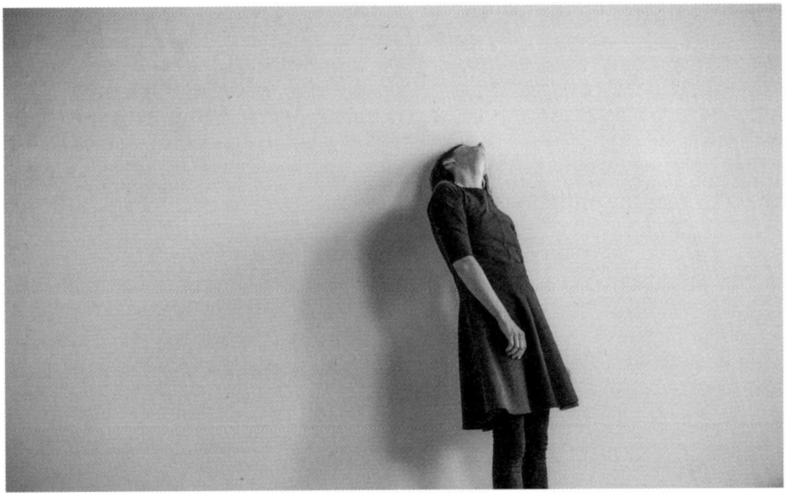

Dancer: Aistė Kriukelytė. Photographer: Dainius Putinas

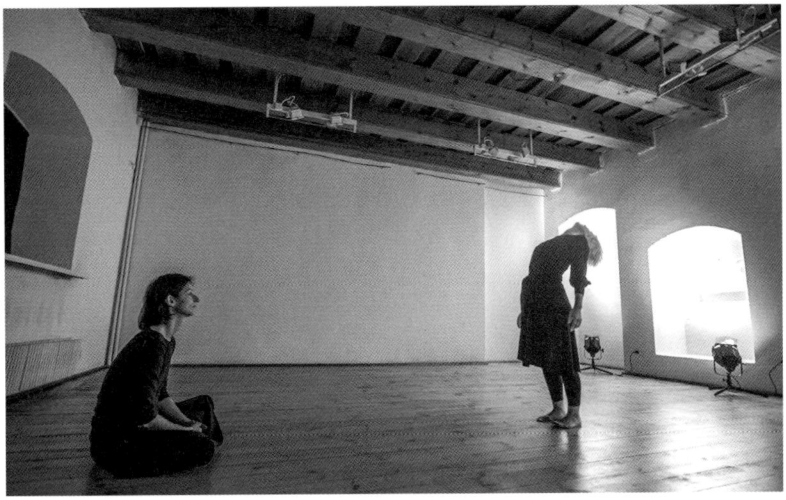

Dancer: Rasa Birietė. Photographer: Dainius Putinas

Chapter 20

Online specifics

I am dancing to Rasa online. I stand up, raise my arms and ... wonder whether they can be seen on the screen. At that moment I cannot see the screen to check. I decide to let it go and accept the possibility that she does not see all of me ... that maybe she does not even see the part of me which feels the most important. Afterwards, she shares her feeling that the camera chooses for her what she will see.

This way, the camera was an additional "player" in the meetings with the spectator. Sometimes it interfered with the internal impulses: for example, I felt an impulse to move forward but this would have taken me out of shot. In real-life situations, when you come closer, the other person can see details, such as your feet, better. In online meetings, if you come too close, the feet may not be seen at all.

One more additional "player" was the music chosen by the spectator. Thus, instead of pure connection with another in silence and following internal impulses from that, we had two additional potential sources of impulses – more options, less clarity. I missed the clarity a little, but it was partly compensated for by the additional energy often brought by the sounds of music.

While listening to Rasa on Zoom, I try to feel my body. I notice being somewhere very far from it – much further away than usual. I realize communicating via screen reduces my attention to myself and to the physical environment around me. I notice myself bending towards the screen, maybe subconsciously trying to hear and to be heard better.

I aimed to learn to relax, to trust that I am seen and heard. Still, even consciously being aware of these things, I found it more difficult to arrive and stay in my body, compared to live meetings. That could be another reason why the connection with the spectator felt weaker. I wonder whether seeing only each other's heads for most of the day makes it more difficult for us to stay grounded, and results in even less attention to our bodies.

In a live meeting, it sometimes feels good to sit together in silence. I found it much harder to have silent moments during online meetings – I felt obliged to say or do something. It was also more difficult to lead the spectator towards a calm and slow state of mind; it remained up to the spectators how and whether they did anything to take themselves out of the everyday noise in the heads.

Eye contact via a screen is very different: if you look a person in the eyes, for them it does not feel as if you are looking at their eyes. This may be an opportunity for people who do not dare to look at other people's eyes, because it is less awkward examining someone else on screen compared to a live encounter. It was unusual to see myself while talking and dancing. For some reason, the feeling was different from seeing myself in the mirror.

In the second phase of the project, we heard the phrase "it was about me" much less often. The most common feedback was *"I felt as if it was me dancing there ..."* and *"According to MY music, you dance completely differently!"*

There were cases when the connection seemed to be as strong and the meeting as touching as live meetings. I guess two factors contributed to this. First, it happened more often with people I already knew. Second, I think it had to do with spectators' relationship to the music: do they see music only as something to cheer them up and give them energy, or does music participate in their lives in more diverse ways – accompanying them also in sadness, anger, fear, and other emotions? It seemed that, in the latter case, there was a greater chance that the music might help us to connect and that the dance might evoke stronger emotions.

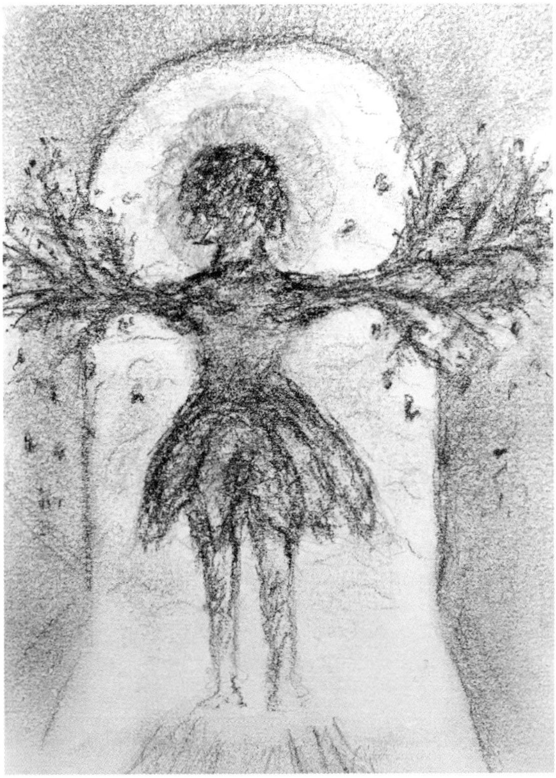

Drawing by Haja Pham.

I dance. A woman on the screen is watching me. Suddenly I realize my dance is not about her. Nor about me. And not even about our connection or the relationship between us. It is about my relationship with people in general.

At times, dancing on screen felt similar to a "usual dance improvisation"; this never happened during the live performances. Maybe this was because of the greater variety of impulses, which more often seduced me to play with the music or camera, and to develop those impulses on my own without checking with the spectator so often. This way, the dance on screen became more of an impulse for creative work, a way to produce choreographic material, and less of a way to establish connection with another.

Final Remarks

A month after the presentation of the first stage of the research, a young woman gave me the drawing shown here. "At one moment I saw you like this," she said.

After the second phase of the project, I watch the video recordings, the session with Rasa that we did without music. I see her dance and my face in the screen while watching her. I see and hear myself talking about the experience. I see Rasa talking. I see my wet hair and remember I didn't have time to dry it. I see my glasses and remember regretting not taking them off – without them, the recording would have been nicer, I thought. I watch another session. And another, in which I dance for a spectator that I didn't know before. I see her face, I hear her music, and I see myself seeing her ... and then dancing. I feel the connection with her again. At this moment I notice my tears coming. Then a new thought comes to my mind – this project is the best present I could give myself.

Chapter 20

Glossary

Spectator: an audience consisting of one person. It depends on the audience how involved they will be in what they see: they can sense all their body and feel part of what is going on, similar to witnessing in the Authentic Movement Discipline, or they can remain detached, as at a sports event.

This research was financed by Dance Research Platform "Bitės", Lithuanian Dance Information Center and Lithuanian Council for Culture.

Video link
A glimpse of the research process

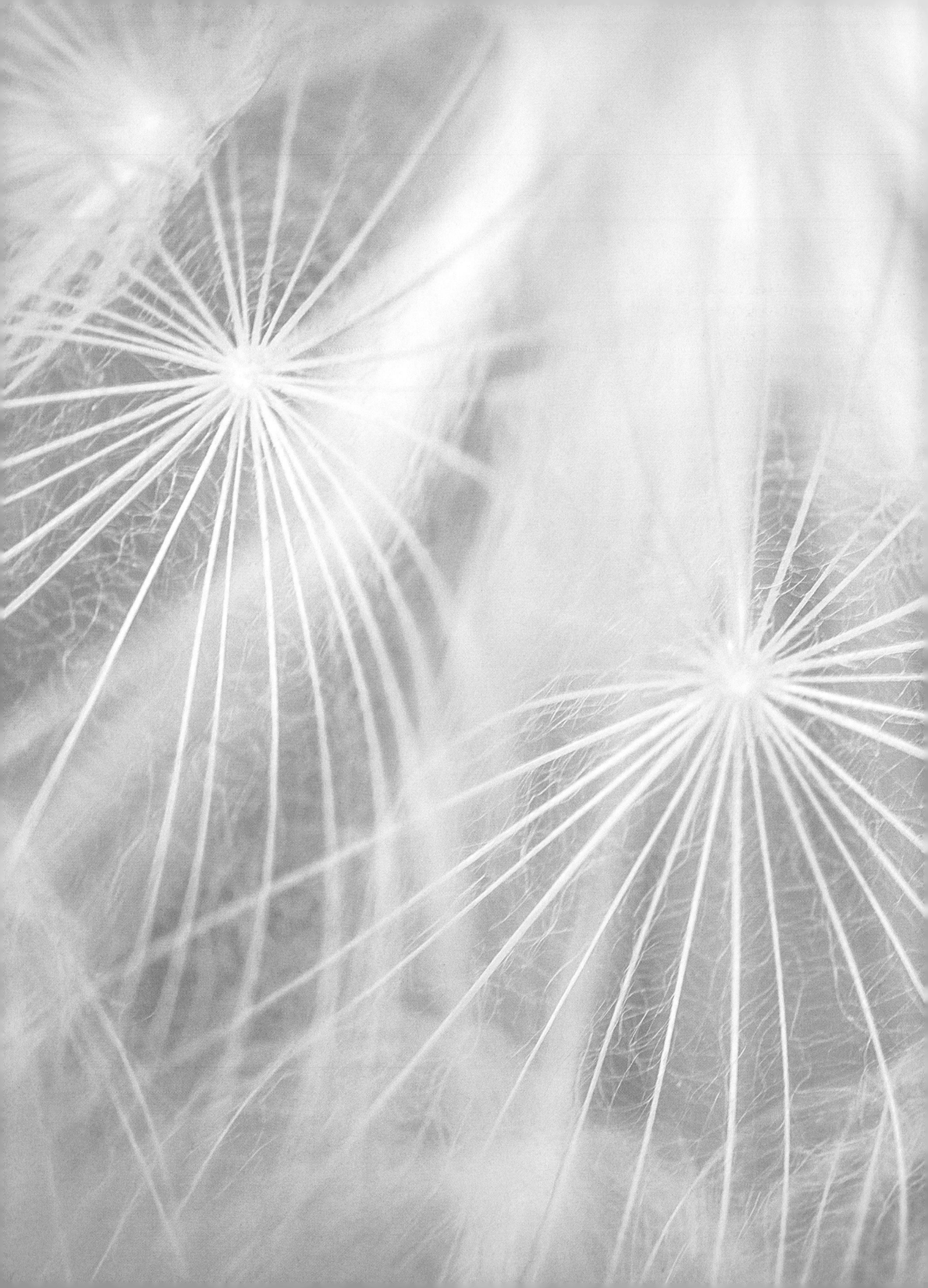

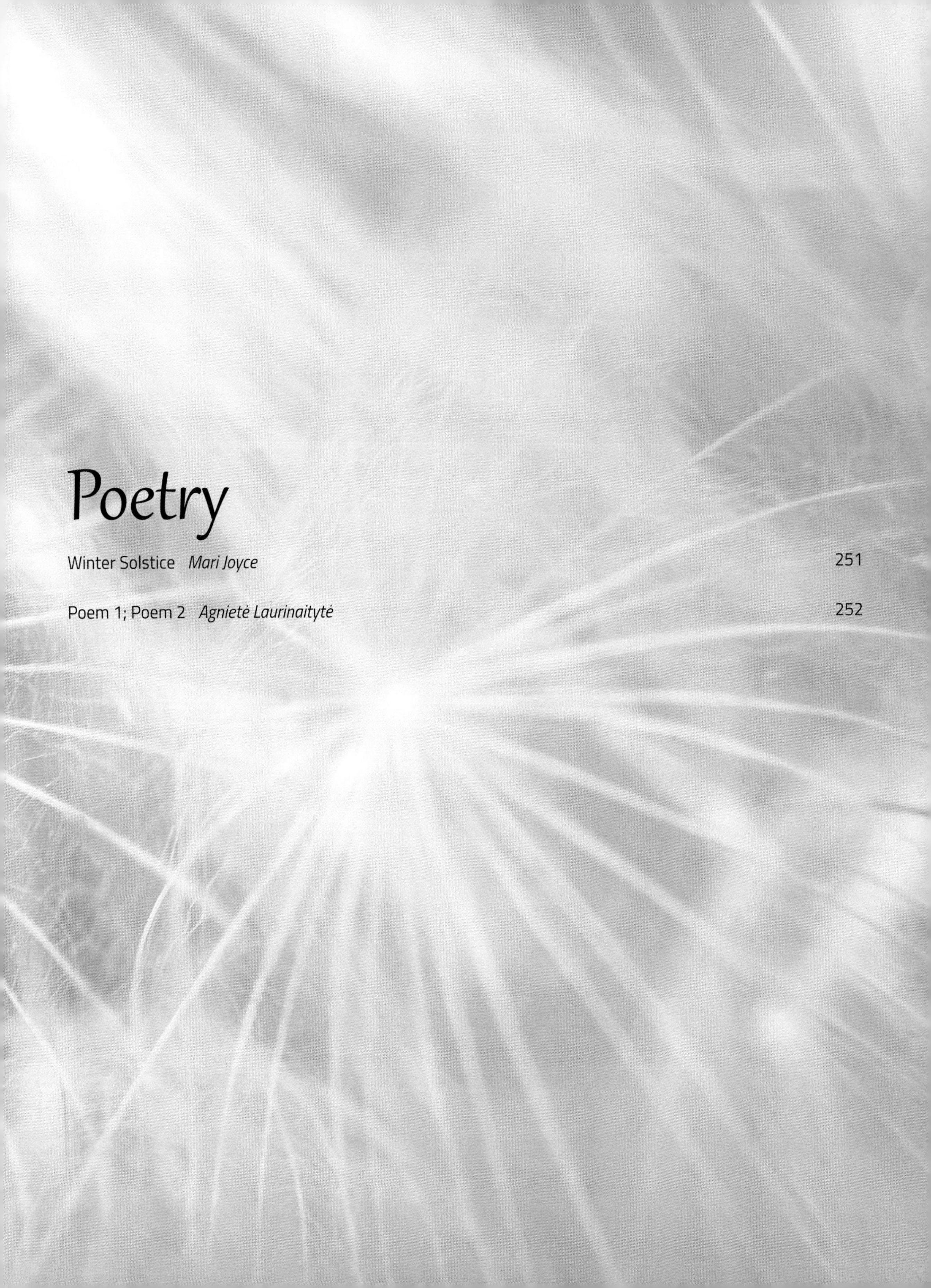

Poetry

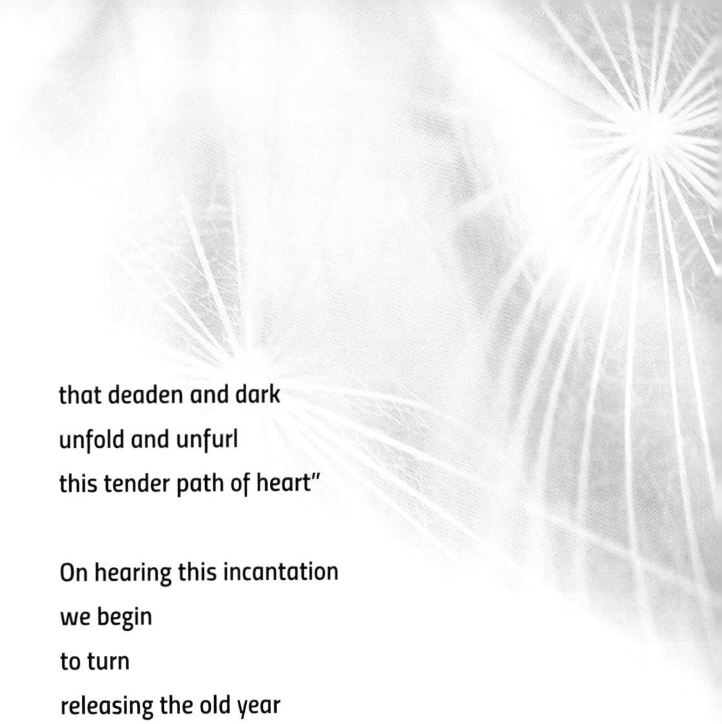

Winter Solstice

Mari Joyce

Stand quietly at years end
witnessing the dance
of emptying
the body
to stillness

The stillpoint of winter

The moment
after the out breath
and receding of tide
when sap's gone inward
deep as marrow

When dreamtime is arising

hope
delicate as sapling
and small seed planted at dusk
whispers this prayer
in urgent tones:

"Touch all obstructions;
witness the layers
that deaden and dark
unfold and unfurl
this tender path of heart"

On hearing this incantation
we begin
to turn
releasing the old year
sighing out the bones

And empty with longing
discover we've rooted over night

Homecoming greets us
effortless and easy
as the dawn's arrival
Eyes open softly
to the morning light

New moon
heart song
Silver seeds
planted at winter solstice

Agnietė Laurinaitytė

(Translated by Jurgita Motiejūnienė)

Poem 1

don't go there
leave behind
the busiest
city street

it's better
to stay here
sit in silence
and be happy

can there be
anything more
exciting
than an awakening heart

when you can almost touch it
with the tips of your fingers
and almost feel it

take off
your old clothing
take off your jewelry
destroy all the castles
which you have built
in the blossoming meadows

wash your face
in unexplainable excitement
coming from your depth
and refuse everything
refuse everything
with which you covered your natural being

there is nothing more precious in the world
than this meeting
my friend

there is nothing more precious

Poem 1 in original Lithuanian

neik ten
palik
tą judriausią
miesto gatvę

geriau
pabūk čia
pasėdėk tyliai
pasidžiauk

argi gali būti
kažkas labiau
jaudinančio
už bundančią širdį

kai savo pirštų galiukais
jau beveik lieti
beveik apčiuopi

nusimesk
senus rūbus nuo savęs
nusiimk papuošalus
sugriauk visas pilis
kurias statei
žydinčiose pievose

nuprausk veidą
nepaaiškinamu jauduliu
kylančiu iš tavo gelmės
ir atsisakyk visko
atsisakyk visko
kuo dengei savo natūralumą

nėra nieko brangesnio pasaulyje
už šį susitikimą
mano drauge

nėra nieko brangesnio

Poem 2

if only you tried
to meet life
like the river meets
those who enter it
like the flower meets
those who smell it
like the tree meets
those who lean on it

without any expectations
without fear
without judgment

what if you dared
to lose yourself right this second

you would find the life
which is you

you would find the life
which is you

and maybe then
maybe then
we would all meet within it

Poem 2 in original Lithuanian

tik jeigu tu pabandytum
sutikti gyvenimą
taip kaip upė sutinka
į ją brendančius
taip kaip gėlė sutinka
ją beuostančius
taip kaip medis sutinka
prie jo besiglaudžiančius

be lūkesčių
be baimės
be vertinimų
jeigu tu imtum ir išdrįstum
dabar šią sekundę pamesti save

tu atrastum gyvenimą
kuris ir esi tu

tu atrastum gyvenimą
kuris ir esi tu

ir galbūt tada
galbūt tada
mes visi susitiktume tame

References

Chapter 1

Adler, J. (2002) *Offering from the Conscious Body: The Discipline of Authentic Movement*. Rochester, VT: Inner Traditions.

Bainbridge Cohen, B. (1993) *Sensing, Feeling, and Action*. Northampton, MA: Contact Editions.

Bainbridge Cohen, B. (2017) "An Introduction to Body-Mind Centering®." https://www.bodymindcentering.com/introduction/ (accessed September 29, 2002).

Eddy, M. (2016) *Mindful Movement – The Evolution of the Somatic Arts and Conscious Action*. Bristol, UK: Intellect Books.

Galbusera, L. and Fuchs, T. (n.d.) "Embodied Understanding: Discovering the Body from Cognitive Science to Psychotherapy." *In-Mind Italia V1-6*. https://www.academia.edu/7192112/Embodied_understanding_Rediscovering_the_body_from_cognitive_science_to_psychotherapy (accessed October 14, 2021).

Hartley, L. (1995) *Wisdom of the Body Moving*. Berkeley, CA: North Atlantic Books.

Hartley, L. (2004) *Somatic Psychology: Body, Mind and Meaning*. London, UK: Whurr/Wiley.

Larisey, K. C. (2012) 'The Wounded Healer: A Jungian Perspective,' *C. G. Jung Society of Atlanta*, Fall, pp. 12–3.

Lovelock, J. (2000) *Gaia: A New Look at Life on Earth*, 3rd edn. Oxford, UK: Oxford University Press.

Porges, S. (2011) *The Polyvagal Theory: Neurophysiological Foundations of Emotions, Attachment, Communication, and Self-Regulation*. London, UK: W. W. Norton & Company.

Stern, D. (1985) *The Interpersonal World of the Infant: A View from Psychoanalysis and Development Psychology*. London, UK: Karnac Books.

Course Modules

Hartley, L. "Infant Movement Development," Module 1, Diploma course, Institute for Integrative Bodywork and Movement Therapy. http://ibmt.co.uk/infant-movement-development/ (accessed September 28, 2020).

Hartley, L. "Body Systems," now titled "Embodied Anatomy and Movement Repatterning." Modules 3 & 4, Diploma course, Institute for Integrative Bodywork and Movement Therapy, UK. Diploma in Integrative Bodywork and Movement Therapy. http://ibmt.co.uk/embodied-anatomy-movement-re-patterning-body-systems-1/ (accessed September 29, 2020).

Activist Groups

Black Lives Matter (2013) https://blacklivesmatter.com/ (accessed September 29, 2020).

Extinction Rebellion (2018) https://extinctionrebellion.uk/the-truth/demands/ (accessed September 29, 2020).

Red Rebels (2019) http://redrebelbrigade.com/ (accessed September 29, 2020).

Chapter 2

Bainbridge Cohen, B. (2008) *Sensing, Feeling, and Action: The Experiential Anatomy of Body-Mind Centering®*. Northampton, MA: Contact Editions.

Brook, A. (2001) *From Conception to Crawling: Foundations for Developmental Movement*. https://anniebrook.com (accessed October 14, 2021).

Cohen, L. (1984) *Various Positions – Hallelujah*. New York: Columbia Records.

Feldman, C. (1998) *Principles of Meditation: The Only Introduction You'll Ever Need*. London, UK: Thorsons.

Levine, P. (1997) *Waking the Tiger: Healing Trauma*. Berkeley, CA: North Atlantic Books.

Liang, Master T. T. (1977) *T'ai Chi Ch'uan for Health and Self-Defense*. New York: Vintage Books.

Pert, C. (1999) *Molecules of Emotion: Why You Feel the Way You Feel*. London, UK: Simon & Schuster.

Chapter 3

Abram, D. (1996) *The Spell of the Sensuous: Perception and Language in a More-Than-Human World*. New York: Pantheon Books.

Adler, J. (1999a) "The Collective Body," in Pallaro, P. *Authentic Movement: Essays by Mary Starks Whitehouse, Janet Adler and Joan Chodorow*. London, UK: Jessica Kingsley.

Adler, J. (1999b) "Who is the Witness?," in Pallaro, P. *Authentic Movement: Essays by Mary Starks Whitehouse, Janet Adler and Joan Chodorow*. London, UK: Jessica Kingsley.

Adler, J. (2002) *Offering from the Conscious Body*. Rochester, VT: Inner Traditions.

Armstrong, J. (1995) "Keepers of the Earth," in Roszak, T. *Ecopsychology: Restoring the Earth, Healing the Mind*. San Francisco: Sierra Club Books

Carrington, D. (2020) "Pandemics Result from Destruction of Nature," *The Guardian*, June 17.

Conger, J. P. (2005) *Jung and Reich: The Body as Shadow*. Berkeley, CA: North Atlantic Books.

Eisenstein, C. (2013) *The More Beautiful World Our Hearts Know is Possible*. Berkeley, CA: North Atlantic Books.

Hartley, L. (2001) *Servants of the Sacred Dream: Re-birthing the Deep Feminine – Psychospiritual Crisis and Healing*. Norfolk, UK: Elmdon Books.

Hartley, L. (2004) *Somatic Psychology*. London, UK: Whurr.

Hartley, L. (2020) "Humanity in a Time of Collective Initiation," *Journal of Dance, Movement and Spiritualities*, 7(1&2) Autumn.

References *continued*

Hauk, M. (2018) "Dreams of Earth: Myth and Planetary Presence While Convening a Virtual Hygeian Dream Temple," in Reger, S. and Hauk, M. *Vibrant Voices: Women, Myth & the Arts*. Brooklyn, NY: Women & Myth Press.

Macy, J. (2007) *World as Lover, World as Self*. Berkeley, CA: Parallax Press.

Næss, A. (1985) In Devall, B. *Deep Ecology*. Layton, UT: Gibbs Smith.

Moore, T. (2005) *Dark Nights of the Soul*. New York: Avery.

Olsen, A. (2002) *Body and Earth*. Lebanon, NH: Middlebury Bicentennial Series.

Rilke, R. M. (2004) *Letters to a Young Poet*, translated by H. Norton. London, UK: W. W. Norton.

Shantideva (1997) *The Way of the Bodhisattva*. Boston: Shambala.

Shaw, M. (2020) *Courting the Wild Twin*. London, UK: Chelsea Green.

Somé, M. (1994) *Of Water and the Spirit: Ritual, Magic, and Initiation in the Life of an African Shaman*. New York: Penguin Books.

Whitehouse, M. (1999) "Physical Movement and Personality," in Pallaro, P. *Authentic Movement: Essays by Mary Starks Whitehouse, Janet Adler and Joan Chodorow*. London: Jessica Kingsley.

Wu-men, H. (1996) "The Gateless Gate," in *The Gateless Barrier*, translated by R. Aitken, p. 4.

Chapter 5

Eliot, T. S. (2001) *The Four Quartets*. London: Faber & Faber.

Emoto, M. (2005) *Hidden Messages in Water*. New York: Atria Books/Simon and Schuster.

Hartley, L. (1995) *Wisdom of the Body Moving: An Introduction to Body-Mind Centering*. Berkeley, CA: North Atlantic Books.

Iyengar, B. K. S. (n.d.) https://www.threeseasonsayurveda.com/post/om-aum (accessed November 10, 2021).

Jenny, H. (1967 / 2001) *Cymatics: A Study of Wave Phenomena and Vibration. A Complete Compilation of the Original Two Volumes by Hans Jenny*. Newmarket, NH: Jeff Volk.

Sanskrit Dictionary (n.d.) "Advaita," "dvandva" *kumbhaka, japa* http://www.sanskritdictionary.com (accessed October 21, 2021).

Van der Wal, J. (2003) "Human Conception: How to Overcome Reproduction? A Phenomenological Approach of Human Fertilization." http://www.embryo.nl (accessed October 14, 2021).

Wikipedia (2021) "James Gimzewski." https://en.wikipedia.org/wiki/James_Gimzewski (accessed October 21, 2021).

Chapter 6

Bainbridge Cohen, B. (2018) *Basic Neurocellular Patterns*. El Sorbante, CA: Burchfield Rose.

Holt, C. (2016) *Pregnant Pause: A Gift for Those Expecting*. Lulu.com.

Huijing, P. (2007) "Myofascial Force Transmission and Spastic Paresis." Special issue, *Journal of Electromyography and Kinesiology*, 17(6).

Leavitt, J. (1986) *Brought to Bed*. New York: Oxford University Press.

Lim, R. (2017) *Placenta – The Forgotten Chakra*. St Petersburg: Valyaeva & Co.

Myers, T. (2001) *Anatomy Trains*. Amsterdam: Elsevier.

Paoletti, S. and Startseva, O. (2012) *Fasciae: Role of Tissues in the Human Body*, 3rd edn. St Petersburg: Nevsky Rakurs.

Rūmī, J. (1997) *A Treasure Trove of Memories*. Moscow: Ganga.

Stecco, C., Gagey, O., Belloni, A., Pozzuoli, A., Porzionato, A., Macchi, V., Aldegheri, R., De Caro, R. and Delmas, V. (2007) "Anatomy of the Deep Fascia of the Upper Limb. Second Part: Study of Innervation," *Morphologie*, 91(292), pp. 38-43.

Still, A. T. (1899) *Philosophy of Osteopathy*. Kirksville, MO: A. T. Still.

Van der Wal, J. (2015) "EMBRYO FA Some Functional Considerations as to Nomenclature in the Domain of the Fascia and Connective Tissue." https://www.embryo.nl/368-Some-functional-considerations-as-to-nomenclature-EN (last accessed October 3, 2020).

Chapter 7

Bainbridge Cohen, B. (2012) *Sensing, Feeling, and Action*, 3rd edn. Northampton, MA: Contact Editions.

Bainbridge Cohen, B. (2016) *Embodying Form and Flow: A Body-Mind Centering® Approach to Movement, Consciousness and Well-Being*. https://www.tanzfabrik-berlin.de/en/events/421 (accessed September 7, 2020).

Hartley, L. (2014) "Embodiment of Spirit: From Embryology to Authentic Movement as Embodied Relational Spiritual Practice," first published as Chapter 1 of *Dance, Somatics and Spiritualities: Contemporary Sacred Narratives*, edited by Amanda Williamson, Glenna Batson, Sarah Whatley, and Rebecca Weber. Bristol, UK, and Chicago: Intellect.

Männer, J. (2013) "Von Anfang an ein Mensch," *Göttinger Tageblatt*, May 11.

Schad, I. (2019) "Wie eine Kettenreaktion". Interview: https://www.hebbel-am-ufer.de/isabelle-schad-interview/ (last accessed September 6, 2020).

Talbott, St. L. (2013) "The Embryo's Eloquent Form". https://bwo.life/mqual/embryo (accessed December 11, 2020).

References *continued*

van der Wal, J., van der Bie, G. (2005) Highlights of a Phenomenological Embryology. https://www.embryo.nl/upload/documents/artikelen-embryosofie/Highlights%20Phenomenological%20Embryology%202005%20EN%20chapter.pdf (accessed September 4, 2020).

van der Wal, J. (2016) *Dynamische Morphologie und Entwicklung der menschlichen Gestalt*, 4th edn. Dornieden: am Goetheanum.

van der Wal, J. (2020) *What the Embryo Has to Say About Togetherness*. www.youtube.com/watch?v=IBMgXLVU1JQ (accessed April 26, 2020).

Chapter 8

Argamakova, T. (n.d.) "Location of Internal Organs During Pregnancy." https://beremennost.net/raspolozhenie-vnutrennikh-organov-priberemennosti (accessed February 1, 2021).

Calais-Germain, B. (2003) *The Female Pelvis: Anatomy and Exercises*. Seattle: Eastland Press.

Hartley, L. (1995) *Wisdom of the Body Moving: An Introduction to Body-Mind Centering*. Berkeley, CA: North Atlantic Books.

Olsen, A., McHose, C. (2004) *Bodystories: A Guide to Experiential Anatomy*. Hanover, NH: University Press of New England.

Chapter 9

Adler, J. (2002) *Offering from the Conscious Body: The Discipline of Authentic Movement*. Rochester, VT: Inner Traditions.

Baring, A. (2013) *The Dream of the Cosmos: A Quest for the Soul*. Dorset, UK: Archive.

Grof, S. (1985) *Beyond the Brain: Birth, Death, and Transcendence in Psychotherapy*. New York: State University of New York Press.

Haines, S. (2015) *Trauma is Really Strange*. London, UK: Singing Dragon.

Hartley, L. (1995) *Wisdom of the Body Moving: An Introduction to Body-Mind Centering*. Berkeley, CA: North Atlantic Books.

Hartley, L. (2004) *Somatic Psychology: Body, Mind and Meaning*. London, UK, and Philadelphia: Whurr.

Hartley, L. (2015) "Choice, Surrender and Transitions in Authentic Movement: Reflections on Personal and Teaching Practice," *Journal of Dance and Somatic Practices*, 7(2).

Hayes, J. (2007) *Performing the Dreams of Your Body: Plays of Animation and Compassion*. London: Archive.

Hayes, J. (2013) *Soul and Spirit in Dance Movement Psychotherapy: A Transpersonal Approach*. London, UK, and Philadelphia: Jessica Kingsley.

Hillman, J. (1979) *The Dream and the Underworld*. London, UK, and New York: Harper & Row.

McNiff, S. (1998) *Trust the Process: An Artist's Guide to Letting Go*. London, UK, and Boston: Shambhala.

McNiff, S. (2004) *Art Heals: How Creativity Cures the Soul*. Boston and London: Shambhala.

Pallaro, P. (ed.) (1999) *Authentic Movement: A Collection of Essays by Mary Starks Whitehouse, Janet Adler, and Joan Chodorow*, vol. 1. London: Jessica Kingsley.

Pallaro, P. (ed.) (2007) *Authentic Movement: Moving the Body, Moving the Self, Being Moved. A Collection of Essays*, vol. 2. London: Jessica Kingsley.

Stromsted, T. (2015) "The Alchemy of Authentic Movement: Awakening Spirit in the Body," in A. Williamson, S. Whately, and G. Batson (eds), *Dance, Somatics and Spiritualities: Contemporary Sacred Narratives, Leading Edge Voices in the Field: Sensory Experiences of the Divine*. Bristol, UK: Intellect Books.

Tufnell, M. (2017) *When I Open My Eyes: Dance, Health, Imagination*. Binstead: Dance Books.

Williamson, A. (2010) "Reflections and Theoretical Approaches to the Study of Spiritualities Within the Field of Somatic Movement Dance Education," *Journal of Dance and Somatic Practices*, 2(1), pp. 35–61.

Chapter 10

Bainbridge Cohen, B. (1984) "Perceiving in Action", *Contact Quarterly*, VIII(2), Spring/Summer 24.

Bainbridge Cohen, B. (2018) *Basic Neurocellular Patterns*. El Sobrante, CA: Burchfield Rose.

Bentzen, M. (2016) *Das neuroaffektive Bilderbuch*. Copenhagen, Denmark: Hans Reitzels.

Carroll, R. (2007) *An Interview with Allan Schore – "the American Bowlby."* Thinking Through the Body. https://web.archive.org/web/20080325110438/http://www.thinkbody.co.uk/papers/interview-with-allan-s.htm (accessed November 25, 2020).

Hartley, L. (1995) *Wisdom of the Body Moving*. Berkeley, CA: North Atlantic Books.

Hartley, L. (2004) *Somatic Psychology*. London and Philadelphia: Whurr.

Rass, E. (2012) *Allan Schore: Schaltstellen der Entwicklung*. Stuttgart: Klett-Cotta.

Siegel, D. [Founder of interpersonal neurobiology]. https://www.drdansiegel.com/interpersonal-neurobiology/ (accessed October 20, 2020).

Siegel, D. (2020) *The Developing Mind*, 3rd edn. New York and London, UK: Guilford Press.

References *continued*

Siegel, D., Hartzell, M. (2009) *Gemeinsam Leben, Gemeinsam Wachsen.* Freiamt im Schwarzwald: Arbor.

Stern, D. (1985) *The Interpersonal World of the Infant.* New York: Basic Books / HarperCollins.

Stern, D. (2011) *Ausdrucksformen der Vitalität.* Frankfurt am Main: Brandes & Apsel.

Van der Kolk, B. (2014) *The Body Keeps the Score: Mind, Brain and the Body in the Transformation of Trauma.* Harmondsworth, UK: Penguin.

Chapter 11

Adler, J. (2002) *Offering from the Conscious Body.* Rochester, VT: Inner Traditions.

Bainbridge Cohen, B. (2018) *Basic Neurocellular Patterns.* El Sobrante, CA: Burchfield Rose.

Dana, D. (2018) *The Polyvagal Theory in Therapy.* New York: Norton.

Greenland, P. (2000) *Hopping Home Backwards.* Leeds, UK: JABADAO.

Hartley, L. (1995) *Wisdom of the Body Moving.* Berkeley, CA: North Atlantic Books.

Heller, L. (2012) *Healing Developmental Trauma.* Berkeley, CA: North Atlantic Books.

Hughes, D. (2009) *Attachment-Focused Parenting: Effective Strategies to Care for Children.* New York: Norton.

Kranowitz, C. (2005) *The Out-of-sync Child.* New York: Perigee.

Mindell, A. (1985) *The River's Way.* Portland, OR: Deep Democracy Exchange.

Rothschild, B. (2000) *The Body Remembers.* New York: Norton.

Van der Kolk, B. (2014) *The Body Keeps the Score.* Harmondsworth, UK: Penguin.

Worth, L., Poynor, H. (2004) *Anna Halprin.* Abingdon, UK: Routledge.

Chapter 12

Bion W. (1959) "Attacks on Linking," *International Journal of Psycho-Analysis*, 40, pp. 308–15. Translated into Russian by Babloyan, Z. (2008), "Attacks on Linking," *Journal of Practical Psychology and Psychoanalysis* (2008), 1. https://psyjournal.ru/articles/napadeniya-na-svyaz (accessed January 3, 2021).

Bion, W. (1962) *Learning from Experience.* London, UK: Karnac Books. Translated into Russian by Cogito-center (2008), *Learning from Experience.* Moscow, Russia: Cogito-center.

Graham, W. (2017) *The Art of Thought.* New York: SOLIS Press.

Grof, S. (1985) *Beyond the Brain: Birth, Death, and Transcendence in Psychotherapy.* Albany, NY: State University of New York Press. Translated into Russian by Kisilev, A. (2018), *Beyond the Brain: Birth, Death, and Transcendence in Psychotherapy.* Moscow, Russia: Ganga.

Hartley, L. (2004) *Somatic Psychology: Body, Mind and Meaning.* London, UK: Whurr.

Jung, C. G. (1963) *Memories, Dreams, Reflections.* New York: Vintage Books. Translated into Russian by Polikarpov, V. (2003) *Memories, Dreams, Reflections.* Moscow, Russia: Harvest LLC.

Kopytin, A. I. (2005) *Diagnostics in Art-Therapy. Method "Mandala."* St Petersburg, Russia: Rech' Publ.

Rogers, C. R. (1986) "Reflection of Feelings," *Person-Centered Review*, 1(4), pp. 375–7.

Rothschild, B. (2005) "The Physiology of Empathy: Negotiating Our Double-Edged Sword," *Journal of Bioenergetic Research*, 34, pp. 44–9.

Winnicott, D. W. (1971) *Playing and Reality.* London: Tavistock. Translated into Russian by Institute of General Humanitarian Research (2002) *Playing and Reality.* Moscow, Russia: Institute of General Humanitarian Research.

Chapter 13

Basch-Kahre, E. (1984) "On Difficulties Arising in Transference and Countertransference when Analyst and Analysand Have Different Socio-cultural Backgrounds," *International Review of Psychoanalysis*, 11(1), pp. 61-7.

Bauer, J. (2009) *Why I Feel What You Feel.* Werner Regen.

Bernstein, P. L. (1984) "The Somatic Countertransference: The Inner Pas de Deux," in P. L. Bernstein (ed.), *Theoretical Approaches in Dance/Movement Therapy*, vol. 2. Dubuque, IA: Kendall/Hunt.

Boadella, D. (1980) "Transference." Transcript of talk given at the Boyesen Center, London, UK. November.

Etchegoyen, R. Horacio (1991) *The Fundamentals of Psychoanalytic Technique.* London, UK, and New York: Karnac Books.

Fiedler, I. (1989) "The Interdependence of Kinesthetic Empathy and Somatic Countertransference in Dance/Movement Therapy." Unpublished master's thesis, University of California, Los Angeles.

Freud, S. (1910) "The Future Prospects of Psycho-analytic Therapy," in J. Strachey (ed.), *The Standard Edition of the Complete Psychological Works of Sigmund Freud*, vol. 11. London, UK: Hogarth Press.

Hartley, L. (2004) *Somatic Psychology: Body, Mind and Meaning.* London, UK: Whurr.

Kaplan, A. G. (1990) *Empathy and its Vicissitudes*, in *Empathy Revisited: Work in Progress*, 40. Wellesley, MA: The Stone Center.

Kohut, H. (1971) *The Analysis of the Self.* New York: International Universities Press.

Pallaro, P. (2008) "Somatic Countertransference: The Therapist in the Relationship," *Journal of Practical Psychology and Psychoanalysis*, 2.

Pick, I. B. (1985) "Working Through the Countertransference," *International Journal of Psychoanalysis*, 66, pp. 157–66.

Schore, A. N. (1994) *Affect Regulation and the Origin of the Self: The Neurobiology of Emotional Development.* Hillsdale, NJ: Lawrence Erlbaum.

Stevens, V. (2005) "Reading the Language of the Right Brain: Fine-tuning the Analyst's Capacity for Creativity Attuned Empathic Resonance," *Psychologist-Psychoanalyst*, 26(2), pp. 9–13.

Winnicott, D. (1958) *Collected Papers: Through Pediatrics to Psychoanalysis.* New York: Basic Books.

Chapter 14

Bainbridge Cohen, B. (2008) *Sensing, Feeling, and Action*, 2nd edn. Northampton, MA: Contact Editions.

Hartley, L. (1995), *Wisdom of the Body Moving.* Berkeley, CA: North Atlantic Books.

Juhan, D. (1992) *Körperarbeit – Die Soma-Psyche Verbindung.* Munich: Knaur. Originally published in 1987 as *Job's Body: A Handbook for Bodywork.* New York: Barrytown.

Ridley, C. (2006) *Stillness – Biodynamic Cranial Practice and the Evolution of Consciousness.* Berkeley, CA: North Atlantic Books.

Seitz, O. (2015) *Verbinden und Loslassen [Connecting and Letting Go – Fascial System Research]*, Berlin. www.odile-seitz.de/_Über: Diplomarbeit pdf.

Chapter 15

Bainbridge Cohen, B. (2012), *Sensing, Feeling, and Action – The Experiental Anatomy of Body-Mind Centering®*, 3rd edn. Northampton, MA: Contact Editions.

Hartley, L. (1995) *Wisdom of the Body Moving – An Introduction to Body-Mind Centering.* Berkeley, CA: North Atlantic Books.

LaPierre, A. (2019–20) "Healing the Relational Matrix," *Foundation Training Manual.* Oslo, Norway: NeuroAffective Touch© Training Institute. https://neuroaffectivetouch.com (accessed October 22, 2021).

LaPierre, A. (2020) "Peter Levine Interviewed by Dr A LaPierre – A Shaman's Scientific Journey," *16 International Body Psychotherapy Journal*, 19(1), Spring/Summer.

Chapter 16

Adler, J. (2002) *Offering from the Conscious Body: The Discipline of Authentic Movement.* Rochester, VT: Inner Traditions.

Bainbridge Cohen, B. (1993) *Sensing, Feeling, and Action: The Experiential Anatomy of Body-Mind Centering.* Northampton, MA: Contact Editions.

Berg, A. L., Bullington, J., Sandahl, C. (2010) "Patients' Perspective of Change Processes in Affect-focused Body Psychotherapy for Generalised Anxiety Disorder," *Body, Movement and Dance in Psychotherapy*, 5(2), pp. 151–69.

Bitzaraki, A., Karkou, V., McAslan, F. (2010) "Dance Movement Psychotherapy with Adults with Chronic Pain: Key Themes in Theory and Practice." Unpublished.

Bojner-Horwitz, E., Kowalski, J., Anderberg, U. M. (2010) "Theatre for, by and with Fibromyalgia Patients: Evaluation of Emotional Expression using Video Interpretation," *The Arts in Psychotherapy*, 37(1), pp. 13–9.

Bral, E., Shaughnessy, M., Eisenman, R. (2002) "Intimacy in People with Chronic Pain," *International Journal of Psychosocial Rehabilitation*, 6, pp. 51–60.

Bullington, J., Nordemar, K., Sjöström-Flanagan, C. (2003) "Meaning out of Chaos: A Way to Understand Chronic Pain," *Nordic College of Caring Sciences*, 17, pp. 325–31.

Bullington, J., Sjöström-Flanagan, C., Nordemar, K., Nordemar, R. (2005) "From Pain Through Chaos Towards New Meaning: Two Case Studies," *The Arts in Psychotherapy*, 32, pp. 261–74.

Cady, M. (2016) "Value of Pain Stories." https://www.instituteforchronicpain.org/treating-common-pain/value-of-pain-stories (accessed February 15, 2021).

Chang, M., Leventhal, F. (1995) "Mobilizing Battered Women: A Creative Step Forward," in Fran Levy (ed.) *Dance and Other Expressive Art Therapies: When Words Are Not Enough.* New York: Routledge, pp. 59–68.

Chodorow, J. (1991) *Dance Therapy and Depth Psychology: The Moving Imagination.* Hove, UK: Routledge.

Defrin, R., Ginzburg, K., Solomon, Z., Polad, E., Bloch, M., Govenzensky, M., Schreiber, S. (2008) "Quantitative Testing of Pain Perception in Subjects with PTSD: Implications for the Mechanism of the Coexistence between PTSD and Chronic Pain," *Pain*, 138, pp. 450–9.

Devereaux, C. (2008) "Untying the Knots: Dance/Movement Therapy with a Family Exposed to Domestic Violence," *American Dance Therapy Journal*, 30, pp. 58–70.

Dosamantes-Beaudry, I. (2003) *The Arts in Contemporary Healing.* Westport, CT: Praeger, pp. 15–8.

Erber, B. T. (2015) "Growing From Pain – A Creative Process," *Pain and Rehabilitation: Journal of the Physiotherapy Pain Association*, 39, pp. 11–6.

Erber, B. T. (forthcoming) *Authentic Movement and Feeling Safe.* Unpublished

References *continued*

doctoral thesis, University of Edinburgh, UK.

Galon, C. (2019) *Trauma-informed Dance Movement Psychotherapy: Understanding the Therapeutic Process and its Components*. Doctoral thesis, Edgehill University, UK. https://research.edgehill.ac.uk/en/studentTheses/trauma-informed-dance-movement-psychotherapy-understanding-the-th (accessed February 15, 2021).

Harris, B. (2011) *Individuation: The Promise in Jung's Legacy and Why Our Culture Has Trouble Accepting It*. C. G. Jung Memorial Lecture, Jung Society of Washington. http://www.jung.org/Bud%20Harris%20article.html (accessed May 23, 2015).

Hartley, L. (1995). *Wisdom of the Body Moving: An Introduction to Body-Mind Centering*. Berkeley, CA: North Atlantic Books.

Hartley, L. (2001) *Servants of the Sacred Dream: Rebirthing the Deep Feminine, Psychospiritual Crisis and Healing*. Norfolk, UK: Elmdon Books.

Hartley, L. (2004) *Somatic Psychology: Body, Mind and Meaning*. London, UK: Whurr.

Hartley, L. (2012) *Authentic Movement and Therapeutic Presence*. Workshop. Norfolk, UK: IBMT Institute.

Holifield, B. (2007 [1998]) "'Against the wall, her beating heart': Working with Somatic Aspects of Transference, Countertransference and Dissociation," in Pallaro, P. (ed.) *Authentic Movement: Moving the Body, Moving the Self, Being Moved*. London, UK: Jessica Kingsley, pp. 137–53.

Jones, G. T., Power, C., Macfarlane, G. J. (2009) "Adverse Events in Childhood and Chronic Widespread Pain in Adult Life: Results from the 1958 British Birth Cohort Study," *Pain*, 143, pp. 92–6.

Jung, C. G. (1959) *The Archetypes and the Collective Unconscious*, 2nd edn. Translated by Hull, R. F. C. London, UK: Routledge.

Keleman, S. (1986) *Bonding: A Somatic-Emotional Approach to Transference*. Berkeley, CA: Center Press.

Levine, P. (1997) *Waking the Tiger: Healing Trauma*. Berkeley, CA: North Atlantic Books.

Levine, P. (2010) *In an Unspoken Voice: How the Body Releases Trauma and Restores Goodness*. Berkeley, CA: North Atlantic Books.

Levine, P., Phillips, M. (2012) *Freedom from Pain: Discover Your Body's Power to Overcome Physical Pain*. Boulder, CO: Sounds True.

Main, C. J., Sullivan, M. J. L., Watson, P. J. (2008) *Pain Management: Practical Applications of the Biopsychosocial Perspective in Clinical and Occupational Settings*, 2nd edn. London, UK: Churchill Livingstone/Elsevier.

Malchiodi, Cathy A. (2008) *Creative Interventions with Traumatized Children*. New York: Gilford Press.

Mallon, B., Tufnell, M., Rubidge, T. (2004) "'When I open my eyes': A Report on a Three-year Project Exploring Body, Imagination and Health." Body Stories, unpublished report. For more information see http://www.mirandatufnell.co.uk/books/whennew.html (accessed November 11, 2021).

McAllister, M. J. (2017a) "Trauma." https://www.instituteforchronicpain.org/understanding-chronic-pain/complications/trauma (accessed January 1, 2021).

McAllister, M. J. (2017b) "What is Central Sensitization?" https://www.instituteforchronicpain.org/understanding-chronic-pain/what-is-chronic-pain/central-sensitization (accessed January 1, 2021).

McFarlane, A. C. (2010) "The Long-term Costs of Traumatic Stress: Intertwined Physical and Psychological Consequences," *World Psychiatry*, 9, pp. 3–10.

Natiello, P. (2001) *The Person-Centred Approach: A Passionate Presence*. Herefordshire, UK: PCCS Books.

National Pain Audit – Final Report (2012). www.nationalpainaudit.org/media/files/NationalPainAudit-2012.pdf (accessed December 27, 2012).

NHS Inform (2021) "Chronic Pain." https://www.nhsinform.scot/illnesses-and-conditions/brain-nerves-and-spinal-cord/chronic-pain (accessed January 1, 2021).

Nijenhuis, E. R. S., Steele, K., Van der Hart, O. (2006) *The Haunted Self: Structural Dissociation and the Treatment of Chronic Traumatization*. London, UK: W. W. Norton & Co.

Ogden, P., Minton, K., Pain, C. (2006) *Trauma and the Body: A Sensorimotor Approach to Psychotherapy*. London, UK: W. W. Norton & Co.

Otis, J. D., Keane, T. M., Kerns, R. D. (2003) "An Examination of the Relationship Between Chronic Pain and Post-traumatic Stress Disorder," *Journal of Rehabilitation Research and Development*, 40(5), pp. 397–406.

Pallaro, P. (ed.) (1999) *Authentic Movement: Essays by Mary Starks Whitehouse, Janet Adler and Joan Chodorow*. London, UK: Jessica Kingsley.

Pallaro, P. (2007) "Somatic Countertransference: The Therapist in Relationship," in Pallaro, P. (ed.) *Authentic Movement*, vol. 2. London, UK: Jessica Kingsley, pp. 176–93.

Porges, S. W. (2011) *The Polyvagal Theory: Neurophysiological Foundations of Emotions, Attachment, Communication, Self-Regulation*. London, UK: W. W. Norton & Co.

Porges, S. W. (2017) *The Pocket Guide to the Polyvagal Theory: The Transformative Power of Feeling Safe*. London, UK: W. W. Norton & Co.

References *continued*

Porges, S. W., Carter, S. (2017) "Polyvagal Theory and the Social Engagement System: Neurophysiological Bridge Between Connectedness and Health," in Gerbarg, P. L., Muskin, P. R., Brown, R. P. (eds) *Complementary and Integrative Treatments in Psychiatric Practice.* Arlington, VA: American Psychiatric Association, pp. 221–40.

Richman, A. (2012) "The Challenges of Working with Complex Trauma," seminar, November 10. London, UK: Confer.

Roth, R. S., Geisser, M. E., Bates, R. (2008) "The Relation of Post-Traumatic Stress Symptoms to Depression and Pain in Patients with Accident-Related Chronic Pain," *The Journal of Pain*, 9(7), pp. 588–96.

Rothschild, B. (2000) *The Body Remembers: The Psychophysiology of Trauma and Trauma Treatment.* London, UK: W. W. Norton & Co.

Sager, P. C. (2008) "Witness Consciousness in the Development of the Individual." MA Dissertation, The Owen Barfield School of Sunbridge College. http://threestonestudio.org/Three_Stone_Studio/Witness_Consciousness.html (accessed August 8, 2014).

Scaer, R. (2007) *The Body Bears the Burden: Trauma, Dissociation and Disease.* New York: Routledge.

Schore, A. N. (2003) *Affect Regulation and the Repair of the Self.* New York: Norton.

Scottish Intercollegiate Guidelines Network (2013) "Management of Chronic Pain: A National Clinical Guide," 136. Edinburgh, UK: SIGN. http://www.sign.ac.uk (accessed October 22, 2021).

Sledjeski, E. M., Speisman, B., Dierker, L. C. (2008) "Does Number of Lifetime Traumas Explain the Relationship between PTSD and Chronic Medical Conditions? Answers from the National Comorbidity Survey-Replication (NCS-R)," *Journal of Behavioural Medicine*, 31, pp. 341–9.

Stern, D. N. (1985) *The Interpersonal World of the Infant: A View from Psychoanalysis and Developmental Psychology.* New York: Basic Books.

Stromsted, T. (2001) "Re-inhabiting the Female Body: Authentic Movement as a Gateway to Transformation," *The Arts in Psychotherapy*, 28, pp. 39–55.

Van der Kolk, B. A., McFarlane, A. C., Weisaeth, L. (eds) (1996) *Traumatic Stress: The Effects of Overwhelming Experience on Body, Mind and Society.* New York: Gilford Press.

Weare, S. (2020) *Rhythm and Safety of Social Engagement: Polyvagal Theory Informed Dance/Movement Therapy.* Expressive Therapies Capstone Theses, 347. Cambridge, MA: Lesley University.

Winnicott, D. W. (1960) *The Maturational Process and the Facilitating Environment.* London, UK: Hogarth Press.

Woodman, M. (1985) *The Pregnant Virgin: A Process of Psychological Transformation.* Toronto, Canada: Inner City Books.

Wuest, J., Ford-Gilboe, M., Merritt-Gray, M., Wilk, P., Campbell, J. C., Lent, B., Varcoe, C., Smye, V. (2010) "Pathways of Chronic Pain in Survivors of Intimate Partner Violence," *Journal of Women's Health*, 19(9), pp. 1665–74.

Chapter 17

Bainbridge Cohen, B. (1993) *Sensing, Feeling, and Action.* Northampton, MA: Contact Editions.

Bovell, A. (2019) *Las cosas que sé que son verdad.* Spain [online]. Punto de vista editores.

Gerhardt, S. (2004) *Why Love Matters.* London, UK, and New York: Routledge.

Hartley, L. (1995) *Wisdom of the Body Moving.* Berkeley, CA: North Atlantic Books.

Levine, P. (2018) *Trauma y Memoria.* Barcelona: Eleftheria.

Levine, P., Kline, M. (2007) *Trauma Through Child's Eyes.* Berkeley, CA: North Atlantic Books.

Linklater, K. (2006) *Freeing the Natural Voice.* Hollywood, CA: Drama Publishers.

Nadeem, S. (2020) *Message for World Theatre Day.* https://www.world-theatre-day.org/fr/pdfs/WTD2020_EN_Message_ShahidNADEEM.pdf (accessed October 26, 2021).

Schwartz, R. (2019) NICABM Webinar. Session with author.

Raine, N. (2010) *Tribes.* New York: Dramatists Play Service.

Shakespeare, W. (1994) *Hamlet*, bilingual version. Madrid: Editorial Cátedra.

Troccoli, P., Santafé, L. (2020) "When Stage Fright Comes for a Visit," in Kapadocha, C. (ed.), *Somatic Voices in Performance Research and Beyond.* Abingdon, UK, and New York: Routledge.

Chapter 18

Bainbridge Cohen, B. (2012) *Sensing, Feeling, and Action: The Experiential Anatomy of Body-Mind Centering®.* Northampton, MA: Contact Editions.

Eddy, M. (2009) "A Brief History of Somatic Practices and Dance: Historical Development of the Field of Somatic Education and its Relationship to Dance," *Journal of Dance & Somatic Practices*, June.

Hay, D. (2000) *My Body, the Buddhist.* Middletown, CT: Wesleyan University Press.

Olsen, A. (2002) *Body and Earth.* Lebanon, NH: University Press of New England.

Olsen, A. (2015) *http://www.body-earth.org/Seven Web-based Somatic Excursions.* http://www.body-earth.org/ (accessed November 1, 2020).

References *continued*

Priklonskaya, V. (2019), interview with author, October 15.

Chapter 19

Adler, J. (2002) *Offering from the Conscious Body: The Discipline of Authentic Movement*. Rochester, VT: Inner Traditions.

Albright, A. C., Gere, D. (2003) *Taken by Surprise: A Dance Improvisation Reader*. Middletown, CT: Wesleyan University Press.

Aposhyan, S. (1999) *Natural Intelligence: Body-mind Integration and Human Development*. Philadelphia: Williams & Wilkins.

Bachelard, G. (1994 [1964]) *The Poetics of Space*. Boston: Beacon Press.

Bacon, J. (2010) "The Voice of Her Body: Somatic Practices as a Basis for Creative Research Methodology," *Journal of Dance and Somatic Practices*, 2, pp. 63–72.

Bainbridge Cohen, B. (2008) *Sensing, Feeling, and Action*. Northampton, MA: Contact Editions.

De Spain, K. (2014) *Landscape of the Now: A Topography of Movement Improvisation*. New York: Oxford University Press.

Deleuze, G. (2012) *Cinema 2: The Time-image*. London, UK: Athlone.

Deleuze, G., Smith, D. W. (2008) *Francis Bacon: The Logic of Sensation*. London, UK: Continuum.

Hartley, L. (2015) "Choice, Surrender and Transitions in Authentic Movement: Reflections on Personal and Teaching Practice," *Journal of Dance and Somatic Practices*, 7, pp. 299–312.

Hartley, L. (2017) "Woman, body, earth and spirit: Journeys of descent through myth, embodiment and movement practice," *Intellect Journals*, 4(1), pp. 15–39.

Hay, D. (2016) *Using the Sky: A Dance*. London, UK: Routledge.

Juhan, D. (2003) *Job's Body: A Handbook for Bodywork*. New York: Barrytown.

Levine, P. (2017). *What Resets Our Nervous System After Trauma?* http://legacyplacesociety.com/wp-content/uploads/2017/10/Levine-What-Resets-Our-Nervous-System-After-Trauma-1.pdf (accessed November 11, 2021), pp. 1–7.

Little, G. (2020) *Mediating Resonant Spaces: Somatic Practice Informing from Within a Solo Dance and Image Making Process*. Unpublished Master's thesis, Trinity Laban Conservatoire of Music and Dance, London, UK.

Nelson, R. (2013) *Practice as Research in the Arts: Principles, Protocols, Pedagogies, Resistances*. Basingstoke, UK: Palgrave Macmillan.

Olsen, A. (2014) *The Place of Dance: A Somatic Guide to Dancing and Dance Making*. Middletown, CT: Wesleyan University Press.

Porges, S. (n.d.) Home of Dr. Stephen Porges. https://www.stephenporges.com/bio (accessed March 25, 2021).

Rethorst, S. (2015) *A Choreographic Mind: Autobodygraphical Writings*. Helsinki, Finland: University of the Arts Helsinki.

Solnit, R. (2006) *A Field Guide to Getting Lost*. London, UK: Canongate.

Speller, J. (2018) *Neurotransmitters*. https://teachmephysiology.com/nervous-system/components/neurotransmitters/ (accessed December 14, 2020).

Starks Whitehouse, M (1999). "The Tao of the Body," in Pallaro, P. *Authentic Movement*. London, UK: Jessica Kingsley.

Tarkovsky, A. (1991) *Sculpting in Time: Reflections on the Cinema*. Translated K. Hunter-Blair. Austin: University of Texas Press.

Voris, A. (2018) *Forming, Returning and Deepening: Dance-making with Authentic Movement*. Unpublished doctoral thesis, University of Chichester, UK.

Chapter 20

Neufeld, G., Maté, G. (2014) *Hold On to Your Kids: Why Parents Need to Matter More Than Peers*. New York: Balantine.

Porges, S. (2018) "Q&A about Freezing, Fainting, and the 'Safe' Sounds of Music Therapy." https://www.everydayhealth.com/wellness/united-states-of-stress/advisory-board/stephen-w-porges-phd-q-a/ (accessed December 31, 2020).

Saul, J., Perel, E. (2019) "Private Drama to Public Healing," https://www.youtube.com/watch?v=TYfqs5gcBjM (accessed September 30, 2020).

Thiran, Y. (2015) "Kinaesthetic Empathy in Spectators of Contemporary Dance." London Contemporary Dance School. https://yanaellethiran.files.wordpress.com/2015/09/np-yanaecc88lle-thiran.pdf (accessed October 26, 2021).

van der Kolk, B. A. (2005) "Developmental Trauma Disorder: Toward a Rational Diagnosis for Children with Complex Trauma Histories," *Psychiatric Annals*, May.

Winerman, L. (2005) "The Mind's Mirror," *Monitor*, 36(9), p. 48.

Index

A

B

C

D

E

Index *continued*

Index *continued*

of related interest

Somatics in Action
A Mindful and Physical Conditioning Tool for Movers
Lauren Kearns
ISBN 978 1 90914 164 3
eISBN 978 1 90914 165 0

The Feldenkrais Method
Learning Through Movement
Staffan Elgelid and Chrish Kresge
ISBN 978 1 91208 569 9
eISBN 978 1 91208 570 5

Dynamic Embodiment of the Sun Salutation?
Pathways to Balancing the Chakras and the Neuroendocrine System
Martha Eddy and Shakti Andrea Smith
ISBN 978 1 91208 599 6
eISBN 978 1 91342 600 2

Embody the Skeleton
A guide for conscious movement
Mark Taylor
ISBN 978 1 91208 509 5
eISBN 978 1 91208 510 1